THE AMERICAN PSYCHIATRIC ASSOCIATION PRACTICE GUIDELINE FOR THE Treatment of Patients With Schizophrenia

THIRD EDITION

Guideline Writing Group

George A. Keepers, M.D., *Chair*

Laura J. Fochtmann, M.D., M.B.I., *Vice-Chair; Methodologist*

Joan M. Anzia, M.D.

Sheldon Benjamin, M.D.

Jeffrey M. Lyness, M.D.

Ramin Mojtabai, M.D.

Mark Servis, M.D.

Art Walaszek, M.D.

Peter Buckley, M.D.

Mark F. Lenzenweger, Ph.D.

Alexander S. Young, M.D., M.S.H.S.

Amanda Degenhardt, M.D.

Systematic Review Group

Laura J. Fochtmann, M.D., M.B.I., *Methodologist*

Seung-Hee Hong

Committee on Practice Guidelines

Daniel J. Anzia, M.D., *Chair*

R. Scott Benson, M.D.

Thomas J. Craig, M.D.

Catherine Crone, M.D.

Annette L. Hanson, M.D.

John M. Oldham, M.D.

Carlos N. Pato, M.D., Ph.D.

Michael J. Vergare, M.D.

Joel Yager, M.D., *Consultant*

Laura J. Fochtmann, M.D., M.B.I., *Consultant*

APA Assembly Liaisons

Daniel Dahl, M.D.

Bhasker Dave, M.D.

Evan Eyler, M.D.

Annette L. Hanson, M.D.

Jason W. Hunziker, M.D.

Marvin Koss, M.D.

Robert M. McCarron, D.O.

John P.D. Shemo, M.D.

APA wishes to acknowledge the contributions of APA staff and former staff (Jennifer Medicus, Seung-Hee Hong, Samantha Shugarman, Michelle Dirst, Kristin Kroeger Ptakowski). APA also wishes to acknowledge the contribution of Amanda S. Eloma, Pharm.D., BCPP, in reviewing information related to medications in the guideline and associated tables. In addition, APA and the Guideline Writing Group especially thank Laura J. Fochtmann, M.D., M.B.I.; Seung-Hee Hong; and Jennifer Medicus for their outstanding work and effort in developing this guideline. APA also thanks the APA Committee on Practice Guidelines (Daniel J. Anzia, M.D., Chair), liaisons from the APA Assembly for their input and assistance, and APA Councils and others for providing feedback during the comment period.

For inquiries about permissions or licensing, please contact Permissions & Licensing, American Psychiatric Association Publishing, 800 Maine Avenue SW, Suite 900, Washington, DC 20024-2812 or submit inquiries online at: www.appi.org/Support/Customer-Information/Permissions.

If you wish to buy 50 or more copies of the same title, please go to www.appi.org/specialdiscounts for more information.

Third Edition

Manufactured in the United States of America on acid-free paper
24 23 22 21 20   5 4 3 2 1

American Psychiatric Association
800 Maine Avenue SW
Suite 900
Washington, DC 20024-2812
www.appi.org

Library of Congress Cataloging-in-Publication Data
Names: American Psychiatric Association, author, issuing body.
Title: The American Psychiatric Association practice guideline for the treatment of patients with schizophrenia / Guideline Writing Group, Systematic Review Group, Committee on Practice Guidelines.
Other titles: Treatment of patients with schizophrenia
Description: Third edition. | Washington, DC : American Psychiatric Association, [2021] | Preceded by: Practice guideline for the treatment of patients with schizophrenia. 2nd ed. c2004. | Includes bibliographical references.
Identifiers: LCCN 2020016573 (print) | LCCN 2020016574 (ebook) | ISBN 9780890424698 (paperback ; alk. paper) | ISBN 9780890424742 (ebook)
Subjects: MESH: Schizophrenia—therapy | Practice Guideline
Classification: LCC RC514 (print) | LCC RC514 (ebook) | NLM WM 203 | DDC 616.89/8—dc23
LC record available at https://lccn.loc.gov/2020016573
LC ebook record available at https://lccn.loc.gov/2020016574

British Library Cataloguing in Publication Data
A CIP record is available from the British Library.

Contents

Acronyms/Abbreviations

ACT   Assertive community treatment

AHRQ   Agency for Healthcare Research and Quality

AIMS   Abnormal Involuntary Movement Scale

ANC   Absolute neutrophil count

APA   American Psychiatric Association

BAP   British Association for Psychopharmacology

BMI   Body mass index

BPRS   Brief Psychiatric Rating Scale

CATIE   Clinical Antipsychotic Trials of Intervention Effectiveness

CBT   Cognitive-behavioral therapy

CBTp   Cognitive-behavioral therapy for psychosis

CDC   Centers for Disease Control and Prevention

CGI   Clinical Global Impression

CI   Confidence interval

CrI   Credible interval

CSC   Coordinated specialty care

CSG   Canadian Schizophrenia Guidelines

CYP   Cytochrome P450

DISCUS   Dyskinesia Identification System: Condensed User Scale

DSM   *Diagnostic and Statistical Manual of Mental Disorders*

DSM-5   *Diagnostic and Statistical Manual of Mental Disorders*, 5th Edition

ECG   Electrocardiography

ECT   Electroconvulsive therapy

FDA   U.S. Food and Drug Administration

FGA   First-generation antipsychotic

GAF   Global Assessment of Functioning

GRADE   Grading of Recommendations Assessment, Development and Evaluation

HIPAA   Health Insurance Portability and Accountability Act

HIV   Human immunodeficiency virus

HR   Hazard ratio

ICD   International Classification of Diseases

IPS   Individual placement and support

LAI   Long-acting injectable

MD   Mean difference

NICE   National Institute for Health and Care Excellence

NMDA   *N*-methyl-D-aspartate

NMS   Neuroleptic malignant syndrome

NNH   Number needed to harm

NNT   Number needed to treat

NQF   National Quality Forum

OR   Odds ratio

PANSS-6   Positive and Negative Syndrome Scale, 6-item version

PANSS-30   Positive and Negative Syndrome Scale, 30-item version

PORT   Schizophrenia Patient Outcomes Research Team

PROMIS   Patient-Reported Outcomes Measurement Information System

RAISE   Recovery After an Initial Schizophrenia Episode

RANZCP   Royal Australian and New Zealand College of Psychiatry

RCT   Randomized controlled trial

REMS   Risk Evaluation and Mitigation Strategy

RR   Relative risk

SANS   Scale for the Assessment of Negative Symptoms

SAPS   Scale for the Assessment of Positive Symptoms

SD   Standard deviation

SFS   Social Functioning Scale

SGA   Second-generation antipsychotic

SIGN   Scottish Intercollegiate Guidelines Network

SMD   Standardized mean difference

SOE   Strength of evidence

SOFAS   Social and Occupational Functioning Assessment Scale

TdP   Torsades de pointes

TMS   Transcranial magnetic stimulation

TRRIP   Treatment Response and Resistance in Psychosis

UKU   Udvalg for Kliniske Undersogelser

VMAT2   Vesicular monoamine transporter 2

WFSBP   World Federation of Societies of Biological Psychiatry

WHODAS 2.0   World Health Organization Disability Schedule 2.0

WHOQOL-BREF   World Health Organization Quality of Life scale

WMD   Weighted mean difference

XR   Extended release

Introduction

Rationale

The goal of this guideline is to improve the quality of care and treatment outcomes for patients with schizophrenia, as defined by the *Diagnostic and Statistical Manual of Mental Disorders*, 5th Edition (DSM-5; American Psychiatric Association 2013a). Since publication of the last American Psychiatric Association (APA) practice guideline (American Psychiatric Association 2004) and guideline watch on schizophrenia (American Psychiatric Association 2009a), there have been many studies on new pharmacological and nonpharmacological treatments for schizophrenia. Additional research has expanded our knowledge of previously available treatments. This practice guideline aims to help clinicians optimize care for their patients by providing evidence-based statements that are intended to enhance knowledge and increase the appropriate use of treatments for schizophrenia.

Schizophrenia is associated with significant health, social, occupational, and economic burdens as a result of its early onset and its severe and often persistent symptoms (American Psychiatric Association 2013a). Worldwide, schizophrenia is one of the top 20 causes of disability (GBD 2017 Disease and Injury Incidence and Prevalence Collaborators 2018). Economic burdens associated with schizophrenia are high (Chapel et al. 2017; Jin and Mosweu 2017), with an estimated cost of more than $150 billion annually in the United States based on 2013 data (Cloutier et al. 2016). Lost productivity due to unemployment and caregiving each account for approximately one-third of total costs, and direct health care costs account for approximately one-quarter of total costs. The lifetime prevalence of schizophrenia is estimated to be approximately 0.7% (McGrath et al. 2008; Moreno-Küstner et al. 2018; van der Werf et al. 2014), although findings vary depending on the study location, demographic characteristics of the sample, the approach used for case finding, the method used for diagnostic confirmation, and the diagnostic criteria used.

Schizophrenia is also associated with increased mortality, with a shortened life span and standardized mortality ratios that are reported to be twofold to fourfold those in the general population (Hayes et al. 2017; Heilä et al. 2005; Hjorthøj et al. 2017; Laursen et al. 2014; Lee et al. 2018; Oakley et al. 2018; Olfson et al. 2015; Tanskanen et al. 2018; Walker et al. 2015). The common co-occurrence of other psychiatric disorders (Plana-Ripoll et al. 2019), including substance use disorders (Hunt et al. 2018), contributes to morbidity and mortality among individuals with schizophrenia. About 4%–10% of persons with schizophrenia die by suicide, with rates that are highest among males in the early course of the disorder (Drake et al. 1985; Heilä et al. 2005; Hor and Taylor 2010; Inskip et al. 1998; Laursen et al. 2014; Nordentoft et al. 2011; Palmer et al. 2005; Popovic et al. 2014; Saha et al. 2007; Tanskanen et al. 2018). Additional causes of death include other unnatural causes, such as accidents and traumatic injuries, and physical conditions, such as cardiovascular, respiratory, and infectious diseases and malignancies, particularly lung cancer (American Psychiatric Association 2013a; Hayes et al. 2017; Heilä et al. 2005; Hjorthøj et al. 2017; Laursen et al. 2014; Lee et al. 2018; Oakley et al. 2018; Olfson et al. 2015; Tanskanen et al. 2018; Walker et al. 2015). Increases in morbidity and mortality related to physical health in individuals with schizophrenia are likely associated with such factors as obesity, diabetes, hyperlipidemia, greater use of cigarettes, reduced engagement in health maintenance (e.g., diet, exercise), and disparities in access to preventive health care and treatment for physical conditions (Bergamo et al. 2014; De Hert et al. 2011; Druss et al. 2000; Janssen et al. 2015; Kisely et al. 2007, 2013; Kugathasan et al. 2018; Lawrence et al. 2010; Moore et al. 2015). Lack of access to adequate psychiatric treatment may also influence mortality (Schoenbaum et al. 2017).

This practice guideline focuses on evidence-based pharmacological and nonpharmacological treatments for schizophrenia. In addition, it includes statements related to assessment and treatment planning, which are an integral part of patient-centered care. Thus, the overall goal of this guideline is to enhance the treatment of schizophrenia for affected individuals, thereby reducing the mortality, morbidity, and significant psychosocial and health consequences of this important psychiatric condition.

Scope of Document

The scope of this document is shaped by *Treatments for Schizophrenia in Adults* (McDonagh et al. 2017), a systematic review commissioned by the Agency for Healthcare Research and Quality (AHRQ) that serves as a principal source of information for this guideline on the basis of its methodological rigor and adherence to accepted standards for systematic reviews. This guideline is focused on the treatment of patients with schizophrenia, and, as such, the statements in this guideline will be relevant to individuals with a diagnosis of schizophrenia. The AHRQ review uses the DSM-5 definition of schizophrenia; however, many of the systematic reviews included studies that used earlier DSM or International Classification of Diseases (ICD) criteria for schizophrenia. Several studies, particularly those assessing harms and psychosocial interventions, also included patients with a schizophrenia spectrum disorder diagnosis. Consequently, discussion of treatment, particularly treatment of first-episode psychosis, may also be relevant to individuals with schizophreniform disorder.

Although many of the studies included in the systematic review also included individuals with a diagnosis of schizoaffective disorder, these data were rarely analyzed separately in a way that would permit unique recommendations to be crafted for this group of patients. In addition, this guideline does not address issues related to identification or treatment of attenuated psychosis syndrome or related syndromes of high psychosis risk, which were not part of the AHRQ systematic review.

Data are also limited on individuals with schizophrenia and significant physical health conditions or co-occurring psychiatric conditions, including substance use disorders. Many of the available studies excluded these individuals from the clinical trial or did not analyze data separately for these patient subgroups. Nevertheless, in the absence of more robust evidence, the statements in this guideline should generally be applicable to individuals with co-occurring conditions, including individuals who receive treatment using integrated collaborative care or inpatient or outpatient medical settings. Although treatment-related costs are often barriers to receiving treatment, and cost-effectiveness considerations are relevant to health care policy, few high-quality studies exist on the cost-effectiveness of treatments for schizophrenia. In addition, costs of treatment typically differ by country and geographic region and vary widely with the health system and payment model. Consequently, cost-effectiveness considerations are outside the scope of this guideline and its recommendations.

Overview of the Development Process

Since the publication of the Institute of Medicine (now known as the National Academy of Medicine) report *Clinical Practice Guidelines We Can Trust* (Institute of Medicine 2011), there has been an increasing focus on using clearly defined, transparent processes for rating the quality of evidence and the strength of the overall body of evidence in systematic reviews of the scientific literature. This guideline was developed using a process intended to be consistent with the recommendations of the Institute of Medicine (2011) and the *Principles for the Development of Specialty Society Clinical Guidelines* of the Council of Medical Specialty Societies (2012). Parameters used for the guideline's systematic review are included with the full text of the guideline; the development process is fully described in the following document available at the APA website: www.psychiatry.org/psychiatrists/practice/clinical-practice-guidelines/guideline-development-process.

Rating the Strengths of Guideline Statements and Supporting Research Evidence

Development of guideline statements entails weighing the potential benefits and harms of each statement and then identifying the level of confidence in that determination. This concept of balancing benefits and harms to determine guideline recommendations and strength of recommendations is a hallmark of Grading of Recommendations Assessment, Development and Evaluation (GRADE), which is used by multiple professional organizations around the world to develop practice guideline recommendations (Guyatt et al. 2013). With the GRADE approach, recommendations are rated by assessing the confidence that the benefits of the statement outweigh the harms and burdens of the statement, determining the confidence in estimates of effect as reflected by the quality of evidence, estimating patient values and preferences (including whether they are similar across the patient population), and identifying whether resource expenditures are worth the expected net benefit of following the recommendation (Andrews et al. 2013).

In weighing the balance of benefits and harms for each statement in this guideline, our level of confidence is informed by available evidence, which includes evidence from clinical trials as well as expert opinion and patient values and preferences. Evidence for the benefit of a particular intervention within a specific clinical context is identified through systematic review and is then balanced against the evidence for harms. In this regard, harms are broadly defined and may include serious adverse events, less serious adverse events that affect tolerability, minor adverse events, negative effects of the intervention on quality of life, barriers and inconveniences associated with treatment, direct and indirect costs of the intervention (including opportunity costs), and other negative aspects of the treatment that may influence decision-making by the patient, the clinician, or both.

Many topics covered in this guideline have relied on forms of evidence such as consensus opinions of experienced clinicians or indirect findings from observational studies rather than research from randomized trials. It is well recognized that there are guideline topics and clinical circumstances for which high-quality evidence from clinical trials is not possible or is unethical to obtain (Council of Medical Specialty Societies 2012). For example, many questions need to be asked as part of an assessment, and inquiring about a particular symptom or element of the history cannot be separated out for study as a discrete intervention. It would also be impossible to separate changes in outcomes due to assessment from changes in outcomes due to ensuing treatment. Research on psychiatric assessments and some psychiatric interventions can also be complicated by multiple confounding factors such as the interaction between the clinician and the patient or the patient's unique circumstances and experiences. The GRADE working group and guidelines developed by other professional organizations have noted that a strong recommendation or *good practice statement* may be appropriate even in the absence of research evidence when sensible alternatives do not exist (Andrews et al. 2013; Brito et al. 2013; Djulbegovic et al. 2009; Hazlehurst et al. 2013). For each guideline statement, we have described the type and strength of the available evidence as well as the factors, including patient preferences, that were used in determining the balance of benefits and harms.

The authors of the guideline determined each final rating, as described in the section "Guideline Development Process," that is endorsed by the APA Board of Trustees. A *recommendation* (denoted by the numeral 1 after the guideline statement) indicates confidence that the benefits of the intervention clearly outweigh harms. A *suggestion* (denoted by the numeral 2 after the guideline statement) indicates greater uncertainty: although the benefits of the statement are still viewed as outweighing the harms, the balance of benefits and harms is more difficult to judge, or the benefits or the harms may be less clear. With a suggestion, patient values and preferences may be more variable, and this can influence the clinical decision that is ultimately made.

Each guideline statement also has an associated rating for the *strength of supporting research evidence*. Three ratings are used: *high*, *moderate*, and *low* (denoted by the letters A, B, and C, respectively). These ratings reflect the level of confidence that the evidence for a guideline statement reflects a true effect based on consistency of findings across studies, directness of the effect on a specific health outcome, precision of the estimate of effect, and risk of bias in available studies (Agency for Healthcare Research and Quality 2014; Balshem et al. 2011; Guyatt et al. 2006).

Proper Use of Guidelines

The APA Practice Guidelines are assessments of current (as of the date of authorship) scientific and clinical information provided as an educational service. The guidelines 1) should not be considered as a statement of the standard of care or inclusive of all proper treatments or methods of care, 2) are not continually updated and may not reflect the most recent evidence because new evidence may emerge between the time information is developed and when the guidelines are published or read, 3) address only the question(s) or issue(s) specifically identified, 4) do not mandate any particular course of medical care, 5) are not intended to substitute for the independent professional judgment of the treating clinician, and 6) do not account for individual variation among patients. As such, it is not possible to draw conclusions about the effects of omitting a particular recommendation, either in general or for a specific patient. Furthermore, adherence to these guidelines will not ensure a successful outcome for every individual, nor should these guidelines be interpreted as including all proper methods of evaluation and care or excluding other acceptable methods of evaluation and care aimed at the same results. The ultimate recommendation regarding a particular assessment, clinical procedure, or treatment plan must be made by the clinician directly involved in the patient's care in light of the psychiatric evaluation, other clinical data, and the diagnostic and treatment options available. Such recommendations should be made in collaboration with the patient, whenever possible, and should incorporate the patient's personal and sociocultural preferences and values in order to enhance the therapeutic alliance, adherence to treatment, and treatment outcomes.

For all of these reasons, APA cautions against the use of guidelines in litigation. Use of these guidelines is voluntary. APA provides the guidelines on an "as is" basis and makes no warranty, expressed or implied, regarding them. APA assumes no responsibility for any injury or damage to persons or property arising out of or related to any use of the guidelines or for any errors or omissions.

Guideline Statement Summary

Assessment and Determination of Treatment Plan

1. APA *recommends* **(1C)** that the initial assessment of a patient with a possible psychotic disorder include the reason the individual is presenting for evaluation; the patient's goals and preferences for treatment; a review of psychiatric symptoms and trauma history; an assessment of tobacco use and other substance use; a psychiatric treatment history; an assessment of physical health; an assessment of psychosocial and cultural factors; a mental status examination, including cognitive assessment; and an assessment of risk of suicide and aggressive behaviors, as outlined in APA's *Practice Guidelines for the Psychiatric Evaluation of Adults* (3rd edition).
2. APA *recommends* **(1C)** that the initial psychiatric evaluation of a patient with a possible psychotic disorder include a quantitative measure to identify and determine the severity of symptoms and impairments of functioning that may be a focus of treatment.
3. APA *recommends* **(1C)** that patients with schizophrenia have a documented, comprehensive, and person-centered treatment plan that includes evidence-based nonpharmacological and pharmacological treatments.

Pharmacotherapy

4. APA *recommends* **(1A)** that patients with schizophrenia be treated with an antipsychotic medication and monitored for effectiveness and side effects.*
5. APA *recommends* **(1A)** that patients with schizophrenia whose symptoms have improved with an antipsychotic medication continue to be treated with an antipsychotic medication.*
6. APA *suggests* **(2B)** that patients with schizophrenia whose symptoms have improved with an antipsychotic medication continue to be treated with the same antipsychotic medication.*
7. APA *recommends* **(1B)** that patients with treatment-resistant schizophrenia be treated with clozapine.*
8. APA *recommends* **(1B)** that patients with schizophrenia be treated with clozapine if the risk for suicide attempts or suicide remains substantial despite other treatments.*
9. APA *suggests* **(2C)** that patients with schizophrenia be treated with clozapine if the risk for aggressive behavior remains substantial despite other treatments.*
10. APA *suggests* **(2B)** that patients receive treatment with a long-acting injectable antipsychotic medication if they prefer such treatment or if they have a history of poor or uncertain adherence.*
11. APA *recommends* **(1C)** that patients who have acute dystonia associated with antipsychotic therapy be treated with an anticholinergic medication.
12. APA *suggests* **(2C)** the following options for patients who have parkinsonism associated with antipsychotic therapy: lowering the dosage of the antipsychotic medication, switching to another antipsychotic medication, or treating with an anticholinergic medication.

---

*This guideline statement should be implemented in the context of a person-centered treatment plan that includes evidence-based nonpharmacological and pharmacological treatments for schizophrenia.

13. APA *suggests* **(2C)** the following options for patients who have akathisia associated with antipsychotic therapy: lowering the dosage of the antipsychotic medication, switching to another antipsychotic medication, adding a benzodiazepine medication, or adding a beta-adrenergic blocking agent.

14. APA *recommends* **(1B)** that patients who have moderate to severe or disabling tardive dyskinesia associated with antipsychotic therapy be treated with a reversible inhibitor of the vesicular monoamine transporter 2 (VMAT2).

Psychosocial Interventions

15. APA *recommends* **(1B)** that patients with schizophrenia who are experiencing a first episode of psychosis be treated in a coordinated specialty care program.*

16. APA *recommends* **(1B)** that patients with schizophrenia be treated with cognitive-behavioral therapy for psychosis (CBTp).*

17. APA *recommends* **(1B)** that patients with schizophrenia receive psychoeducation.*

18. APA *recommends* **(1B)** that patients with schizophrenia receive supported employment services.*

19. APA *recommends* **(1B)** that patients with schizophrenia receive assertive community treatment if there is a history of poor engagement with services leading to frequent relapse or social disruption (e.g., homelessness; legal difficulties, including imprisonment).*

20. APA *suggests* **(2B)** that patients with schizophrenia who have ongoing contact with family receive family interventions.*

21. APA *suggests* **(2C)** that patients with schizophrenia receive interventions aimed at developing self-management skills and enhancing person-oriented recovery.*

22. APA *suggests* **(2C)** that patients with schizophrenia receive cognitive remediation.*

23. APA *suggests* **(2C)** that patients with schizophrenia who have a therapeutic goal of enhanced social functioning receive social skills training.*

24. APA *suggests* **(2C)** that patients with schizophrenia be treated with supportive psychotherapy.*

Guideline Statements and Implementation

Assessment and Determination of Treatment Plan

STATEMENT 1: Assessment of Possible Schizophrenia

APA *recommends* **(1C)** that the initial assessment of a patient with a possible psychotic disorder include the reason the individual is presenting for evaluation; the patient's goals and preferences for treatment; a review of psychiatric symptoms and trauma history; an assessment of tobacco use and other substance use; a psychiatric treatment history; an assessment of physical health; an assessment of psychosocial and cultural factors; a mental status examination, including cognitive assessment; and an assessment of risk of suicide and aggressive behaviors, as outlined in APA's *Practice Guidelines for the Psychiatric Evaluation of Adults* (3rd edition).

Implementation

The importance of the psychiatric evaluation cannot be underestimated because it serves as the initial basis for a therapeutic relationship with the patient and provides information that is crucial to differential diagnosis, shared decision-making about treatment, and educating patients and family members about such factors as illness course and prognosis. APA's *Practice Guidelines for the Psychiatric Evaluation of Adults*, 3rd edition (American Psychiatric Association 2016a) describe recommended and suggested elements of assessment for any individual who presents with psychiatric symptoms (Table 1). These elements are by no means comprehensive, and additional areas of inquiry will become apparent as the evaluation unfolds, depending on the responses to initial questions, the presenting concerns, the observations of the clinician during the assessment, the complexity and urgency of clinical decision-making, and other aspects of the clinical context. In many circumstances, aspects of the evaluation will extend across multiple visits (American Psychiatric Association 2016a).

The specific approach to the interview will depend on many factors, including the patient's ability to communicate, degree of cooperation, level of insight, illness severity, and ability to recall historical details (American Psychiatric Association 2016a). Such factors as the patient's health literacy (Clausen et al. 2016) and cultural background (Lewis-Fernández et al. 2016) can also influence the patient's understanding or interpretation of questions. Typically, a psychiatric evaluation involves a direct interview between the patient and the clinician (American Psychiatric Association 2016a). The use of open-ended empathic questions about the patient's current life circumstances and reasons for evaluation can provide an initial picture of the individual and serve as a way of establishing rapport. Such questions can be followed up with additional structured inquiry about history, symptoms, or observations made during the assessment.

Throughout the assessment process, it is important to gain an understanding of the patient's goals, their view of the illness, and preferences for treatment. This information will serve as a starting point for person-centered care and shared decision-making with the patient, family, and other persons of support (Dixon et al. 2016; Hamann and Heres 2019). It will also provide a framework for recovery, which has been defined as "a process of change through which individuals improve their health and wellness, live self-directed lives, and strive to reach their full potential" (Substance Abuse

TABLE 1. **Recommended aspects of the initial psychiatric evaluation**

History of present illness
- Reason that the patient is presenting for evaluation, including current symptoms, behaviors, and precipitating factors
- Current psychiatric diagnoses and psychiatric review of systems

Psychiatric history
- Hospitalization and emergency department visits for psychiatric issues, including substance use disorders
- Psychiatric treatments (type, duration, and, where applicable, doses)
- Response and adherence to psychiatric treatments, including psychosocial treatments, pharmacotherapy, and other interventions such as electroconvulsive therapy or transcranial magnetic stimulation
- Prior psychiatric diagnoses and symptoms, including
  - Hallucinations (including command hallucinations), delusions, and negative symptoms
  - Aggressive ideas or behaviors (e.g., homicide, domestic or workplace violence, other physically or sexually aggressive threats or acts)
  - Suicidal ideas, suicide plans, and suicide attempts, including details of each attempt (e.g., context, method, damage, potential lethality, intent) and attempts that were aborted or interrupted
  - Intentional self-injury in which there was no suicide intent
  - Impulsivity

Substance use history
- Use of tobacco, alcohol, and other substances (e.g., vaping, marijuana, cocaine, heroin, hallucinogens) and any misuse of prescribed or over-the-counter medications or supplements
- Current or recent substance use disorder or change in use of alcohol or other substances

Medical history
- Whether or not the patient has an ongoing relationship with a primary care health professional
- Allergies or drug sensitivities
- All medications the patient is currently taking or has recently taken and the side effects of these medications (i.e., both prescribed and nonprescribed medications, herbal and nutritional supplements, and vitamins)
- Past or current medical illnesses and related hospitalizations
- Relevant past or current treatments, including surgeries, other procedures, or complementary and alternative medical treatments
- Sexual and reproductive history
- Cardiopulmonary status
- Past or current neurological or neurocognitive disorders or symptoms
- Past physical trauma, including head injuries
- Past or current endocrinological disease
- Past or current infectious disease, including sexually transmitted diseases, HIV, tuberculosis, hepatitis C, and locally endemic infectious diseases such as Lyme disease
- Past or current sleep abnormalities, including sleep apnea
- Past or current symptoms or conditions associated with significant pain and discomfort
- Additional review of systems, as indicated

Family history
- Including history of suicidal behaviors or aggressive behaviors in biological relatives

Personal and social history
- Preferred language and need for an interpreter
- Personal/cultural beliefs, sociocultural environment, and cultural explanations of psychiatric illness
- Presence of psychosocial stressors (e.g., financial, housing, legal, school/occupational, or interpersonal/relationship problems; lack of social support; painful, disfiguring, or terminal medical illness)
- Exposure to physical, sexual, or emotional trauma
- Exposure to violence or aggressive behavior, including combat exposure or childhood abuse
- Legal or disciplinary consequences of past aggressive behaviors

Examination, including mental status examination

- General appearance and nutritional status
- Height, weight, and body mass index (BMI)
- Vital signs
- Skin, including any stigmata of trauma, self-injury, or drug use
- Coordination and gait
- Involuntary movements or abnormalities of motor tone
- Sight and hearing
- Speech, including fluency and articulation
- Mood, degree of hopelessness, and level of anxiety
- Thought content, process, and perceptions, including current hallucinations, delusions, negative symptoms, and insight
- Cognition
- Current suicidal ideas, suicide plans, and suicide intent, including active or passive thoughts of suicide or death
    - If current suicidal ideas are present, assess patient's intended course of action if current symptoms worsen; access to suicide methods, including firearms; possible motivations for suicide (e.g., attention or reaction from others, revenge, shame, humiliation, delusional guilt, command hallucinations); reasons for living (e.g., sense of responsibility to children or others, religious beliefs); and quality and strength of the therapeutic alliance
- Current aggressive ideas, including thoughts of physical or sexual aggression or homicide
    - If current aggressive ideas are present, assess specific individuals or groups toward whom homicidal or aggressive ideas or behaviors have been directed in the past or at present, access to firearms, and impulsivity, including anger management issues

Source.   Adapted from APA's *Practice Guidelines for the Psychiatric Evaluation of Adults,* 3rd Edition. Arlington VA, American Psychiatric Association, 2016. Copyright © 2016 American Psychiatric Association. Used with permission.

and Mental Health Services Administration 2012a, p. 3). Consequently, discussions of goals should be focused beyond symptom relief and may include goals related to schooling, employment, living situation, relationships, leisure activities, and other aspects of functioning and quality of life. Questions about the patient's views may help determine whether the patient is aware of having an illness and whether the patient has other explanations for symptoms that are helpful to them (Saks 2009). Patients may have specific views about such topics as medications, other treatment approaches, mechanical restraints, or involuntary treatment based on prior treatment experiences. They may also be able to delineate strategies that have been helpful for them in coping with or managing their symptoms in the past (Cohen et al. 2017). Some patients will have completed a psychiatric advance directive (Murray and Wortzel 2019), which is important to review with the patient if it exists.

In addition to direct interview, patients may be asked to complete electronic or paper-based forms that ask about psychiatric symptoms or key aspects of the history (American Psychiatric Association 2016a). When available, prior medical records, electronic prescription databases, and input from other treating clinicians can add further details to the history or corroborate information obtained in the interview (American Psychiatric Association 2016a).

Family members, friends, and other individuals involved in the patient's support network can be an important part of the patient's care team and valuable sources of collateral information about the reason for evaluation, the patient's past history, and current symptoms and behavior (American Psychiatric Association 2016a). Outreach to family, friends, and others in the support network will typically occur with the patient's permission. In situations in which the patient is given the opportunity and does not object, necessary information can be shared with family members or other persons involved in the patient's care or payment for care (Office for Civil Rights 2017b). For example, if a relative or person of support is present with the patient at an appointment, the clinician may discuss information about medications or give education about warning signs of a developing emergency.

In some instances, however, patients may ask that family or others not be contacted. When this is the case, patients can usually identify someone whom they trust to provide additional information, and they are often willing to reconsider contact as treatment proceeds. It is also useful to discuss the reasons that the patient has concerns about contacts with family members or other important people in the patient's life. For example, a patient may wish to avoid burdening a loved one, may have felt unsupported by a particular family member in the past, or may be experiencing delusional beliefs that involve a family member or friend. The patient may also want to limit the information that clinicians receive about past or recent treatment, symptoms, or behaviors. Even when a patient does not want a specific person to be contacted, the clinician may listen to information provided by that individual, as long as confidential information is not provided to the informant (American Psychiatric Association 2016a). Also, to prevent or lessen a serious and imminent threat to the health or safety of the patient or others, *The Principles of Medical Ethics* (American Psychiatric Association 2013f) and the Health Insurance Portability and Accountability Act of 1996 (HIPAA; Office for Civil Rights 2017b) permit clinicians to disclose necessary information about a patient to family members, caregivers, law enforcement, or other persons involved with the patient as well as to jails, prisons, and law enforcement officials having lawful custody of the patient. HIPAA also permits health care providers to disclose necessary information to the patient's family, friends, or other persons involved in the patient's care or payment for care when such disclosure is judged to be in the best interests of the patient and the patient either is not present or is unable to agree or object to a disclosure because of incapacity or emergency circumstances. Examples of such circumstances are not limited to unconsciousness and may also include such circumstances as temporary psychosis or intoxication with alcohol or other substances (Office for Civil Rights 2017b).

Although it is beyond the scope of this guideline to discuss the differential diagnosis and evaluation of psychotic disorders, many features and aspects of clinical course will enter into such a determination in addition to psychotic symptoms per se. Clinicians should also be mindful that biases can influence assessment and diagnosis, with disparities in diagnosis based on race being particularly common (Olbert et al. 2018; Schwartz and Blankenship 2014). The clinician should be alert to features of the history, including family, developmental, and academic history, that may suggest specific conditions or a need for additional physical or laboratory evaluation. Examples of conditions that can mimic schizophrenia in their initial presentation include neurosyphilis, Huntington's disease, Wilson's disease, and anti-*N*-methyl-D-aspartate (NMDA) receptor encephalitis (Lieberman and First 2018). Individuals with 22q11.2 deletion syndrome have a substantially increased risk of developing schizophrenia (Bassett et al. 2017; McDonald-McGinn et al. 2015; Van et al. 2017). In addition, the presence of a 22q11.2 deletion is associated with an increased likelihood of neurocognitive and physical health impairments (McDonald-McGinn et al. 2015; Moberg et al. 2018; Swillen and McDonald-McGinn 2015), which has implications for treatment (Fung et al. 2015; Mosheva et al. 2019). Psychotic symptoms can also occur in the context of other neurological and systemic illnesses, with or without delirium, and such acute states can at times be mistaken for an acute exacerbation of schizophrenia. Furthermore, because a significant fraction of individuals with psychosis will have a shift in diagnosis over time, the diagnosis may need to be reevaluated as new information about the patient's illness course and symptoms becomes available (Bromet et al. 2011). Specialty consultation can be helpful in establishing and clarifying diagnosis (Coulter et al. 2019), particularly if the illness symptoms or course appear to be atypical or if the patient is not responding to treatment.

A thorough history is also important for identifying the presence of co-occurring psychiatric conditions or physical disorders that need to be addressed in treatment planning (American Psychiatric Association 2016a; Firth et al. 2019). For example, individuals with serious mental illness have higher rates of smoking, higher rates of heavy smoking, and lower rates of smoking cessation than do community samples (Cook et al. 2014; de Leon and Diaz 2005; Myles et al. 2012; Wium-Andersen et al. 2015). Furthermore, the use of cannabis may be more frequent in individuals with schizophrenia (Koskinen et al. 2010) and associated with greater symptom severity or earlier onset of psychosis (Carney et al. 2017; Large et al. 2011). Other substance use disorders, if present, can also produce or exacerbate symptoms of psychosis (American Psychiatric Association 2016a; Large et al. 2014). Thus, as part of the initial evaluation, it is important to determine whether the patient uses tobacco, cannabis, or other substances such as alcohol, caffeine, cocaine, opioids, sedative-hypnotic agents, stimulants, 3,4-methylenedioxymethamphetamine (MDMA), solvents, androgenic steroids, hallucinogens, or synthetic substances (e.g., "bath salts," K2, Spice). The route by which substances are used (e.g., ingestion, smoking, vaping, intranasal, intravenous) is similarly important to document.

Mortality is increased in individuals with schizophrenia (Brown et al. 2000; Fazel et al. 2014; Olfson et al. 2015), and the average life span is shortened by a decade or more, with much of this decrease related to increased rates of co-occurring physical conditions (Laursen et al. 2013; Saha et al. 2007; Walker et al. 2015). Adverse health effects of smoking also contribute to an increased risk of mortality among individuals with schizophrenia (Lariscy et al. 2018; Reynolds et al. 2018; Tam et al. 2016). Many other conditions are more frequent in individuals with serious mental illness in general (Janssen et al. 2015; McGinty et al. 2016) and schizophrenia in particular (Henderson et al. 2015), including, but not limited to, poor oral health (Kisely et al. 2015), hepatitis C infection (Chasser et al. 2017; Hauser and Kern 2015; Hughes et al. 2016), HIV infection (Hobkirk et al. 2015; Hughes et al. 2016), cancer (Olfson et al. 2015), sleep apnea (Myles et al. 2016; Stubbs et al. 2016b), obesity (Janssen et al. 2015), diabetes mellitus (Vancampfort et al. 2016a), metabolic syndrome (Vancampfort et al. 2015), and cardiovascular disease (Correll et al. 2017c). These disorders, if present, can contribute to mortality or reduced quality of life, and some may be induced or exacerbated by psychiatric medications. Laboratory tests and physical examination as part of the initial evaluation can help to identify common co-occurring conditions and can serve as a baseline for subsequent monitoring during treatment (Table 2).

As part of the initial evaluation, it is also useful to inquire about the course and duration of symptoms prior to treatment (i.e., duration of untreated psychosis) (Penttilä et al. 2014; Register-Brown and Hong 2014; Santesteban-Echarri et al. 2017) and whether the patient has received any mental health treatment. If the patient has received treatment previously, it is important to ask about a broad range of treatments and other approaches to addressing the patient's symptoms and functioning and to specifically ask about the full range of treatment settings (e.g., outpatient, partial hospitalization, inpatient) and approaches that the patient has found helpful or problematic (American Psychiatric Association 2016a). Although most patients will comment on prior medications, psychotherapy, or psychiatric hospitalizations if asked about treatment history, specific questions may be needed to gather details of such treatments. Prompting may be needed to learn information about the patient's experiences with other interventions such as psychosocial rehabilitation, supported employment, assertive community treatment (ACT), court-ordered treatment, treatment while incarcerated, substance use treatments, neuromodulatory therapies (e.g., electroconvulsive therapy [ECT], transcranial magnetic stimulation [TMS]), 12-step programs, self-help groups, spiritual healers, and complementary or alternative treatment approaches. Pharmacy databases and patients' lists of active medications are not likely to include long-acting injectable (LAI) medications (e.g., antipsychotics, naltrexone, buprenorphine) or implants (e.g., buprenorphine, contraceptive agents), over-the-counter medications, herbal products, or nutritional supplements. For each specific type of intervention that the patient has received, it is helpful to learn more about the duration, mode of delivery (e.g., formulation, route, and dose for medications; format, type, and frequency of treatment for psychotherapy), response (including tolerability, changes in quality of life, level of functioning, and symptom response/remission), and degree of adherence.

The psychosocial history reviews the stages of the patient's life and may include attention to perinatal events, delays in developmental milestones, academic history and performance (including learning difficulties, special education interventions, or disciplinary actions), relationship and sexual history, interpersonal functioning (including in social and family roles, such as parenting), occupational history (including military history), legal history, and identification of major life events (e.g., parental loss, divorce, traumatic experiences, migration history) and psychosocial

TABLE 2. Suggested physical and laboratory assessments for patients with schizophrenia

	Initial or baseline assessments[a]	Follow-up assessments[b]
Assessments to monitor physical status and detect concomitant physical conditions		
Vital signs	Pulse, blood pressure	Pulse, blood pressure, temperature as clinically indicated
Body weight and height	Body weight, height, BMI[c]	BMI[c] every visit for 6 months and at least quarterly thereafter
Hematology	CBC, including ANC	CBC, including ANC if clinically indicated (e.g., patients treated with clozapine)
Blood chemistries	Electrolytes, renal function tests, liver function tests, TSH	As clinically indicated
Pregnancy	Pregnancy test for women of childbearing potential	
Toxicology	Drug toxicology screen, if clinically indicated	Drug toxicology screen, if clinically indicated
Electrophysiological studies	EEG, if indicated on the basis of neurological examination or history	
Imaging	Brain imaging (CT or MRI, with MRI being preferred), if indicated on the basis of neurological examination or history[d]	
Genetic testing	Chromosomal testing, if indicated on the basis of physical examination or history, including developmental history[e]	
Assessments related to other specific side effects of treatment		
Diabetes[f]	Screening for diabetes risk factors,[g] fasting blood glucose[h]	Fasting blood glucose or hemoglobin A1C at 4 months after initiating a new treatment and at least annually thereafter[h]
Hyperlipidemia	Lipid panel[i]	Lipid panel[i] at 4 months after initiating a new antipsychotic medication and at least annually thereafter
Metabolic syndrome	Determine whether metabolic syndrome criteria are met[j]	Determine whether metabolic syndrome criteria are met[j] at 4 months after initiating a new antipsychotic medication and at least annually thereafter
QTc prolongation	ECG before treatment with chlorpromazine, droperidol, iloperidone, pimozide, thioridazine, or ziprasidone[k] or in the presence of cardiac risk factors[l]	ECG with significant change in dose of chlorpromazine, droperidol, iloperidone, pimozide, thioridazine, or ziprasidone[k] or with the addition of other medications that can affect QTc interval in patients with cardiac risk factors[l] or elevated baseline QTc intervals
Hyperprolactinemia	Screening for symptoms of hyperprolactinemia[m] Prolactin level, if indicated on the basis of clinical history	Screening for symptoms of hyperprolactinemia at each visit until stable, then yearly if treated with an antipsychotic known to increase prolactin[m] Prolactin level, if indicated on the basis of clinical history

	Initial or baseline assessments[a]	Follow-up assessments[b]
Assessments related to other specific side effects of treatment *(continued)*		
Antipsychotic-induced movement disorders	Clinical assessment of akathisia, dystonia, parkinsonism, and other abnormal involuntary movements, including tardive dyskinesia[n] Assessment with a structured instrument (e.g., AIMS, DISCUS) if such movements are present	Clinical assessment of akathisia, dystonia, parkinsonism, and other abnormal involuntary movements, including tardive dyskinesia, at each visit[n] Assessment with a structured instrument (e.g., AIMS, DISCUS) at a minimum of every 6 months in patients at high risk of tardive dyskinesia[o] and at least every 12 months in other patients[p] as well as if a new onset or exacerbation of preexisting movements is detected at any visit

[a]APA's *Practice Guidelines for the Psychiatric Evaluation of Adults,* 3rd edition (American Psychiatric Association 2016a) recommends that the initial psychiatric evaluation of a patient include assessment of whether or not the patient has an ongoing relationship with a primary care health professional. Preventive care and other tests, such as screening for hepatitis C or HIV, are expected to occur as a part of routine primary care. Nevertheless, determining whether a patient is receiving primary care and inquiring about the patient's relationship with their primary care practitioner can be a starting point for improved access to quality health care and preventive services.

[b]Although this practice guideline recommends that patients treated with antipsychotic medications be monitored for physical conditions and side effects on a regular basis, there are no absolute criteria for frequency of monitoring. Occurrence of conditions and side effects may be influenced by the patient's history, preexisting conditions, and use of other medications in addition to antipsychotic agents. Thus, decisions about monitoring patients for physical conditions, specific side effects, or abnormalities in laboratory test results will necessarily depend on the clinical circumstances. In general, assessments related to physical conditions and specific medication-related side effects will be done at the time of initiating or changing antipsychotic medications or when adding other medications that contribute to these side effects.

[c]BMI may be calculated by using the formula weight in kg/(height in m)^2 or the formula $703 \times$ weight in lb/(height in inches)^2 or by using a BMI calculator available from the National Heart, Lung, and Blood Institute (www.nhlbi.nih.gov/health/educational/lose_wt/BMI/bmicalc.htm). A person with a BMI of 25–29.9 is considered overweight, and one with a BMI of 30 or higher is considered obese. In addition to BMI, waist circumference can be used as an indicator of risk (>35 inches for women and >40 inches for men). Except for patients with a BMI of <18.5, an increase in BMI of 1 unit would suggest a need for intervention by monitoring weight more closely, engaging the patient in a weight management program, using an adjunctive treatment to reduce weight, or changing the antipsychotic medication.

[d]Factors that suggest a possible need for imaging include focal neurological signs, new onset of seizures, later age at symptom onset, symptoms suggestive of intracranial pathology (e.g., chronic or severe headaches, nausea, vomiting), and symptoms suggestive of autoimmune encephalitis (e.g., rapid progression of working memory deficits over less than 3 months; decreased or altered level of consciousness, lethargy, or personality change; Graus et al. 2016). In the absence of such indications, decisions about imaging should consider that the yield of routine brain imaging is low, with <1% of studies showing potentially serious incidental findings or abnormalities that would influence treatment (Cunqueiro et al. 2019; Falkenberg et al. 2017; Forbes et al. 2019; Gibson et al. 2018). On the other hand, routine imaging is a low-risk procedure, and a negative finding can be reassuring to patients and to families. If imaging is ordered, it is rarely necessary to delay other treatment or hospitalization while awaiting imaging results.

[e]Factors that may suggest a possible need for chromosomal testing (e.g., to identify abnormalities such as 22q11.2 deletion syndrome) include mild dysmorphic features, hypernasal speech, developmental delays, intellectual impairments, learning difficulties, and congenital heart defects (Bassett and Chow 1999; Miller et al. 2010).

[f]The U.S. Food and Drug Administration has requested that all manufacturers of second-generation antipsychotic medications (SGAs) include a warning in their product labeling regarding hyperglycemia and diabetes mellitus. Although precise risk estimates for hyperglycemia-related adverse events are not available for each agent, epidemiological studies suggested an increased risk of treatment-emergent adverse events with SGAs, including extreme hyperglycemia. In some patients, this hyperglycemia was associated with ketoacidosis, hyperosmolar coma, or death.

[g]Factors that indicate an increased risk for undiagnosed diabetes include a BMI >25, a first-degree relative with diabetes, habitual physical inactivity, being a member of a high-risk ethnic population (African American, Hispanic, American Indian, Asian American, Pacific Islander), history of cardiovascular disease, hypertension (≥140/90 mmHg or on therapy for hypertension), high-density lipoprotein cholesterol (HDL-C) <35 mg/dL (0.90 mmol/L) and/or triglyceride level >250 mg/dL (2.82 mmol/L), polycystic ovary syndrome (in women), having had gestational diabetes, and other clinical conditions associated with insulin resistance (e.g., severe obesity, acanthosis nigricans) (American Diabetes Association 2018). Symptoms of possible diabetes include frequent urination, excessive thirst, extreme hunger, unusual weight loss, increased fatigue, irritability, and blurry vision.

[h]When screening for the presence of diabetes, criteria for diagnosis include a fasting blood glucose higher than 125 mg/dL, where fasting is defined as no caloric intake for at least 8 hours (American Diabetes Association 2018). Alternatively, a hemoglobin A1C of 6.5% or greater can be used. Other acceptable approaches for diagnosis of diabetes include an oral glucose tolerance test or a random blood glucose of at least 200 mg/dL in conjunction with a hyperglycemic crisis or classic symptoms of hyperglycemia. With all of these approaches, results should be confirmed by repeat testing unless unequivocal hyperglycemia is present. In patients with hemoglobinopathies or conditions associated with increased red blood cell turnover (e.g., second- or third-trimester pregnancy, hemodialysis, recent blood loss, transfusion, erythropoietin therapy), fasting blood glucose should be used rather than hemoglobin A1C. An abnormal value of fasting blood glucose or hemoglobin A1C suggests a need for medical consultation. More frequent monitoring may be indicated in the presence of weight change, symptoms of diabetes, or a random measure of blood glucose >200 mg/dL.

[i]Additional information on screening and management of patients with lipid disorders can be found in the *AHA/ACC/AACVPR/AAPA/ABC/ACPM/ADA/AGS/APhA/ASPC/NLA Guideline on the Management of Blood Cholesterol* (Grundy et al. 2018).

[j]Metabolic syndrome is currently defined by the presence of at least three of the following five risk factors: elevated waist circumference (defined for the United States and Canada as >102 cm [40.2 inches] for men and >88 cm [34.6 inches] for women); elevated triglycerides of ≥150 mg/dL (or drug treatment for elevated triglycerides, such as fibrates, nicotinic acid, or high-dose omega-3 fatty acids); reduced HDL-C of <40 mg/dL in men or <50 mg/dL in women (or drug treatment for reduced HDL-C, such as fibrates or nicotinic acid); elevated blood pressure (BP) with systolic BP ≥130 mmHg and/or diastolic BP ≥85 mmHg (or antihypertensive treatment in a patient with a history of hypertension); and elevated fasting glucose ≥100 mg/dL (or drug treatment for elevated glucose) (Alberti et al. 2009).

[k]Using an adverse drug event causality analysis intended to evaluate the risk of sudden death when taking a specific medication (Woosley et al. 2017), the listed drugs have been categorized as prolonging the QT interval and being clearly associated with a known risk of torsades de pointes, even when taken as recommended (Woosley et al. 2009).

[l]In this context, risk factors include non-modifiable (e.g., congenital long QT syndrome, age, sex, family history of sudden cardiac death, personal or family history of structural or functional heart disease, personal history of drug-induced QT prolongation, metabolizer status) and modifiable risk factors (e.g., starvation; bradycardia; risk or presence of hypokalemia, hypomagnesemia, or hypocalcemia; excess dose or rapid intravenous infusion of QTc interval–prolonging drugs; simultaneous use of multiple drugs that prolong QTc intervals; or factors affecting drug metabolism such as drug-drug interactions, acute or chronic kidney disease, or hepatic impairment) (Funk et al. 2018).

[m]Screening should assess changes in libido, menstrual changes, or galactorrhea in women, and changes in libido or in erectile or ejaculatory function in men.

[n]Assessment can occur through clinical examination or through the use of a structured evaluative tool such as the Abnormal Involuntary Movement Scale (AIMS; Guy 1976; Munetz and Benjamin 1988) or the Dyskinesia Identification System: Condensed User Scale (DISCUS; Kalachnik and Sprague 1993). For a copy of the AIMS, see www.aacap.org/App_Themes/AACAP/docs/member_resources/toolbox_for_clinical_practice_and_outcomes/monitoring/AIMS.pdf, and for a copy of the DISCUS, see https://portal.ct.gov/-/media/DDS/Health/hcsma20002b.pdf.

[o]Patients at increased risk for developing abnormal involuntary movements include individuals older than 55 years; women; individuals with a mood disorder, substance use disorder, intellectual disability, or central nervous system injury; individuals with high cumulative exposure to antipsychotic medications, particularly high-potency dopamine D_2 receptor antagonists; and patients who experience acute dystonic reactions, clinically significant parkinsonism, or akathisia (Carbon et al. 2017, 2018; Miller et al. 2005; Solmi et al. 2018a). Abnormal involuntary movements can also emerge or worsen with antipsychotic cessation.

[p]Frequency of monitoring for involuntary movements in individuals receiving treatment with an antipsychotic medication is also subject to local regulations in some jurisdictions.

Abbreviations. AIMS=Abnormal Involuntary Movement Scale; ANC=absolute neutrophil count; BMI=body mass index; CBC=complete blood count; CT=computed tomography; DISCUS=Dyskinesia Identification System: Condensed User Scale; ECG=electrocardiography; EEG=electroencephalogram; MRI=magnetic resonance imaging; QTc=corrected QT interval; TSH=thyroid-stimulating hormone.

stressors (e.g., financial, housing, legal, school/occupational, or interpersonal/relationship problems; lack of social support; painful, disfiguring, or terminal medical illness) (American Psychiatric Association 2016a; Barnhill 2014; MacKinnon et al. 2016; Smith et al. 2019). Information about the patient's family constellation and persons who provide support will serve as a foundation for working collaboratively with the patient and their support network. The cultural history also emphasizes relationships, both familial and nonfamilial, and the role of important cultural and religious influences on the patient's life (Aggarwal and Lewis-Fernández 2015; American Psychiatric Association 2013a; Lewis-Fernández et al. 2016).

The mental status examination is an integral part of the initial assessment. A full delineation of the mental status examination is beyond the scope of this document, and detailed information on conducting the examination is available elsewhere (American Psychiatric Association 2016a; Barnhill 2014; MacKinnon et al. 2016; Smith et al. 2019; Strub and Black 2000). However, for individuals with possible schizophrenia, a detailed inquiry into hallucinations and delusions will often identify psychotic experiences in addition to the presenting concerns. Negative symptoms and cognitive impairment are common and influence outcomes (Bowie et al. 2006; Green 2016; Jordan et al. 2014; Rabinowitz et al. 2012; Santesteban-Echarri et al. 2017) but may go undetected without specific attention during the evaluation. Negative symptoms also can be difficult to differentiate from lack of interest or reduced motivation due to depression, medication side effects, substance use, or neurological conditions.

Insight is also impaired in a significant proportion of individuals with schizophrenia (Mohamed et al. 2009) and can manifest as a decreased awareness of having a disorder, symptoms, consequences of illness, or a need for treatment (Mintz et al. 2003). Consequently, inquiring about the patient's degree of insight and judgment will provide information relevant to risk assessment, treatment outcomes, and adherence (Mintz et al. 2003; Mohamed et al. 2009).

Risk assessment is another essential part of the initial psychiatric evaluation (American Psychiatric Association 2004). It requires synthesizing information gathered in the history and mental status examination and identifying modifiable risk factors for suicidal or aggressive behaviors that can serve as targets of intervention in constructing a plan of treatment. Suicidal ideas are common in individuals who have had a psychotic experience (Bromet et al. 2017). Death due to suicide has been estimated to occur in about 4%–10% of individuals with schizophrenia (Drake et al. 1985; Heilä et al. 2005; Hor and Taylor 2010; Inskip et al. 1998; Laursen et al. 2014; Nordentoft et al. 2011; Palmer et al. 2005; Popovic et al. 2014; Tanskanen et al. 2018; Yates et al. 2019), yielding a greater than tenfold increase in standardized mortality ratios (Saha et al. 2007). Among individuals with schizophrenia, suicide attempts and suicide may be more common early in the course of the illness (Popovic et al. 2014) and can occur even before initial treatment for psychosis (Challis et al. 2013).

In individuals with schizophrenia, many of the risk factors that contribute to the risks of suicidal or aggressive behaviors are the same as factors increasing risk in other disorders. For example, in individuals with schizophrenia, an increased risk of suicidal or aggressive behaviors has been associated with male sex, expressed suicidal ideation, a history of attempted suicide or other suicide-related behaviors, and the presence of alcohol use disorder or other substance use disorder (Cassidy et al. 2018; Challis et al. 2013; Fazel et al. 2009a, 2014; Fleischhacker et al. 2014; Hawton et al. 2005; Hor and Taylor 2010; Østergaard et al. 2017; Pompili et al. 2007; Popovic et al. 2014; Roché et al. 2018; Sariaslan et al. 2016; Singh et al. 2012; Swanson et al. 2006; Witt et al. 2013, 2014). Firearm access is an additional contributor to suicide risk (Alban et al. 2018; Anestis and Houtsma 2018; Siegel and Rothman 2016). Additional factors that have been identified as increasing risk for suicide among individuals with schizophrenia include depressive symptoms, hopelessness, agitation or motor restlessness, fear of mental disintegration, recent loss, recency of diagnosis or hospitalization, repeated hospitalizations, high intelligence, young age, and poor adherence to treatment (Cassidy et al. 2018; Fleischhacker et al. 2014; Hawton et al. 2005; Lopez-Morinigo et al. 2014; Pompili et al. 2007; Popovic et al. 2014; Randall et al. 2014). It is not clear whether preserved insight is associated with an increase in suicide risk among individuals with schizophrenia (Hor and Taylor 2010) or whether this is an apparent increase that is mediated by other factors such as hopelessness (López-Moríñigo et al. 2012).

Although reduced risk of suicide was associated with hallucinations in one meta-analysis (Hawton et al. 2005), the presence of auditory command hallucinations may confer increased risk (Harkavy-Friedman et al. 2003; Wong et al. 2013). Command hallucinations can also be relevant when assessing individuals for a risk of aggressive behaviors (McNiel et al. 2000; Swanson et al. 2006), although the relationship between experiencing commands and acting on them is complex (Braham et al. 2004). Persecutory delusions may also contribute to risk of aggression, particularly in the absence of treatment or in association with significant anger (Coid et al. 2013; Keers et al. 2014; Swanson et al. 2006).

Among individuals with psychotic illnesses, prior suicidal threats, angry affect, impulsivity, hostility, recent violent victimization, childhood sexual abuse, medication nonadherence, and a history of involuntary treatment were also associated with an increased risk of aggressive behavior (Buchanan et al. 2019; Large and Nielssen 2011; Reagu et al. 2013; Swanson et al. 2006; Witt et al. 2013, 2014). Other factors associated with a risk of aggression are similar to findings in individuals without psychosis and include male sex, young age, access to firearms, the presence of substance use, traumatic brain injury, a history of attempted suicide or other suicide-related behaviors, and prior aggressive behavior, including that associated with legal consequences (Buchanan et al. 2019; Cassidy et al. 2018; Fazel et al. 2009a, 2009b, 2014; Fleischhacker et al. 2014; Large and Nielssen 2011; Monuteaux et al. 2015; Østergaard et al. 2017; Popovic et al. 2014; Roché et al. 2018; Sariaslan et al. 2016; Short et al. 2013; Singh et al. 2012; Swanson et al. 2006; Witt et al. 2013, 2015).

Balancing of Potential Benefits and Harms in Rating the Strength of the Guideline Statement

Benefits

In an individual with a possible psychotic disorder, a detailed assessment is important in establishing a diagnosis, recognizing co-occurring conditions (including substance use disorders, other psychiatric disorders, and other physical health disorders), identifying psychosocial issues, and developing a plan of treatment that can reduce associated symptoms, morbidity, and mortality.

Harms*

Some individuals may become anxious, suspicious, or annoyed if asked multiple questions during the evaluation. This could interfere with the therapeutic relationship between the patient and the clinician. Another potential consequence is that time used to focus on a detailed assessment (as outlined in the *Practice Guidelines for the Psychiatric Evaluation of Adults*, 3rd edition; American Psychiatric Association 2016a) could reduce time available to address other issues of importance to the patient or of relevance to diagnosis and treatment planning.

Patient Preferences

Although there is no specific evidence on patient preferences related to assessment in individuals with a possible psychotic disorder, clinical experience suggests that the majority of patients are cooperative with and accepting of these types of questions as part of an initial assessment.

---

*Harms may include serious adverse events; less serious adverse events that affect tolerability; minor adverse events; negative effects of the intervention on quality of life; barriers and inconveniences associated with treatment; and other negative aspects of the treatment that may influence decision-making by the patient, the clinician, or both.

Balancing of Benefits and Harms

The potential benefits of this guideline statement were viewed as far outweighing the potential harms. This recommendation is also consistent with the APA *Practice Guidelines for the Psychiatric Evaluation of Adults*, 3rd edition (American Psychiatric Association 2016a). The level of research evidence is rated as low because there is minimal research on the benefits and harms of assessing these aspects of history and examination as part of an initial assessment. Nevertheless, expert opinion suggests that conducting such assessments as part of the initial psychiatric evaluation improves the diagnosis and treatment planning in individuals with a psychiatric disorder. For additional details, see the *Practice Guidelines for the Psychiatric Evaluation of Adults*. For additional discussion of the research evidence, see Appendix C, Statement 1.

Differences of Opinion Among Writing Group Members

There were no differences of opinion. The writing group voted unanimously in favor of this recommendation.

Review of Available Guidelines From Other Organizations

Relevant guidelines from the following organizations were reviewed: British Association for Psychopharmacology (BAP), Canadian Psychiatric Association and Schizophrenia Society of Canada, National Institute for Health and Care Excellence (NICE), Royal Australian and New Zealand College of Psychiatry (RANZCP), Scottish Intercollegiate Guidelines Network (SIGN), World Federation of Societies of Biological Psychiatry (WFSBP), and Schizophrenia Patient Outcomes Research Team (PORT). Information from them is generally consistent with this guideline statement. Other guidelines on the treatment of schizophrenia incorporate recommendations related to the need for a comprehensive initial assessment (Addington et al. 2017a; National Institute for Health and Care Excellence 2014), including identification of prior and current psychiatric symptoms and diagnoses (Addington et al. 2017a; Hasan et al. 2015; National Institute for Health and Care Excellence 2014), assessment of tobacco use (Addington et al. 2017a; National Institute for Health and Care Excellence 2014), assessment of substance use (Addington et al. 2017a; Barnes et al. 2011; Crockford and Addington 2017; Galletly et al. 2016; National Institute for Health and Care Excellence 2014), physical health history and examination (Addington et al. 2017a; National Institute for Health and Care Excellence 2014), assessment of psychosocial factors (Addington et al. 2017a; Galletly et al. 2016; National Institute for Health and Care Excellence 2014), and mental status examination (Addington et al. 2017a), including assessment of the risk of harm to self or others (Addington et al. 2017a; Hasan et al. 2015; National Institute for Health and Care Excellence 2014). Several other guidelines also provide information on the circumstances in which an electrocardiogram is suggested (Barnes et al. 2011; National Institute for Health and Care Excellence 2014; Pringsheim et al. 2017).

Quality Measurement Considerations

For patients with psychotic disorders, including schizophrenia, several components of the initial psychiatric evaluation have potential relevance for quality measure development, although such quality measures do not exist at present. A first step toward development of scientifically sound quality measures is identification of discrete indicators that signal the delivery of high-quality care. This step may be challenging to accomplish given the breadth of content within the initial psychiatric assessment and the difficulty in ascertaining evaluation details from chart or administrative data. However, it may still be possible to use available evidence and expert-recommended consensus to develop and specify electronic and clinical data registry quality measures. Additionally, as discussed in the APA *Practice Guidelines for the Psychiatric Evaluation of Adults*, 3rd edition (American Psychiatric Association 2016a), quality improvement efforts at the local level could assess whether specific aspects of the evaluation such as a risk assessment were completed while still allowing flexibility in the documentation of findings.

STATEMENT 2: Use of Quantitative Measures

APA *recommends* **(1C)** that the initial psychiatric evaluation of a patient with a possible psychotic disorder include a quantitative measure to identify and determine the severity of symptoms and impairments of functioning that may be a focus of treatment.

Implementation

APA's *Practice Guidelines for the Psychiatric Evaluation of Adults*, 3rd edition (American Psychiatric Association 2016a) provides a general description of the use of quantitative measures as part of the initial psychiatric evaluation. In the assessment of a patient with a possible psychotic disorder, quantitative measures can also be used to help detect and determine the severity of psychosis and associated symptoms. The intent of using a quantitative measure is not to establish a diagnosis but rather to complement other aspects of the screening and assessment process. Depending on the measure, it can aid in treatment planning by providing a structured replicable way to document the patient's baseline symptoms. It can also help to determine which symptoms should be the target of intervention on the basis of such factors as frequency of occurrence, magnitude, potential for associated harm to the patient or others, and associated distress to the patient.

As treatment proceeds, use of quantitative measures allows more precise tracking of whether nonpharmacological and pharmacological treatments are having their intended effect or whether a shift in the treatment plan is needed. This record of a patient's response to treatment is of particular value when the treatment is nonstandard (e.g., combination of antipsychotics) or expensive. It can also provide helpful information about the actual effects of prior treatments. In addition, patients' ratings can be compared with family members' impressions of treatment effects to clarify the longitudinal course of the patient's illness.

Much of the treatment-related research in psychiatry has used clinician-rated scales to determine patient outcomes; however, patient-rated scales are typically less time-consuming to administer than clinician-rated scales. In addition, they provide important insights into the patient's experience that support person-centered care. The use of anchored, self-rated scales with criteria to assess the severity and frequency of symptoms can also help patients become more informed self-observers. However, correlations between patient- and clinician-rated scales are often modest (Harvey 2011; Spitz et al. 2017), suggesting that both types of quantitative measures provide useful information. If a mismatch is noted in the self-assessment of patients as compared with assessments of other observers, this may provide information relevant to outcomes. The accuracy of self-assessments of ability, skills, performance, or decisions (also termed introspective accuracy) is a better predictor of everyday functional deficits than objective measures of neurocognitive or social cognitive performance (Silberstein and Harvey 2019).

The exact frequency at which measures are warranted will depend on clinical circumstances. Use of quantitative measures over time will help assure that key elements of information are collected to guide treatment (Lewis et al. 2019). Consequently, it is preferable to use a consistent approach to quantitative measurement for a given patient because each rating scale defines and measures psychosis and other symptoms differently.

Although recommending a particular scale, patient- or clinician-rated, is outside the scope of this practice guideline, a number of objective, quantitative rating scales to monitor clinical status in schizophrenia are available (American Psychiatric Association 2013a; Rush et al. 2008). The Clinician-Rated Dimensions of Psychosis Symptom Severity (American Psychiatric Association 2013b), which is included in DSM-5 for further research and clinical evaluation, contains eight domains that are rated on a scale from 0 (not present) to 4 (present and severe) on the basis of symptoms in the prior 7 days. A 6-item version of the Positive and Negative Syndrome Scale (PANSS-6; Bech et al. 2018; Østergaard et al. 2018b) consists of the PANSS items for delusions, conceptual disorganization, hallucinations, blunted affect, social withdrawal, and lack of spontaneity and flow of conversation (Kay et al. 1987). Data on the PANSS-6 suggest that it correlates highly with scores on the 30-item version of the Positive and Negative Syndrome Scale (PANSS-30; Østergaard et al. 2018a, 2018b). Furthermore, the PANSS-6 is sensitive to changes with treatment and able to identify symptom remission with a high degree of accuracy (Østergaard et al. 2018a, 2018b) if individuals who are performing ratings are appropriately trained (Opler et al. 2017). Clinician-rated scales may also be selected to assess specific clinical presentations, such as using the Bush-Francis Catatonia Rating Scale for individuals with catatonic features (Bush et al. 1996a). Other clinician-rated scales are commonly used for monitoring psychopathology in research but are likely to be too lengthy for routine clinical use. These include the PANSS-30 (Kay et al. 1987), the Scale for the Assessment of Negative Symptoms (SANS; Andreasen 1984a), the Scale for the Assessment of Positive Symptoms (SAPS; Andreasen 1984b), and the Brief Psychiatric Rating Scale (BPRS; https://mha.ohio.gov/Portals/0/assets/HealthProfessionals/About MH and Addiction Treatment/First Episode Psychosis/Brief-Psychiatric-Rating-Scale.pdf) (Leucht et al. 2005; Overall and Gorham 1962; Ventura et al. 1993).

In terms of patient-rated scales, the DSM-5 Self-Rated Level 1 Cross-Cutting Symptom Measure—Adult (American Psychiatric Association 2013c) includes a total of 23 items in 13 domains, with only 2 items related to psychosis. Nevertheless, it may be useful for identifying and tracking symptoms other than psychosis, including those related to co-occurring disorders. DSM-5 also includes 36-item self- and proxy-administered versions of the World Health Organization Disability Schedule 2.0 (WHODAS 2.0) for assessing functioning difficulties due to health and mental health conditions (American Psychiatric Association 2013d; Üstün et al. 2010). Other options for assessing functioning include the Social and Occupational Functioning Assessment Scale (SOFAS; American Psychiatric Association 2000) and the Personal and Social Performance scale (Morosini et al. 2000). Several versions of Patient-Reported Outcomes Measurement Information System (PROMIS) scales, which address social roles and functioning, are also available (www.healthmeasures.net/explore-measurement-systems/promis). The use of ratings from other informants is particularly helpful in assessing the patient's level of functioning because individuals with schizophrenia often have a different view of their functioning than do family members or others involved in their lives (Harvey 2011).

For a nonspecific measure of quality of life, patients can be asked to rate their overall (physical and mental) quality of life in the past month on a scale from 0 ("about as bad as dying") to 10 ("life is perfect") (Unützer et al. 2002). In individuals with chronic mental illness, the Satisfaction With Life Scale (Diener et al. 1985) has been developed and used to assess life satisfaction and quality of life. Quality of life can also be measured using a scale developed by the World Health Organization, the WHOQOL-BREF (Skevington et al. 2004; WHOQOL Group 1998) (http://depts.washington.edu/seaqol/WHOQOL-BREF). The Centers for Disease Control and Prevention Healthy Days Measure (HRQOL-14) and Healthy Days Core Module (HRQOL-4) (www.cdc.gov/hrqol/hrqol14_measure.htm) have also been used in general population samples to assess physical and emotional symptoms as related to an individual's perceived sense of well-being (Moriarty et al. 2003).

Rating scales should always be implemented in a way that supports developing and maintaining the therapeutic relationship with the patient. Reviewing scale results with the patient can help foster a collaborative dialogue about progress toward symptom improvement, functioning gains, and recovery goals. Such review may help clinicians, patients, families, and other support persons recognize that improvement is taking place or, conversely, identify issues that need further attention.

If more than one quantitative measure is being used, it is important to minimize duplication of questions and avoid overwhelming the patient with an excessive number of scales to complete. In addition, when choosing among available quantitative measures, objectives of scale use (e.g., screening, documenting baseline symptoms, ongoing monitoring) should be considered. Optimal scale properties (e.g., sensitivity, specificity) will differ depending on the desired purpose, but assessments of scale validity and reliability are typically conducted cross-sectionally in research contexts.

Because many scales ask the patient to rate symptoms over several weeks, they may not be sensitive to change. This can be problematic in acute care settings, where treatment adjustments and symptom improvement can occur fairly quickly. Some symptom-based quantitative measures focus either on symptom frequency over the observation period or on symptom severity. Although these features often increase or decrease in parallel, that is not invariably the case. Other quantitative measures ask the patient to consider both symptom frequency and severity, which can also make the findings difficult to interpret.

Other factors that can affect the statistical reliability and validity of rating scale measures include comorbid illnesses and patient age, language, race, ethnicity, cultural background, literacy, and health literacy. These factors and others can lead patients to misinterpret questions or bias the ratings that they record, either unintentionally (e.g., to please the clinician with their progress) or intentionally (e.g., to obtain controlled substances, to support claims of disability). Thus, the answers to questions and the summative scores on quantitative measures need to be interpreted in the context of the clinical presentation.

The type and extent of quantitative measures used will also be mediated by the clinical setting, the time available for evaluation, and the urgency of the situation. In some clinical contexts, such as a planned outpatient assessment, patients may be asked to complete electronic- or paper-based quantitative measures, either prior to the visit or on arrival at the office (Allen et al. 2009; Harding et al. 2011). Between or prior to visits, electronic approaches (e.g., mobile phone applications, clinical registries, patient portal sites in electronic health records) may also facilitate obtaining quantitative measurements (Lewis et al. 2019; Palmier-Claus et al. 2012; K. Wang et al. 2018). In other clinical contexts, such as acute inpatient settings, electronic modes of data capture may be more cumbersome, and patients may need more assistance in completion of scales. As an alternative, printed versions of scales may be completed by the patient or a proxy or administered by the clinician. In other clinical circumstances, however, printed or electronic versions of quantitative scales may not be readily available or information may not be available to complete all scale items. In emergency settings, use of a quantitative rating scale may need to be postponed until the acute crisis has subsided or until the patient's clinical status permits a detailed examination.

Although available information suggests that ambulatory patients are generally cooperative, some individuals may be unwilling to complete quantitative measures (Narrow et al. 2013). Severe symptoms, co-occurring psychiatric conditions, low health literacy, reading difficulties, or cognitive impairment may limit some patients' ability to complete self-report instruments (Harding et al. 2011; Valenstein et al. 2009; Zimmerman et al. 2011). In these circumstances, it may be necessary to place greater reliance on collateral sources of information such as family members, other treating health professionals, or staff members of community residence programs, if applicable. If collateral sources of information are not immediately available, treatment may also need to proceed, with adjustments in the plan, if indicated, as additional knowledge is gained. If time constraints are present, the clinician may wish to focus on rating of relevant target symptoms (e.g., on a Likert scale). In emergent circumstances, safety of the patient and others must take precedence; the initial assessment may need to be brief, with a more detailed assessment and incorporation of quantitative measures once the acute clinical situation has been stabilized.

Balancing of Potential Benefits and Harms in Rating the Strength of the Guideline Statement

Benefits

Clinical decision-making, including but not limited to diagnosis and treatment planning, requires a careful and systematic assessment of the type, frequency, and magnitude of psychiatric symptoms as well as an assessment of the impact of those symptoms on the patient's day-to-day functioning and quality of life. Intuitively, and by analogy with other medical specialties in which treatment is guided by standardized measurement (e.g., of physiological signs or laboratory tests), the use of a systematic and quantifiable approach to assessment would seemingly produce better patient outcomes and greater standardization of care across patients. As electronic health records become more commonly used, electronic capture of quantitative measures can facilitate use of computerized decision-support systems in guiding evidence-based treatment, catalyzing additional improvements in outcomes and quality of care.

Use of a quantitative measure as part of the initial evaluation can establish baseline information on the patient's symptoms and level of functioning and can help determine specific targets of treatment in the context of shared decision-making. When administered through paper-based or electronic self-report and as compared with a clinical interview, a quantitative measure may help the clinician to conduct a more consistent and comprehensive review of the multiplicity of symptoms that the patient may be experiencing. Using systematic measures may also increase the efficiency of asking routine questions and allow more time for clinicians to focus on symptoms of greatest severity or issues of most concern to the patient. Such measures may also facilitate collection of information from the patient's family or other collateral informants on factors such as symptoms or functioning. When used on a longitudinal basis, quantitative measures can help determine whether nonpharmacological and pharmacological treatments are having their intended effect or whether a shift in the treatment plan is needed to address symptoms, treatment-related side effects, level of distress, functioning impairments, or potential for harm to the patient or others.

Without the use of a consistent quantitative measure, recall biases may confound the ability of patients and clinicians to compare past and current levels or patterns of symptoms and functioning. When patients have had substantial improvements in symptoms and functioning, it can be easy to focus on the improvements and overlook residual symptoms or side effects of treatment that are contributing to ongoing impairment or reduced quality of life. Thus, ongoing use of quantitative assessments may foster identification of residual symptoms or impairments and early detection of illness recurrence. Systematic use of quantitative measures can also facilitate communication among treating clinicians and can serve as a basis for enhanced management of populations of patients as well as individual patients. Although mobile apps may be capable of assisting with quantitative measurement, there is no current evidence on which to base recommendations about use of mobile apps in the treatment of schizophrenia.

Harms

The harms of using a quantitative measure include the time required for administration and review. The amount of time available for an initial psychiatric evaluation is typically constrained by clinician availability, cost, and other factors. Under such circumstances, time that is used to obtain quantitative measures could introduce harms by reducing time available to address other issues of importance to the patient or of relevance to clinical decision-making. Overreliance on quantitative measures may also cause other aspects of the patient's symptoms and clinical presentation to be overlooked.

Some patients may view quantitative measures as impersonal or may feel annoyed by having to complete detailed scales, particularly if done frequently. If a patient feels negatively about quantitative measures, this could alter the therapeutic alliance. In addition, some patients may have difficulty completing self-report scales or may interpret questions incorrectly. Patients may also provide inaccurate information about their symptoms, and relying on inaccurate information can have a negative impact on clinical decision-making, including recommendations for treatment.

Systematic use of measures may require changes in workflow or staffing to distribute scales, increase time needed to review results with the patient, or lead to unreimbursed costs (e.g., to integrate measures into electronic health record systems, to pay to use copyrighted versions of scales).

Patient Preferences

Clinical experience suggests that the majority of patients are cooperative with and accepting of quantitative measures as part of an initial or subsequent assessment. Most patients will be able to appreciate the ways in which the use of quantitative measures will be of benefit to them. For example, in the testing of the DSM-5 Cross-Cutting Symptom Measure as part of the DSM-5 field trials, quantitative measures were found to be acceptable to patients (Clarke et al. 2014; Mościcki et al. 2013), and only a small fraction of individuals felt that measurement of symptoms would not be helpful to their treating clinician (Mościcki et al. 2013).

The fact that the clinician is using a systematic approach to address the patients' symptoms and functioning sends a positive message that could improve the therapeutic relationship. Especially in developed countries, patients are used to and expect digital, computerized information exchange, including for health-related monitoring and communication. For these patients, the use of quantitative measures within the context of an electronic health record, mobile app, or other computerized technology may be more convenient.

Balancing of Benefits and Harms

The potential benefits of this guideline statement were viewed as far outweighing the potential harms. This recommendation is also consistent with Guideline VII, "Quantitative Assessment," in the APA's *Practice Guidelines for the Psychiatric Evaluation of Adults*, 3rd edition (American Psychiatric Association 2016a). Although quantitative measures have been used for reporting purposes as well as research, the level of research evidence for this recommendation is rated as low because it remains unclear whether routine use of these scales in clinical practice improves overall outcomes. Nonetheless, expert opinion suggests that use of quantitative measures will enhance clinical decision-making and improve treatment outcomes. For additional discussion of the research evidence, see Appendix C, Statement 2.

There is minimal research on the harms of using quantitative measures as part of the psychiatric evaluation as compared with assessment as usual. However, expert opinion suggests that harms of assessment are minimal compared with the benefits of such assessments in improving identification and assessment of psychiatric symptoms. For additional details, see the APA's *Practice Guidelines for the Psychiatric Evaluation of Adults*, 3rd edition (American Psychiatric Association 2016a).

Differences of Opinion Among Writing Group Members

There were no differences of opinion. The writing group voted unanimously in favor of this recommendation.

Review of Available Guidelines From Other Organizations

Multiple guidelines from other organizations were reviewed (Addington et al. 2017a, 2017b; Barnes et al. 2011; Buchanan et al. 2010; Crockford and Addington 2017; Galletly et al. 2016; Hasan et al. 2012, 2013, 2015; National Institute for Health and Care Excellence 2014; Norman et al. 2017; Pringsheim et al. 2017; Scottish Intercollegiate Guidelines Network 2013). None of these guidelines specifically recommend using quantitative measures as part of the initial assessment in individuals with schizophrenia, but several guidelines (Barnes et al. 2011; Galletly et al. 2016) do recommend use of rating scales under some circumstances at baseline or as part of ongoing monitoring.

Quality Measurement Considerations

There is insufficient consensus on the most appropriate quantitative measures (i.e., rating scales) to use in assessing individuals with psychotic disorders, including schizophrenia. Nevertheless, data do support the use of clinician-reported, symptom-based ratings to guide treatment. Patient-rated scales may be clinically useful in identifying patient concerns or subjective experiences (e.g., medication side effects). On the basis of these potential benefits, a process-focused internal or health system–based quality improvement measure could determine rates of quantitative measure use, and quality improvement initiatives could be implemented to increase the frequency with which such measures are used in individuals with schizophrenia.

STATEMENT 3: Evidence-Based Treatment Planning

APA *recommends* (1C) that patients with schizophrenia have a documented, comprehensive, and person-centered treatment plan that includes evidence-based nonpharmacological and pharmacological treatments.

Implementation

When treating individuals with schizophrenia, a person-centered treatment plan should be developed, documented in the medical record, and updated with the patient at appropriate intervals. A person-centered treatment plan can be recorded as part of an evaluation note or progress note and does not need to adhere to a defined development process (e.g., face-to-face multidisciplinary team meeting) or format (e.g., time-specified goals and objectives). Depending on the urgency of the initial clinical presentation, the availability of laboratory results, and other sources of information, the initial treatment plan may need to be augmented over several visits as more details of history and treatment response are obtained.

As treatment proceeds, the treatment plan will require iterative reevaluation and adjustment prompted by such factors as inadequate treatment response, difficulties with tolerability or adherence, impairments in insight, changes in presenting issues or symptoms, or revisions in diagnosis. In adapting treatment to the needs of the individual patient, tailoring of the treatment plan may also be needed on the basis of sociocultural or demographic factors, with an aim of enhancing quality of life or aspects of functioning (e.g., social, academic, occupational). Factors that influence medication metabolism (e.g., age, sex, body weight, renal or hepatic function, smoking status, use of multiple concurrent medications) may also require adjustments to the treatment plan in terms of either typical medication doses or frequency of monitoring. For most individuals with schizophrenia, it is challenging to piece together a coherent picture of the patient's longitudinal course from medical records. Thus, it is important to note the rationale for any changes in the treatment plan as well as the specific changes that are being made because an accurate history of past and current treatments and responses to them is a key part of future treatment planning.

Aims of Treatment Planning

The overarching aims of treatment planning are 1) to promote and maintain recovery, 2) to maximize quality of life and adaptive functioning, and 3) to reduce or eliminate symptoms. To achieve these aims, it is crucial to identify the patient's aspirations, goals for treatment, and treatment-related preferences. Depending on prevailing state laws, psychiatric advance directives are one approach to encouraging patients to contemplate and state their preferences about treatment choices (Easter et al. 2017; Kemp et al. 2015; Shields et al. 2014; Wilder et al. 2010). For patients who have completed a psychiatric advance directive, wellness recovery action plan (Copeland 2000), or individualized crisis prevention or safety plan (Stanley and Brown 2012, 2019; Stanley et al. 2018), these documents will be important to review with the patient when crafting a person-centered approach to care. Discussions with the patient, other treating health professionals, family members, and others involved in the patient's life can each be vital in developing a full picture of the patient and formulating a person-centered treatment plan, using shared decision-making whenever possible. The patient and others may express opinions about specific treatment approaches or identify practical barriers to the patient's ability to participate in treatment, such as lack of insight, cognitive impairments, disorganization, or inadequate social resources.

Elements of the Treatment Plan

Depending on the clinical circumstances and input from the patient and others, a comprehensive and person-centered treatment plan will typically delineate treatments aimed at improving functioning, reducing positive and negative symptoms, and addressing co-occurring psychiatric symptoms or disorders. In each of these respects, it is essential to consider both nonpharmacological and pharmacological treatment approaches and recognize that a combination of nonpharmacological and pharmacological treatments will likely be needed to optimize outcomes. Other elements of the treatment plan may include the following:

- determining the most appropriate treatment setting
- delineating plans for addressing risks of harm to self or others (if present)
- addressing barriers to adherence
- engaging family members and others involved in the patient's life
- providing information to patients, family members, and others involved in the patient's life about treatment options, early symptoms of relapse, need for ongoing monitoring, coping strategies, case management services, and community resources, including peer-support programs
- incorporating goals of treatment related to
    - social support networks
    - interpersonal, family, or intimate relationships
    - parenting status
    - living situation
    - past trauma or victimization
    - school or employment
    - financial considerations, including disability income support, when indicated
    - insurance status
    - legal system involvement
- identifying additional needs for
    - history or mental status examination
    - physical examination (either by the evaluating clinician or by another health professional)
    - laboratory testing, imaging, electrocardiography (ECG), or other clinical studies (if indicated on the basis of the history, examination, and planned treatments)
- collaborating with other treating clinicians (including provision of integrated care) to avoid fragmentation of treatment efforts and assure that co-occurring substance use disorders and physical health conditions are managed

Engagement of Family Members and Other Persons of Support

Discussions with the patient, family members, and others will typically occur as part of the initial assessment (see Statement 1), and additional input will be needed as treatment proceeds and the treatment plan is updated. Family members and others involved in the patient's life may also express specific concerns about the individual's symptoms or behaviors, which, if present, should be documented and addressed. Most individuals welcome involvement of family members and other persons of support (Cohen et al. 2013; Drapalski et al. 2018; Mueser et al. 2015), and family members can be an important part of the care team. Family members can also be provided with educational materials or directed to organizations that offer education to family members and other persons of support (Mental Health America 2019; National Alliance on Mental Illness 2019a).

Strategies to Promote Adherence

Strategies to promote adherence are always important to consider when developing a patient-centered treatment plan (Ferrando et al. 2014). Maintaining adherence to treatment is often challenging

(Acosta et al. 2012; Shafrin et al. 2016; Valenstein et al. 2006), and poor adherence is associated with poor outcomes, including increased risks of relapse, rehospitalization, suicidal and aggressive behaviors, and mortality (Bowtell et al. 2018; Cassidy et al. 2018; Goff et al. 2017; Hawton et al. 2005; Hui et al. 2018; Kishi et al. 2019; Leucht et al. 2012; Thompson et al. 2018; Tiihonen et al. 2018; Vermeulen et al. 2017; Witt et al. 2013). Treatment planning to address adherence will depend on the specific contributing factors and whether reduced adherence is related to medication use, missed appointments, or other aspects of treatment. Issues that may influence adherence include, but are not limited to, lack of awareness of illness, forgetting to take doses, difficulties managing complex regimens (e.g., due to cognitive impairment, frequency of doses, or number of medications), side effects that are of particular importance to the patient (e.g., weight gain, akathisia, sexual dysfunction, effects on cognition), financial barriers (e.g., cost, insurance coverage), perceived risks and benefits of treatment, insufficient understanding of medication benefits for symptoms that are important to the patient, ambivalence or suspiciousness of medications or treatment in general, lack of a perceived need for treatment (e.g., due to feeling good or not viewing self as ill; due to personal, religious, or cultural beliefs), co-occurring conditions (e.g., depression; alcohol, cannabis, or other substance use disorder), high levels of hostility, persecutory delusions, prior difficulties with adherence, prior experiences with treatment (e.g., effectiveness, side effects), limited geographic availability or accessibility of services, financial or insurance constraints on medications or visits, difficulties in the therapeutic relationship, lack of support from significant others for treatment, cultural or family beliefs about illness or treatment, and perceptions of stigma about having an illness and taking medication (Acosta et al. 2012; Ascher-Svanum et al. 2006; Czobor et al. 2015; Foglia et al. 2017; García et al. 2016; Haddad et al. 2014; Hartung et al. 2017; Hatch et al. 2017; Higashi et al. 2013; Kane et al. 2013; MacEwan et al. 2016a; Mueser et al. 2015; Pyne et al. 2014; Shafrin et al. 2016; Velligan et al. 2017; Volavka et al. 2016; Wade et al. 2017). Adherence with appointments can also be influenced by financial barriers, difficulties scheduling visits around work or school schedules, or issues with transportation or with childcare. Addressing these barriers as part of the treatment plan will require active collaboration and problem-solving between the clinician and patient, often with input from the patient's family and others involved in the patient's' life (Mueser et al. 2015).

When assessing adherence, it is important to take a patient-centered approach in inquiring in a nonjudgmental way whether the individual has experienced difficulties with taking medication (Haddad et al. 2014). Obtaining information from patient diaries, patient-completed rating scales, pharmacy records, family members, or other collateral sources of information can be useful supplements to subjective patient reporting (Acosta et al. 2012; Haddad et al. 2014; Hatch et al. 2017; Kane et al. 2013). Tablet counts, monitoring using electronic pill bottle caps, and drug formulations with implanted sensors have also been used to assess adherence with antipsychotic medications (Acosta et al. 2012; Haddad et al. 2014). It can also be useful to obtain medication blood levels. Levels of clozapine have been best studied, but blood levels of other antipsychotic medications are also available. Although the utility of routine therapeutic monitoring is unclear for antipsychotic medications other than clozapine, blood levels may help in establishing whether a patient is taking the medication (Hiemke et al. 2018; Horvitz-Lennon et al. 2017; Lopez and Kane 2013; Lopez et al. 2017; McCutcheon et al. 2018; Predmore et al. 2018). Urine levels of antipsychotic medications can also be used to assess for adherence (Velligan et al. 2006).

In terms of enhancing adherence, a wide range of approaches have been tried. However, evidence on the most effective techniques remains limited (Hartung et al. 2017), and different approaches will likely be needed for different patients. A checklist that includes barriers, facilitators, and motivators for adherence has been developed and may be helpful in promoting discussion and identifying adherence-related factors in individual patients (Pyne et al. 2014). In addition to conducting ongoing monitoring of adherence as treatment proceeds, it can be helpful to focus on optimizing treatment efficacy, addressing side effects and concerns about treatment, adjusting dosing to minimize side effects while maintaining efficacy, providing information about the illness and its treatments, engaging in shared decision-making, fostering a strong therapeutic alliance, and engaging family members and other community and social supports, as appropriate (Acosta et al. 2012; Haddad et al. 2014; Hamann and Heres 2019; Kane et al. 2013; Rezansoff et al. 2017).

For some patients, the formulation of the antipsychotic medication may influence adherence (see Statement 4, Table 3). For example, rapidly dissolving tablets, oral concentrates, or LAI formulations may be preferable for patients who have difficulty swallowing pills or who are ambivalent about medications and inconsistent in swallowing them. For individuals who have difficulty remembering to take medication, LAI formulations of medications can be used, oral medication regimens can be simplified to reduce the number of pills or daily doses, watches or cell phone alarms can be used as reminders to take medications, pillboxes may be filled with the week's medication, and family or significant others may be enlisted to assist with medication if cognitive impairments are present. Another approach that can be used to improve adherence is behavioral tailoring, which involves cuing oneself to take medications by incorporating adherence into one's daily routine (Kreyenbuhl et al. 2016; Mueser et al. 2002). If financial issues with medications are affecting adherence, reassessment of the treatment regimen may be needed, or patients' assistance programs may be pursued (e.g., through pharmaceutical company programs or a discount program such as GoodRx, www.goodrx.com). When a patient does not appear for appointments or is nonadherent in other ways, assertive outreach such as telephone calls or secure messages may be helpful in reengaging the patient in treatment.

Addressing Risks for Suicidal and Aggressive Behavior

Identifying risk factors and estimating risks for suicidal and aggressive behaviors are essential parts of psychiatric evaluation (American Psychiatric Association 2016a and as described in detail in Statement 1, subsection "Implementation"). Despite identification of these risk factors, it is not possible to predict whether an individual patient will engage in aggressive behaviors or attempt or die by suicide. However, when an increased risk for such behaviors is present, it is important that the treatment plan reevaluates the setting of care and implements approaches to target and reduce modifiable risk factors. Although demographic and historical risk factors are static, potentially modifiable risk factors may include poor adherence, core symptoms of schizophrenia (e.g., hallucinations, delusions), co-occurring symptoms (e.g., depression, hopelessness, hostility, impulsivity), and co-occurring diagnoses (e.g., depression, alcohol use disorder, other substance use disorders). Additional elements of the treatment plan can address periods of increased risk (e.g., shortly after diagnosis, during incarceration, subsequent to hospital discharge).

Addressing Tobacco Use and Other Substance Use Disorders

Individuals with schizophrenia have high rates of nicotine dependence (Centers for Disease Control and Prevention 2020; Cook et al. 2014; de Leon and Diaz 2005; Dickerson et al. 2018; Hartz et al. 2014; Myles et al. 2012; Smith et al. 2014; Wium-Andersen et al. 2015), cannabis use (Brunette et al. 2018; Hartz et al. 2014; Hunt et al. 2018; Koskinen et al. 2010; Nesvåg et al. 2015; Toftdahl et al. 2016), and use of alcohol and other substances (Brunette et al. 2018; Hartz et al. 2014; Hunt et al. 2018; Nesvåg et al. 2015; Toftdahl et al. 2016). Smoking is a major contributor to increased mortality in individuals with serious mental illness (Reynolds et al. 2018; Tam et al. 2016), and the adverse health consequences of smoking are well documented (Lariscy et al. 2018; U.S. Department of Health and Human Services 2014; Van Schayck et al. 2017). Thus, smoking cessation is recommended for any individual who smokes. Some studies have assessed smoking cessation approaches targeted to individuals with mental illnesses, but specific evidence in patients with schizophrenia is still limited (Sharma et al. 2017). Thus, smoking cessation approaches will typically follow guidelines for the general population (National Cancer Institute 2019; SAMHSA-HRSA Center of Excellence for Integrated Health Solutions 2018; Siu et al. 2015; Van Schayck et al. 2017; Verbiest et al. 2017). Although quit rates may be lower in individuals with schizophrenia than in the general population (Lum et al. 2018; Streck et al. 2020), health education and motivational interviewing approaches can be helpful in those who are ambivalent about stopping cigarette use (Levounis et al. 2017) or who have had prior unsuccessful attempts at smoking cessation.

Rates of cannabis use and other substance use are also increased among individuals with schizophrenia (Hartz et al. 2014; Hunt et al. 2018; Swartz et al. 2006). Cannabis use has been associated with an increased incidence (Nielsen et al. 2017; Vaucher et al. 2018) and earlier onset (Donoghue et al. 2014; Helle et al. 2016; Kelley et al. 2016; Large et al. 2011) of schizophrenia, and it may also contribute to a higher burden of symptoms (Carney et al. 2017; Oluwoye et al. 2018). Other substance use disorders are associated with a poorer prognosis in individuals with schizophrenia (Brunette et al. 2018; Conus et al. 2017; Weibell et al. 2017) and, as noted previously, can contribute to risk of suicide or aggressive behavior. Thus, it is important for the treatment plan to address substance use disorders when they are present. Screening, Brief Intervention, and Referral to Treatment (SBIRT) can be integrated into a range of clinical settings (Agerwala and McCance-Katz 2012; SAMHSA-HRSA Center of Excellence for Integrated Health Solutions 2019). Often, a comprehensive integrated treatment model is suggested in which the same clinicians or team of clinicians provide treatment for schizophrenia as well as treatment of substance use disorders. However, if an integrated treatment is unavailable, the treatment plan should address both disorders with communication and collaboration among treating clinicians. For patients who do not recognize the need for treatment of a substance use disorder, a stagewise motivational approach can be pursued (Catley et al. 2016; Levounis et al. 2017).

Addressing Other Concomitant Psychiatric Symptoms and Diagnoses

Depressive symptoms are common in individuals with schizophrenia and should be addressed as part of treatment planning. The approach to treating depression will be grounded in a careful differential diagnosis that considers the possible contributions of demoralization, negative symptoms of schizophrenia, side effects of antipsychotic medications, substance intoxication or withdrawal, physical health condition, or a co-occurring major depressive episode. Depressive symptoms that occur during an acute episode of psychosis often improve as psychotic symptoms respond to treatment.

Evidence on the use of antidepressants to treat depression in individuals with schizophrenia comes from multiple trials, many of which have small sample sizes or factors that increase the risk of bias in the findings (Dondé et al. 2018; Gregory et al. 2017; Helfer et al. 2016). Nevertheless, a meta-analysis suggests that the addition of antidepressant medications results in small beneficial effects on symptoms of depression, quality of life, and response rates as well as on positive symptoms, negative symptoms, and overall symptoms (Helfer et al. 2016). These effects were more prominent in patients with more severe depressive symptoms. Furthermore, antidepressant treatment did not appear to be associated with exacerbation of psychosis or significant differences in adverse effects (Helfer et al. 2016). Nonpharmacological treatments for depression in schizophrenia have been less well studied but could also be incorporated into treatment planning (Dondé et al. 2018; Opoka and Lincoln 2017).

Treatments for posttraumatic stress disorder (Brand et al. 2018; Sin et al. 2017b) and anxiety (Howells et al. 2017) in individuals with schizophrenia have been less well studied. Nevertheless, many individuals with schizophrenia will have experienced violent victimization (de Vries et al. 2019; Morgan et al. 2016; Roy et al. 2014) or childhood adversity (Bonoldi et al. 2013; Schalinski et al. 2019; Trotta et al. 2015; Varese et al. 2012), and the impact of these experiences needs to be considered as part of a patient-centered treatment plan (Center for Substance Abuse Treatment 2014). When anxiety symptoms are present in individuals with schizophrenia, the possible contributions of psychotic symptoms, medication side effects, substance intoxication or withdrawal, or co-occurring anxiety disorders may suggest an approach to treatment. Given the relative safety of adjunctive antidepressant medications in individuals with schizophrenia and depression, these medications may be considered if otherwise indicated to treat posttraumatic stress disorder or an anxiety disorder. On the other hand, studies on the use of benzodiazepines in schizophrenia are limited (Dold et al.

2012), and long-term use of benzodiazepines may be associated with increased risk of poorer outcomes, including side effects (Dold et al. 2013; Fond et al. 2018; Fontanella et al. 2016; Tiihonen et al. 2016) or misuse (Maust et al. 2019). Nonpharmacological treatments for posttraumatic stress disorder in individuals with schizophrenia have been less well studied but may have modest benefits and do not appear to have significant adverse effects as compared with usual care (Brand et al. 2018; Sin et al. 2017b).

In terms of the use of stimulants to treat preexisting attention-deficit/hyperactivity disorder in individuals with schizophrenia, available evidence is also very limited but suggests a potential for worsening of psychotic symptoms as well as potential for development of a stimulant use disorder (Sara et al. 2014; Solmi et al. 2019). Thus, if stimulant medications are used, monitoring for these possible adverse effects is warranted as part of the treatment plan.

Addressing Other Concomitant Health Conditions

As described in Statement 1, other health conditions are more frequent in individuals with serious mental illness in general (Firth et al. 2019; Janssen et al. 2015; McGinty et al. 2016) and schizophrenia in particular (Henderson et al. 2015). Such disorders include but are not limited to poor oral health (Kisely et al. 2015), hepatitis C infection (Chasser et al. 2017; Hauser and Kern 2015; Hughes et al. 2016), HIV infection (Hobkirk et al. 2015; Hughes et al. 2016), cancer (Olfson et al. 2015), sleep apnea (Myles et al. 2016; Stubbs et al. 2016b), obesity (Janssen et al. 2015), diabetes mellitus (Vancampfort et al. 2016a), metabolic syndrome (Vancampfort et al. 2015), and cardiovascular disease (Correll et al. 2017c). These disorders, if present, can contribute to mortality or reduced quality of life, and some may be induced or exacerbated by psychiatric medications. Impairments in renal and hepatic function, if present, can influence treatment recommendations.

Table 2 (see Statement 1) provides a discussion of suggested physical and laboratory assessments for patients with schizophrenia as part of initial evaluation and follow-up assessments. Such assessments are important for prevention, early recognition, and treatment of abnormalities such as glucose dysregulation, hyperlipidemia, and metabolic syndrome. It is important that patients have access to primary care clinicians who can work with the psychiatrist to diagnose and treat concurrent physical health conditions (American Psychiatric Association 2016a), but the psychiatrist may also provide ongoing monitoring and treatment of common medical conditions in conjunction with primary care clinicians (Druss et al. 2018).

Pregnancy and Postpartum Period

Women with childbearing potential and at risk for pregnancy should be assisted in obtaining effective contraception if pregnancy is not desired. For women who are planning to become pregnant or who are pregnant or in the postpartum period, it is essential to collaborate with the patient, her obstetrician-gynecologist or other obstetric practitioner, and, if involved, her partner or other persons of support. For women who are breastfeeding, collaboration with the infant's pediatrician is similarly important. The overall goal is to develop a plan of care aimed at optimizing outcomes for both the patient and her infant. In addition, during pregnancy and postpartum, frequent reassessment will be needed to determine whether any modifications to the treatment plan are indicated.

As with any decisions related to the use of psychiatric medications prior to conception, during pregnancy, or while breastfeeding, it is essential to consider the potential benefits of treatment as well as the potential harms of untreated illness and the potential for negative fetal or neonatal effects. Untreated or inadequately treated maternal psychiatric illness can result in poor adherence to prenatal care, inadequate nutrition, increased alcohol or tobacco use, and disruptions to the family environment and mother-infant bonding (ACOG Committee on Practice Bulletins—Obstetrics 2008; American Academy of Pediatrics and the American College of Obstetricians and Gynecologists 2017; Tosato et al. 2017). For women with childbearing potential, decisions about medications and advice about contraceptive practices should consider the potential effects if pregnancy were to occur. Some medications are best avoided in women with childbearing potential; for example, valproic acid should be avoided because of its teratogenic effects (Briggs et al. 2017) and association with maternal metabolic syndrome.

All psychotropic medications studied to date cross the placenta, are present in amniotic fluid, and enter human breast milk (American Academy of Pediatrics and the American College of Obstetricians and Gynecologists 2017). In addition, the period from the third through the eighth week of gestation is associated with greatest risk for teratogenesis (American Academy of Pediatrics and the American College of Obstetricians and Gynecologists 2017). If a woman becomes pregnant while taking an antipsychotic medication, consideration should be given to consulting an obstetrician-gynecologist or maternal/fetal medicine subspecialist in addition to discussion with the prescribing clinician before indicated psychotropic medications are stopped to determine whether the risks of stopping the medication outweigh any possible fetal risks (American Academy of Pediatrics and the American College of Obstetricians and Gynecologists 2017; U.S. Food and Drug Administration 2011a). For many women, the eighth week of gestation will already have passed before obstetric care begins, and stopping medication will not avoid or reduce teratogenic risk. Thus, for a woman with schizophrenia, the benefits of continued treatment with antipsychotic medications in minimizing relapse will generally outweigh the potential for fetal risk (Briggs et al. 2017).

Knowledge of the effects of antipsychotic medications is limited to observational and registry-based studies. Although limited information is known about newer second-generation antipsychotic medications (SGAs), first-generation antipsychotic medications (FGAs) have been in wide use for more than 40 years, and older SGAs have been available for several decades. The available data suggest that these medications have minimal risk in terms of teratogenic or toxic effects on the fetus (ACOG Committee on Practice Bulletins—Obstetrics 2008; Briggs et al. 2017; Chisolm and Payne 2016). There does appear to be a risk of withdrawal symptoms or neurological effects of antipsychotic medications in the newborn if an antipsychotic medication is used in the third trimester (Briggs et al. 2017; U.S. Food and Drug Administration 2011a). Symptoms may include agitation, abnormally increased or decreased muscle tone, tremor, sleepiness, severe difficulty breathing, and difficulty in feeding (Briggs et al. 2017; U.S. Food and Drug Administration 2011a). Nevertheless, tapering of antipsychotic medication late in pregnancy is not advisable because of the associated risk of relapse. In some newborns, the symptoms subside within hours or days and do not require specific treatment; other newborns may require longer hospital stays (U.S. Food and Drug Administration 2011a). The possibility of these effects signals the importance of close monitoring of the newborn in conjunction with the infant's pediatrician. As noted above, however, the benefits of treatment for the mother and the longer-term benefits of treatment for the infant (e.g., enhanced mother-infant bonding, better adherence to prenatal care and nutrition, lesser rates of prenatal alcohol or tobacco use) will generally favor continuing and not tapering antipsychotic treatment.

A number of other considerations are relevant when treating women with an antipsychotic medication during pregnancy. In general, symptoms should be managed with the lowest effective dose, although it is preferable to maintain efficacy using a single medication at a higher dose rather than using multiple medications at lower doses (American Academy of Pediatrics and the American College of Obstetricians and Gynecologists 2017). If a patient's symptoms are well controlled on a specific medication, it is usually not advisable to switch to a different antipsychotic medication, even if more safety information is available for a different drug (Chisolm and Payne 2016). Changing medications exposes the fetus to two different medications and also increases possibilities for symptom relapse in the patient.

As with all women who are pregnant, regular prenatal care is essential to ensuring optimal maternal-fetal outcomes (American Academy of Pediatrics and the American College of Obstetricians and Gynecologists 2017; American College of Obstetricians and Gynecologists 2018). Close monitoring for symptom recurrence and for side effects is important during pregnancy and in the postpartum period because the physiological alterations of pregnancy may affect the absorption, distribution, metabolism, and elimination of medications and may necessitate adjustments in medication doses (ACOG Committee on Practice Bulletins—Obstetrics 2008; Chisolm and Payne 2016). Women who are taking antipsychotic medications are also at increased risk of obesity and hyperglycemia, and folate supplementation to reduce risks of neural tube defects and assessment for diabetes during pregnancy are important elements of prenatal care (Briggs et al. 2017).

In terms of breastfeeding, limited information is available, but infants may be exposed to clinically significant levels of medication in breast milk, and the long-term effects of such exposure are not known (Sachs et al. 2013). Accordingly, mothers who wish to breastfeed their infants should review the potential benefits of breastfeeding as well as potential risks in the context of shared decision-making (American College of Obstetricians and Gynecologists' Committee on Obstetric Practice and the Breastfeeding Expert Work Group 2016; Sachs et al. 2013), with associated monitoring of growth and development by the infant's pediatrician (Sachs et al. 2013).

Additional information related to the use of antipsychotic medications during pregnancy and while breastfeeding can be found at the websites of the U.S. Food and Drug Administration (FDA; www.fda.gov), REPROTOX (www.reprotox.org), the Teratogen Information System (TERIS; www.depts.washington.edu/terisweb/teris), and the U.S. National Library of Medicine's LactMed (www.ncbi.nlm.nih.gov/books/NBK501922). For women who have been treated with an SGA during pregnancy, enrolling in the National Pregnancy Registry for Atypical Antipsychotics is suggested (MGH Center for Women's Mental Health 2019).

Determining a Treatment Setting

In determining a treatment setting, considerations for individuals with schizophrenia are similar to those for individuals with other diagnoses. Thus, in general, patients should be cared for in the least restrictive setting that is likely to be safe and to allow for effective treatment. If inpatient care is deemed essential, efforts should be made to hospitalize patients voluntarily. However, if hospitalization is deemed essential but is not accepted voluntarily by the patient, state or jurisdictional requirements for involuntary hospitalization should be followed. Indications for hospitalization usually include the patient posing a serious threat of harm to self or others or being unable to care for himself or herself and needing constant supervision or support as a result. Other possible indications for hospitalization include psychiatric or other medical problems that make outpatient treatment unsafe or ineffective or new onset of psychosis that warrants initial inpatient stabilization to promote reduction of acute symptoms and permit engagement in treatment.

For individuals with schizophrenia and other significant health issues, determination of a treatment setting will require weighing the pluses and minuses of possible settings to identify the optimal location for care. For example, individuals who require significant medical or surgical interventions or monitoring that are not typically available on a psychiatric inpatient service will likely be better served on a general hospital unit or in an intensive care setting with input from consultation-liaison psychiatrists. Considerable efforts may be needed to help staff who are unfamiliar with psychotic disorders engage with the patient (Freudenreich et al. 2019). In other circumstances, management of the patient on an inpatient psychiatric service in collaboration with consultants of other medical specialties will be optimal.

Less restrictive settings may be indicated when a patient does not meet criteria for inpatient treatment but requires more monitoring or assistance than is available in routine outpatient care. Such settings and programs may include ACT (Substance Abuse and Mental Health Services Administration 2008), assisted outpatient treatment, intensive outpatient treatment, partial hospitalization, and day hospitalization.

Involuntary Treatment Considerations

Under some circumstances, individuals may not wish to participate in treatment or take medications, even if they have severe symptoms. In states where psychiatric advance directives are available, patients may be able to state their preferences about treatment choices while they have capacity in the event of future decompensation and an inability to participate in decision-making. Even in the absence of a psychiatric advance directive, patients can often be helped to accept pharmacological treatment over time and with psychotherapeutic interactions that are aimed toward identifying subjectively distressing symptoms that have previously responded to treatment. Family members and other persons of support can also be helpful in encouraging the patient to engage in treatment.

Prevailing state laws will determine other steps to take if an individual lacks capacity but requires treatment. Some states have processes by which pharmacological treatment may be administered involuntarily, whereas in other states a judicial hearing may be needed to obtain permission to treat a patient who lacks capacity.

For a small subgroup of patients with repeated relapses, rehospitalizations, or even reincarcerations associated with nonadherence or impairments in insight, involuntary outpatient commitment may warrant inclusion in the treatment plan to improve adherence, prevent psychiatric deterioration, enhance outcomes, and promote recovery (American Psychiatric Association 2015; Gaynes et al. 2015; Harris et al. 2019; Segal et al. 2017a, 2017b; Swartz et al. 2017). Involuntary outpatient commitment (which also may be referred to as assisted outpatient treatment, mandated community treatment, outpatient court-ordered treatment, or a community treatment order) is increasingly available but varies among countries (Burns et al. 2013; Harris et al. 2019) and jurisdictions within the United States (Meldrum et al. 2016) in its criteria and implementation. Effective implementation requires adequate resources and individualized treatment planning (American Psychiatric Association 2015) if psychiatric (Gaynes et al. 2015; Harris et al. 2019; Segal et al. 2017a; Swartz et al. 2017) and physical health (Segal et al. 2017b) benefits are to be realized. As with any form of involuntary treatment, decisions about involuntary outpatient commitment require balancing ethical considerations related to patient autonomy and self-determination with considerations about the individual's best interest (American Psychiatric Association 2015).

Addressing Needs of Patients With Schizophrenia in Correctional Settings

Rates of serious mental illness, including schizophrenia, are higher in correctional settings (e.g., prisons, jails, police lockups, detention facilities) than in the general population (Al-Rousan et al. 2017; Bebbington et al. 2017; Bradley-Engen et al. 2010; Hall et al. 2019; Steadman et al. 2009). Careful assessment and treatment planning are essential when individuals with schizophrenia are in correctional settings. Although some aspects of treatment may need to be adjusted to conform with unique aspects of correctional settings (Tamburello et al. 2018), many individuals experience gaps in care during incarceration (Fries et al. 2013; Reingle Gonzalez and Connell 2014; Wilper et al. 2009), and access should be preserved to essential elements of treatment, including antipsychotic medications (American Psychiatric Association 2009b) and treatment for concomitant substance use disorders (American Psychiatric Association 2007).

While in the correctional system, individuals with schizophrenia may be withdrawn or disorganized or behave in a disruptive manner. These behaviors may result in disciplinary infractions, which may lead the individual with schizophrenia to be placed in a locked-down setting. Such units are often called *administrative segregation*, *disciplinary segregation*, or *restricted housing units* (Krelstein 2002; Semenza and Grosholz 2019) and have been conceptualized as having three main characteristics: social isolation, sensory deprivation, and confinement (Zubek et al. 1969). Each of these elements can vary significantly, but inmates typically spend an average of 23 hours per day in a cell, have limited human interaction and minimal or no access to programs, and are maintained in an environment that is designed to exert maximum control over the person, which has raised broader ethical considerations about the long-term use of such settings (Ahalt and Williams 2016; Ahalt et al. 2017; American Psychiatric Association 2017, 2018; American Public Health Association 2013; Cloud et al. 2015; National Commission on Correctional Health Care 2016).

Inmates' responses to the segregation experience differ, and relevant scientific literature is sparse (Kapoor and Trestman 2016; O'Keefe et al. 2013). In addition, mental health clinicians working in such facilities frequently report that inmates without preexisting serious mental disorders develop irritability, anxiety, and other dysphoric symptoms when housed in these units for long periods of time (Metzner 2002). Difficulties in providing appropriate and adequate access to mental health care and treatment are especially problematic in any segregation environment and are related to logistical issues that frequently include inadequate office space and limited access to inmates because of security issues (Metzner 2003; Metzner and Fellner 2010). In addition, because of their inherently punitive structure, such units typically provide very little support or access to relevant treatment modalities or a therapeutic milieu. Furthermore, rates of self-injury and suicide appear to be higher in such settings than elsewhere in the correctional system (Baillargeon et al. 2009b; Glowa-Kollisch et al. 2016; Kaba et al. 2014; Way et al. 2005). Consequently, persons with schizophrenia should generally not be placed in a 23-hour/day lockdown for behaviors that are directly related to schizophrenia because such an intervention is likely to exacerbate rather than reduce psychotic symptoms, as well as increase rather than reduce disruptive behaviors (American College of Correctional Physicians 2013; American Psychiatric Association 2016b, 2017; American Public Health Association 2013; National Commission on Correctional Health Care 2016).

Individuals with schizophrenia, like other individuals with serious mental illness, are at increased risk for symptom relapse and gaps in treatment on release from a correctional setting. Services are often needed to reduce the likelihood of recidivism and maintain continuity of care for treatment of schizophrenia and concomitant disorders (e.g., substance use disorders, other medical conditions). Thus, discharge planning is a crucial aspect of care for inmates with schizophrenia, particularly for those who have been incarcerated for significant periods of time. Often, inmates with schizophrenia have been alienated from systems of care and psychosocial supports prior to arrest, and this estrangement is compounded by incarceration. As a result, inmates will likely need assistance around the time of discharge, which can encompass various domains, including housing, treatment needs, financial support, and obtaining supplemental security income/social security disability and related Medicaid benefits (American Psychiatric Association 2009c; Angell et al. 2014; Baillargeon et al. 2009a, 2010; Draine et al. 2010; Gertner et al. 2019; Morrissey et al. 2016; Wenzlow et al. 2011).

Balancing of Potential Benefits and Harms in Rating the Strength of the Guideline Statement

Benefits

Development and documentation of a comprehensive, person-centered treatment plan assures that the clinician has considered the available nonpharmacological and pharmacological options for treatment and has identified those treatments that are best suited to the needs of the individual patient, with a goal of improving overall outcome. It may also assist in forming a therapeutic relationship, eliciting patient preferences, permitting education about possible treatments, setting expectations for treatment, and establishing a framework for shared decision-making. Documentation of a treatment plan promotes accurate communication among all those caring for the patient and can serve as a reminder of prior discussions about treatment.

Harms

The only identifiable harm from this recommendation relates to the time spent in discussion and documentation that may reduce the opportunity to focus on other aspects of the evaluation.

Patient Preferences

Clinical experience suggests that patients are cooperative with and accepting of efforts to establish treatment plans.

Balancing of Benefits and Harms

The potential benefits of this guideline statement were viewed as far outweighing the potential harms. The level of research evidence is rated as low because no information is available on the harms of such an approach. There is also minimal research on whether developing and documenting a specific treatment plan improves outcomes as compared with assessment and documentation as usual. However, indirect evidence, including expert opinion, supports the benefits of comprehensive treatment planning. For additional discussion of the research evidence, see Appendix C, Statement 3.

Differences of Opinion Among Writing Group Members

There were no differences of opinion. The writing group voted unanimously in favor of this recommendation.

Review of Available Guidelines From Other Organizations

Information from other guidelines (Addington et al. 2017a, 2017b; Barnes et al. 2011; Buchanan et al. 2010; Crockford and Addington 2017; Galletly et al. 2016; Hasan et al. 2012, 2013, 2015; National Institute for Health and Care Excellence 2014; Norman et al. 2017; Pringsheim et al. 2017; Scottish Intercollegiate Guidelines Network 2013) is generally consistent with this guideline statement in either explicitly or implicitly recommending development of a person-centered treatment plan that includes evidence-based nonpharmacological and pharmacological treatments.

Quality Measurement Considerations

It is not known whether psychiatrists and other mental health professionals typically document a comprehensive and person-centered treatment plan that includes evidence-based nonpharmacological and pharmacological treatments, and there is likely to be variability. Although a well-defined and scientifically sound quality measure could be developed to assess for the implementation of an evidence-based treatment plan that meets consensus-based features of person-centered care, clinical judgment would still be needed to determine whether a documented treatment plan is comprehensive and adapted to individual needs and preferences. Manual review of charts to evaluate for the presence of such a person-centered treatment plan would be burdensome and time-consuming to implement.

A quality measure could assess the presence or absence of text in the medical record that would reflect treatment planning. When considering the development of such quality measures, there should be a thorough examination of the potential for unintended negative consequences, such as increased documentation burden or overuse of standardized language that meets the quality measure criteria but would inaccurately reflect what occurred in practice.

Pharmacotherapy

STATEMENT 4: Antipsychotic Medications

APA *recommends* **(1A)** that patients with schizophrenia be treated with an antipsychotic medication and monitored for effectiveness and side effects.*

---

*This guideline statement should be implemented in the context of a person-centered treatment plan that includes evidence-based nonpharmacological and pharmacological treatments for schizophrenia.

Implementation

Selection of an Antipsychotic Medication

General Principles

In the treatment of schizophrenia, antipsychotic medication is one important component. The choice of an antipsychotic agent depends on many factors that are specific to an individual patient. Thus, before initiating treatment with antipsychotic medication, it is recommended that as part of selecting a medication, the treating clinician gather information on the patient's treatment-related preferences and prior treatment responses and then discuss with the patient the potential benefits and risks of medication as compared with other management options. Many patients will wish family members or other persons of support to be involved in this discussion. The depth of this discussion will, of course, be determined by the patient's condition. Even with agitated patients and patients with thought disorder, however, the therapeutic alliance will be enhanced if the patient and physician can identify target symptoms (e.g., anxiety, poor sleep, and, for patients with insight, hallucinations and delusions) that are subjectively distressing and that antipsychotics can ameliorate. Mentioning the possibility of acute side effects (e.g., dizziness, sedation, restlessness) helps patients identify and report side-effect occurrence and also may help maintain a therapeutic alliance. Patients with schizophrenia often have attentional and other cognitive impairments that may be more severe during an acute illness exacerbation, so it is helpful to return to the topic of identification of target symptoms and discussion of acute and longer-term side effects on multiple occasions as treatment proceeds.

An evidence-based ranking of FGAs and SGAs or an algorithmic approach to antipsychotic selection is not possible because of the significant heterogeneity in clinical trial designs, the limited numbers of head-to-head comparisons of antipsychotic medications, and the limited clinical trial data for a number of the antipsychotic medications. By the same token, it is not possible to note a preference for either SGAs or FGAs. Although there may be clinically meaningful distinctions in response to and tolerability of different antipsychotic medications in an individual patient, there is no definitive evidence that one antipsychotic will have consistently superior efficacy compared with another, with the possible exception of clozapine. Although data in first-episode schizophrenia are more limited, there appears to be no difference in response among the SGAs that have been studied (McDonagh et al. 2017; Zhu et al. 2017). Furthermore, there is no reliable strategy to predict response or risk of side effects with one agent compared with another. Consequently, the choice of a particular antipsychotic agent will typically occur in the context of discussion with the patient about the likely benefits and possible side effects of medication options and will incorporate patient preferences; the patient's past responses to treatment (including symptom response and tolerability); the medication's side-effect profile (see Table 6); the presence of physical health conditions that may be affected by medication side effects; and other medication-related factors such as available formulations, potential for drug-drug interactions, receptor binding profiles, and pharmacokinetic considerations (Tables 3–9).

TABLE 3. Antipsychotic medications: available oral and short-acting intramuscular formulations and dosing considerations[a,b]

	Trade name[c]	Available U.S. formulations (mg, unless otherwise noted)	Initial dose (mg/day)	Typical dose range (mg/day)	Maximum daily dose (mg/day)	Comments[d,e,f,g]
First-generation antipsychotics						
Chlorpromazine	Thorazine	Tablet: 10, 25, 50, 100, 200 Short-acting injection (HCl): 25/mL (1 mL, 2 mL)	25–100	200–800	Oral: 1,000–2,000	IM dosing is typically 25–50 mg per upper outer quadrant of gluteal with 200 mg/day maximum. Do not inject subcutaneously. Use much lower IM doses than oral doses because oral first-pass metabolism is significant.
Fluphenazine	Prolixin	Tablet: 1, 2.5, 5, 10 Oral concentrate: 5/mL (120 mL) Elixir: 2.5/5 mL (60 mL) Short-acting injection (HCl): 2.5/mL (10 mL)	2.5–10	6–20	Oral: 40 IM: 10	Short-acting IM dose is 33%–50% of oral dose. Dilute oral concentrate immediately before use to ensure palatability and stability.
Haloperidol	Haldol	Tablet: 0.5, 1, 2, 5, 10, 20 Oral concentrate: 2/mL (5 mL, 15 mL, 120 mL) Short-acting injection (lactate): 5/mL (1 mL, 10 mL)	1–15	5–20	Oral:100 IM: 20	2–5 mg IM can be given every 4–8 hours.
Loxapine	Loxitane	Capsule: 5, 10, 25, 50 Aerosol powder breath-activated inhalation: 10	20	60–100[h]	Oral: 250 Aerosol: 10	Oral inhalation formulation (Adasuve) to treat agitation requires REMS program because of potential for bronchospasm.
Molindone	Moban	Tablet: 5, 10, 25	50–75	30–100[g]	225	
Perphenazine	Trilafon	Tablet: 2, 4, 8, 16	8–16	8–32	64	CYP2D6 poor metabolizers will have higher blood concentrations.
Pimozide	Orap	Tablet: 1, 2	0.5–2	2–4	10	Pimozide does not have an FDA indication for schizophrenia but is sometimes used off-label or to treat delusional disorders such as delusional parasitosis. Avoid concomitant use of CYP1A2 or CYP3A4 inducers or inhibitors. Perform CYP2D6 genotyping if doses greater than 4 mg/day are used. In poor CYP2D6 metabolizers, do not give more than 4 mg/day and do not increase dose earlier than 14 days.

The APA Practice Guideline for the Treatment of Patients With Schizophrenia

	Trade name[c]	Available U.S. formulations (mg, unless otherwise noted)	Initial dose (mg/day)	Typical dose range (mg/day)	Maximum daily dose (mg/day)	Comments[d,e,f,g]
First-generation antipsychotics *(continued)*						
Thioridazine	Mellaril	Tablet: 10, 25, 50, 100	150–300	300–800[g]	800	Use is associated with dose-related QTc prolongation. Baseline ECG and serum potassium level are recommended. Avoid use if QTc interval is >450 msec or with concomitant use of drugs that prolong the QTc interval or inhibit CYP2D6. Reserve use for patients who do not show an acceptable response to adequate courses of treatment with other antipsychotic drugs.
Thiothixene	Navane	Capsule: 1, 2, 5, 10	6–10	15–30	60	Smoking may reduce levels via CYP1A2 induction.
Trifluoperazine	Stelazine	Tablet: 1, 2, 5, 10	4–10	15–20	50	Smoking may reduce levels via CYP1A2 induction.
Second-generation antipsychotics						
Aripiprazole	Abilify	Tablet: 2, 5, 10, 15, 20, 30 Tablet, disintegrating; 10, 15 Tablet with ingestible event marker (Mycite): 2, 5, 10, 15, 20, 30 Solution: 1/mL (150 mL)	10–15	10–15	30	Adjust dose if a poor CYP2D6 metabolizer or with concomitant use of a CYP3A4 inhibitor, CYP3A4 inducer, or CYP2D6 inhibitor. Tablet and oral solution may be interchanged on a mg-per-mg basis, up to 25 mg. Doses using 30 mg tablets should be exchanged for 25 mg oral solution. Orally disintegrating tablets (Abilify Discmelt) are bioequivalent to the immediate-release tablets (Abilify). Mycite tablet cannot be split or crushed.
Asenapine	Saphris	Tablet, sublingual: 2.5, 5, 10	10	20	20	Consider dose adjustment in smokers and with concomitant use of CYP1A2 inhibitors. Do not split, crush, or swallow. Place under tongue and allow to dissolve completely. Do not eat or drink for 10 minutes after administration to ensure absorption.

	Trade name[c]	Available U.S. formulations (mg, unless otherwise noted)	Initial dose (mg/day)	Typical dose range (mg/day)	Maximum daily dose (mg/day)	Comments[d,e,f,g]
Second-generation antipsychotics (continued)						
Asenapine	Secuado	Transdermal system: 3.8 mg/24 hours, 5.7 mg/24 hours, 7.6 mg/24 hours	3.8	3.8–7.6	7.6	Consider dose adjustment in smokers and with concomitant use of CYP1A2 inhibitors. A dose of 3.8 mg/24 hours corresponds to 5 mg twice daily of sublingual asenapine; 7.6 mg/24 hours corresponds to 10 mg twice daily of sublingual asenapine. Apply to clean, dry, and intact skin on the upper arm, upper back, abdomen, or hip; rotate sites when applying a new transdermal system. Do not cut. Do not apply external heat sources to the transdermal system.
Brexpiprazole	Rexulti	Tablet: 0.25, 0.5, 1, 2, 3, 4	1	2–4	4	Adjust dose if a poor CYP2D6 metabolizer or with concomitant use of moderate/strong CYP2D6 inhibitors, strong CYP3A4 inhibitors, or strong CYP3A4 inducers.
Cariprazine	Vraylar	Capsule: 1.5, 3, 4.5, 6	1.5	1.5–6	6[i]	Adjust dose with concomitant use of a strong CYP3A4 inhibitor or inducer.
Clozapine	Clozaril, FazaClo, Versacloz	Tablet: 25, 50, 100, 200 Tablet, disintegrating: 12.5, 25, 100, 150, 200 Oral suspension: 50/mL (100 mL)	12.5–25	300–450[e]	900	Prescribers must complete clozapine REMS education (www.clozapinerems.com) and follow requirements for a baseline CBC and ANC and for ANC monitoring before and during treatment. When initiating clozapine, increase in 25–50 mg/day increments for 2 weeks, then further increments not exceeding 100 mg up to twice weekly. For treatment interruptions of 2 or more days, restart at 12.5 mg once or twice daily. Retitration can occur more rapidly than with initial treatment. With treatment interruptions of more than 30 days, recommendations for initial titration and monitoring frequency should be followed. Adjust dose with concomitant use of strong CYP1A2 inhibitors and with strong CYP3A4 inducers. Smoking reduces clozapine levels via CYP1A2 induction. Clozapine levels can be informative in making dose adjustments.[j]

TABLE 3. Antipsychotic medications: available oral and short-acting intramuscular formulations and dosing considerations[a,b] *(continued)*

	Trade name[c]	Available U.S. formulations (mg, unless otherwise noted)	Initial dose (mg/day)	Typical dose range (mg/day)	Maximum daily dose (mg/day)	Comments[d,e,f,g]
Second-generation antipsychotics *(continued)*						
Iloperidone	Fanapt	Tablet: 1, 2, 4, 6, 8, 10, 12	2	12–24	24	Titrate slowly (no more than 4 mg/day increase in dose). Follow initial titration approach if more than 3-day gap in treatment. Adjust dose with concomitant use of strong CYP2D6 or CYP3A4 inhibitors and reduce dose by 50% in CYP2D6 poor metabolizers.
Lurasidone	Latuda	Tablet: 20, 40, 60, 80, 120	40	40–120	160	Administer with food (≥350 calories). Adjust dose for concomitant use of moderate to strong CYP3A4 inhibitors or inducers.
Olanzapine	Zyprexa	Tablet: 2.5, 5, 7.5, 10, 15, 20 Tablet, disintegrating: 5, 10, 15, 20 Short-acting IM powder for solution: 10/2 mL	5–10	10–20	20[k]	Short-acting IM formulation is used primarily for agitation, with usual dose of 2.5–10 mg IM and maximum dosage of 30 mg/day. Administer IM slowly, deep into muscle. Do not use subcutaneously. Concomitant use of IM olanzapine with parenteral benzodiazepines is not recommended because of potential for excessive sedation and cardiorespiratory depression. Smokers may require a 30% greater daily dose than nonsmokers because of CYP1A2 induction. Women may need lower daily doses. Approximately 40% of an oral dose is removed by first-pass metabolism as compared with IM dose. IM elimination half-life is ~1.5 times greater in the elderly. Oral dissolving tablet dissolves rapidly in saliva and may be swallowed with or without liquid. Olanzapine may be administered with or without food/meals.
Paliperidone	Invega	Tablet, extended release: 1.5, 3, 6, 9	6	3–12	12	If exceeding 6 mg daily, increases of 3 mg/day are recommended at intervals of more than 5 days, up to a maximum of 12 mg/day. Uses OROS; do not split or crush tablet. Use of extended-release tablet is not recommended with preexisting severe gastrointestinal narrowing disorders. Tablet shell is expelled in the stool.

TABLE 3. Antipsychotic medications: available oral and short-acting intramuscular formulations and dosing considerations[a,b] (continued)

	Trade name[c]	Available U.S. formulations (mg, unless otherwise noted)	Initial dose (mg/day)	Typical dose range (mg/day)	Maximum daily dose (mg/day)	Comments[d,e,f,g]
Second-generation antipsychotics (continued)						
Quetiapine	Seroquel	Tablet, immediate release: 25, 50, 100, 200, 300, 400 Tablet, extended release: 50, 150, 200, 300, 400	Immediate release: 50 Extended release: 300	400–800	800	Dosage is once daily for extended release and divided dosing for immediate release. Do not split or crush extended-release tablets. Immediate-release tablets are marginally affected by food, whereas extended-release tablets are significantly affected by a high-fat meal. Give extended-release tablets without food or with <300 calories. Retitrate for gap in treatment of more than 1 week. Adjust dose for concomitant use of strong CYP3A4 inhibitors or inducers.
Risperidone	Risperdal	Tablet: 0.25, 0.5, 1, 2, 3, 4 Tablet, disintegrating: 0.25, 0.5, 1, 2, 3, 4 Oral solution: 1/mL (30 mL)	2	2–8	8[l]	Use lower initial doses and slower titration rates with CrCl <30 mL/min or severe hepatic impairment (Child-Pugh class C). Fraction of free risperidone is increased with hepatic impairment, and the initial starting dose is 0.5 mg twice daily, which may be increased in increments of 0.5 mg or less, administered twice daily. With renal or hepatic impairment, increase in intervals of 1 week or more for doses >1.5 mg twice daily. Adjust dose with concomitant use of inducers or inhibitors of CYP2D6. Check labeling for compatible liquids with oral solution. Do not split or crush oral disintegrating tablets. Inform patients with phenylketonuria that oral disintegrating tablets contain phenylalanine.
Ziprasidone	Geodon	Capsule: 20, 40, 60, 80 Solution reconstituted, IM: 20	40	80–160	320	Give capsules with >500 calories of food. No data suggest improved efficacy at higher doses. See labeling for reconstitution and storage of IM formulation. Short-acting IM formulation is used primarily for agitation, with usual dosage of 20 mg/day and maximum dosage of 40 mg/day.

[a]This table and subsequent medication-related tables include information compiled from multiple sources. Detailed information on such issues as dose regimen, dose adjustments, medication administration procedures, handling precautions, and storage can be found in product labeling. It is recommended that readers consult product labeling information for authoritative information on these medications.

TABLE 3. Antipsychotic medications: available oral and short-acting intramuscular formulations and dosing considerations[a,b] (continued)

[b]Long-acting injectable formulations of antipsychotic medications are described separately in Tables 7, 8, and 9. Droperidol is a first-generation antipsychotic medication but is not included because it is available only in a parenteral formulation for short-term use, primarily for treatment of agitation or postoperative nausea and vomiting. Pimavanserin is a second-generation antipsychotic but is not included because it is FDA indicated for the treatment of hallucinations and delusions associated with Parkinson's disease psychosis (Nuplazid [10 and 34 mg pimavanserin] 2018; Nuplazid [17 mg pimavanserin] 2018). Mesoridazine and triflupromazine were previously marketed in the United States but are no longer available. Other antipsychotic medications and other formulations of the listed medications may be available in Canada.

[c]The most common U.S. trade names are included for reference only. At the time of publication, some of these products may be manufactured only as generic products.

[d]Elderly patients with dementia-related psychosis treated with antipsychotics are at an increased risk of death compared with placebo, and an FDA black box warning applies to all antipsychotic medications. Antipsychotic agents with an indication for augmentation treatment in major depressive disorder (e.g., aripiprazole, brexpiprazole) have an additional black box warning related to increased risk of suicidal thinking/behaviors.

[e]May be taken without regard to food or other medications unless specifically noted.

[f]Tablets can be crushed or split unless specifically noted.

[g]As described by Pugh et al. (1973), Child-Pugh class A corresponds to a Child-Pugh score of 5–6, class B corresponds to a Child-Pugh score of 7–9, and class C corresponds to a Child-Pugh score of 10–15.

[h]Usually given in divided doses.

[i]Up to 9 mg/day has been studied in clinical trials.

[j]Clozapine levels should be drawn after at least 3 days on a stable dose and about 12 hours after the last dose. Levels associated with efficacy show individual variation, but efficacy typically begins at a level above 250 ng/mL, with the most efficacy seen at levels higher than 350 ng/mL.

[k]Olanzapine has been used at higher dosages, typically up to 30 mg/day, although some case series describe use of up to 60 mg/day.

[l]Dosages of risperidone up to 16 mg/day have been studied in clinical trials; however, doses >6 mg for twice-daily dosing do not appear to confer additional benefit and have a higher incidence of extrapyramidal symptoms than do lower doses.

Abbreviations. ANC=absolute neutrophil count; CBC=complete blood count; CrCl=creatinine clearance; CYP=cytochrome P450; ECG=electrocardiography; HCl=hydrochloride; OROS=osmotic-controlled release oral delivery system; QTc=corrected QT interval; REMS=risk evaluation and mitigation strategy.

Source. Hiemke et al. 2018; Koytchev et al. 1996; Lexicomp 2019; Micromedex 2019; Mountjoy et al. 1999; Procyshyn et al. 2019.

Package insert references. Abilify 2017, 2019; Abilify Maintena 2018; Abilify Mycite 2017; Aripiprazole orally disintegrating tablets 2018; Aripiprazole solution 2016; Aristada 2019; Aristada Initio 2019; Chlorpromazine hydrochloride injection 2010, 2016; Chlorpromazine hydrochloride tablets 2018; Clozapine 2017; Clozaril 2017; Fanapt 2017; FazaClo 2017; Fluphenazine decanoate injection 2018; Fluphenazine hydrochloride elixir 2016; Fluphenazine hydrochloride injection 2010; Fluphenazine hydrochloride solution, concentrate 2010; Fluphenazine hydrochloride tablets 2016; Geodon 2018; Haldol decanoate injection 2019; Haldol lactate injection 2019; Haloperidol 2008; Haloperidol lactate injection 2011; Haloperidol lactate oral solution 2016; Haloperidol tablets 2015; Invega 2018, 2019; Invega Sustenna 2018a, 2018b; Invega Trinza 2018a, 2018b; Latuda 2018; Loxapac 2014; Loxitane 2017; Moban 2017; Molindone hydrochloride tablets 2014, 2018; Navane 2010; Orap 2014, 2019; Perphenazine 2016, 2017; Perseris 2018; Rexulti 2019; Risperdal 2019; Risperdal Consta 2019; Risperidone orally disintegrating tablets 2019; Saphris 2017; Seroquel 2019; Seroquel XR 2019; Thioridazine hydrochloride 2016; Trifluoperazine 2017; Vraylar 2019; Zyprexa 2018a, 2018b; Zyprexa Relprevv 2018.

TABLE 4. Antipsychotic medications: pharmacokinetics/pharmacodynamics of oral and short-acting intramuscular formulations

	Trade name	Oral bio-availability	Time to peak level	Protein binding	Metabolic enzymes/transporters	Metabolites	Elimination half-life in adults	Excretion	Hepatic impairment[a]	Renal impairment
First-generation antipsychotics										
Chlorpromazine	Thorazine	32%	2.8 hours	90%–99%	CYP2D6 (major), CYP1A2 (minor), CYP3A4 (minor) substrate	NOR2CPZ, NOR2CPZ SULF, and 3-OH CPZ	Biphasic: initial 2 hours, terminal 30 hours	Primarily renal (<1% as unchanged drug)	Use with caution	Use with caution; not dialyzable
Fluphenazine	Prolixin	2.7%	Oral: 2 hours IM: 1.5–2 hours	99%	CYP2D6 (major) substrate	7-hydroxy-fluphenazine, fluphenazine sulfoxide	4.4–16.4 hours	Renal and fecal; exact proportion unclear	Contraindicated by manufacturer	Use with caution
Haloperidol	Haldol	60%–70%	Oral: 2–6 hours IM: 20 minutes	89%–93%	CYP2D6 (major), CYP3A4 (major), CYP1A2 (minor) substrate; 50%–60% glucuronidation	Hydroxymetabolite-reduced haloperidol	14–37 hours	15% fecal, 30% renal (1% as unchanged drug)	No dose adjustments noted	No dose adjustments noted
Loxapine	Loxitane	99%	1.5–3 hours	97%	CYP1A2 (minor), CYP2D6 (minor), CYP3A4 (minor) substrate; P-glycoprotein inhibitor	N-desmethyl loxapine (amoxapine), 8-hydroxyloxapine	Biphasic: initial 5 hours, terminal 19 hours	Renal and fecal	No dose adjustments noted	No dose adjustments noted
Molindone	Moban	Unclear	1.5 hours	76%	CYP2D6 substrate	Multiple	1.5 hours	Renal and fecal	Use with caution	No dose adjustments noted
Perphenazine	Trilafon	20%–40%	Perphenazine: 1–3 hours 7-hydroxyperphenazine: 2–4 hours	91%–99%	CYP2D6 (major), CYP1A2 (minor), CYP2C19 (minor), CYP2C9 (minor), CYP3A4 (minor) substrate	7-hydroxyperphenazine (responsible for 70% of the activity)	Perphenazine: 9–12 hours 7-hydroxyperphenazine: 10–19 hours	5% fecal, 70% renal	Contraindicated in liver damage	Use with caution

TABLE 4. Antipsychotic medications: pharmacokinetics/pharmacodynamics of oral and short-acting intramuscular formulations (continued)

	Trade name	Oral bioavailability	Time to peak level	Protein binding	Metabolic enzymes/ transporters	Metabolites	Elimination half-life in adults	Excretion	Hepatic impairment[a]	Renal impairment[a]
First-generation antipsychotics (continued)										
Pimozide	Orap	≥50%	6–8 hours	99%	CYP1A2 (major), CYP2D6 (major), CYP3A4 (major) substrate	Unknown activity: 4-bis-(4-fluorophenyl) butyric acid, 1-(4-piperidyl)-2-benzimidazolinone	55 hours	Primarily renal	Use with caution	Use with caution
Thioridazine	Mellaril	25%–33%	1–4 hours	96%–99%	CYP2D6 (major) substrate and moderate inhibitor, CYP2C19 (minor) substrate	Mesoridazine (twice as potent as thioridazine), sulforidazine	21–24 hours	Minimal renal	Use with caution	No dose adjustments noted
Thiothixene	Navane	~50%; erratic absorption	1–2 hours	90%	CYP1A2 (major) substrate	None noted	34 hours	Feces (unchanged drug and metabolites)	No dose adjustments noted	No dose adjustments noted
Trifluoperazine	Stelazine	Erratic absorption	1.5–6 hours	90%–99%	CYP1A2 (major) substrate	N-desmethyltrifluoperazine, 7-hydroxytrifluoperazine, and other metabolites	3–12 hours	Renal	Contraindicated in hepatic disease	No dose adjustments noted
Second-generation antipsychotics										
Aripiprazole	Abilify	87%	3–5 hours	>99%	CYP2D6 (major), CYP3A4 (major) substrate	Dehydroaripiprazole	75 hours, 94 hours dehydroaripiprazole 146 hours in poor CYP2D6 metabolizers	55% fecal, 25% renal	No dose adjustments noted	No dose adjustments noted

TABLE 4. Antipsychotic medications: pharmacokinetics/pharmacodynamics of oral and short-acting intramuscular formulations *(continued)*

	Trade name	Oral bio-availability	Time to peak level	Protein binding	Metabolic enzymes/transporters	Metabolites	Elimination half-life in adults	Excretion	Hepatic impairment[a]	Renal impairment
Second-generation antipsychotics *(continued)*										
Asenapine	Saphris	35%	0.5–1.5 hours	95%	CYP1A2 (major), CYP2D6 (minor), CYP3A4 (minor) substrate; glucuronidation by UGT1A4; CYP2D6 weak inhibitor	Inactive: N(+)-glucuronide, N-desmethyl-asenapine, and N-desmethyl-asenapine N-carbamoyl glucuronide	24 hours	40% fecal, 50% renal	Contraindicated in severe hepatic impairment (Child-Pugh class C)	No dose adjustments noted
Asenapine	Secuado	Not applicable	Not available	95%	CYP1A2 (major), CYP2D6 (minor), CYP3A4 (minor) substrate; glucuronidation by UGT1A4; CYP2D6 weak inhibitor	Inactive: N(+)-glucuronide, N-desmethyl-asenapine, and N-desmethyl-asenapine N-carbamoyl glucuronide	24 hours	40% fecal, 50% renal	Contraindicated in severe hepatic impairment (Child-Pugh class C)	No dose adjustments noted
Brexpiprazole	Rexulti	95%	4 hours	>99%	CYP3A4 (major), CYP2D6 (major) substrate	Inactive: DM-3411	91 hours	46% fecal, 25% renal	Moderate to severe impairment (Child-Pugh class B or C): use maximum dosage of 2 mg/day in MDD and 3 mg/day in schizophrenia	CrCl <60 mL/minute: use maximum dosage of 2 mg/day in MDD and 3 mg/day in schizophrenia

TABLE 4. Antipsychotic medications: pharmacokinetics/pharmacodynamics of oral and short-acting intramuscular formulations *(continued)*

	Trade name	Oral bio-availability	Time to peak level	Protein binding	Metabolic enzymes/ transporters	Metabolites	Elimination half-life in adults	Excretion	Hepatic impairment[a]	Renal impairment
Second-generation antipsychotics *(continued)*										
Cariprazine	Vraylar	High	3–6 hours	91%–97%	CYP3A4 (major), CYP2D6 (minor) substrate	Desmethyl cariprazine (DCAR), didesmethyl cariprazine (DDCAR)	Cariprazine: 2–4 days DCAR: 1–2 days DDCAR: 1–3 weeks	21% renal	Severe impairment (Child-Pugh class C): not recommended	CrCl <30 mL/minute: not recommended
Clozapine	Clozaril, FazaClo, Versacloz	27%–60%	2.2–2.5 hours (range: 1–6 hours)	97%	CYP1A2 (major), CYP2A6 (minor), CYP2C19 (minor), CYP2C9 (minor), CYP2D6 (minor), CYP3A4 (minor) substrate	N-desmethyl-clozapine (active), hydroxylated and N-oxide derivatives (inactive)	4–66 hours (steady state 12 hours)	30% fecal, 50% renal	Significant impairment: dose reduction may be necessary	Significant impairment: dose reduction may be necessary
Iloperidone	Fanapt	96%	2–4 hours	92%–97%	CYP2D6 (major), CYP3A4 (minor) substrate, CYP3A4 weak inhibitor	P88 P95	Extensive metabolizers: iloperidone 18 hours, P88 26 hours, P95 23 hours Poor metabolizers: iloperidone 33 hours, P88 37 hours, P95 31 hours	~20% fecal, ~50% renal	Moderate impairment: use with caution Severe impairment: not recommended	No dose adjustments noted

TABLE 4. Antipsychotic medications: pharmacokinetics/pharmacodynamics of oral and short-acting intramuscular formulations (*continued*)

	Trade name	Oral bio-availability	Time to peak level	Protein binding	Metabolic enzymes/ transporters	Metabolites	Elimination half-life in adults	Excretion	Hepatic impairment[a]	Renal impairment
Second-generation antipsychotics (*continued*)										
Lurasidone	Latuda	9–19%	1–3 hours	99%	CYP3A4 (major) substrate, CYP3A4 weak inhibitor	ID-14283, ID-14326 (active); ID-20219, ID-20220 (inactive)	Lurasidone 18–40 hours ID-14283: 7.5–10 hours	~80% fecal, ~9% renal	Moderate to severe hepatic impairment (Child-Pugh class B and class C): use 20 mg/ day initially, with maximum dose of 80 mg/ day and 40 mg/day, respectively	For CrCl <50 mL/minute: initial 20 mg/day, maximum dose 80 mg/ day
Olanzapine	Zyprexa	>57%	Oral: 6 hours IM: 15–45 minutes	93%	CYP1A2 (major), CYP2D6 (minor) substrate; metabolized via direct glucuronidation	10-N-glucuronide, 4-N-desmethyl olanzapine (inactive)	30 hours	30% fecal, 57% renal	Use with caution	Not removed by dialysis

The APA Practice Guideline for the Treatment of Patients With Schizophrenia

TABLE 4. Antipsychotic medications: pharmacokinetics/pharmacodynamics of oral and short-acting intramuscular formulations *(continued)*

	Trade name	Oral bio-availability	Time to peak level	Protein binding	Metabolic enzymes/ transporters	Metabolites	Elimination half-life in adults	Excretion	Hepatic impairment[a]	Renal impairment
Second-generation antipsychotics *(continued)*										
Paliperidone	Invega	28%	24 hours	74%	P-glycoprotein/ ABCB1, CYP2D6 (minor), CYP3A4 (minor) substrate	Activity unclear: M1, M9, M10, M11, M12, M16	23 hours; 24–51 hours with renal impairment (CrCl <80 mL/minute)	11% fecal, 80% renal	Mild to moderate: no adjustment necessary; Severe: not studied	Not recommended for CrCl <10 mL/minute; for CrCl 10–49 mL/minute and CrCl 50–79 mL/minute, use maximum dosage of 3 mg/day and 6 mg/day, respectively
Quetiapine	Seroquel	100%	Immediate release: 1.5 hours Extended release: 6 hours	83%	CYP3A4 (major), CYP2D6 (minor) substrate	Active: norquetiapine, 7-hydroxyquetiapine Inactive: quetiapine sulfoxide (major), parent acid metabolite	Quetiapine: 6–7 hours Norquetiapine: 12 hours	20% fecal, 73% renal	Immediate release: initial 25 mg/day dose, increase by 25–50 mg/day to effective dose Extended release: initial 50 mg/day, increase by 50 mg/day to effective dose	No dose adjustments noted

TABLE 4. Antipsychotic medications: pharmacokinetics/pharmacodynamics of oral and short-acting intramuscular formulations *(continued)*

	Trade name	Oral bio-availability	Time to peak level	Protein binding	Metabolic enzymes/transporters	Metabolites	Elimination half-life in adults	Excretion	Hepatic impairment[a]	Renal impairment
Second-generation antipsychotics *(continued)*										
Risperidone	Risperdal	Absolute: 70% Tablet relative to oral solution: 94%	1 hour	90%	CYP2D6 (major), CYP3A4 (minor), P-glycoprotein/ABCB1 substrate, N-dealkylation (minor), CYP2D6 weak inhibitor	Active: 9-hydroxy-risperidone	Risperidone: 3–20 hours 9-hydroxy-risperidone: 21–30 hours	14% fecal, 70% renal	Mild or moderate impairment (Child-Pugh class A or B): reduce dose Severe impairment (Child-Pugh class C): initial 0.5 mg twice a day, increase by no more than 0.5 mg twice a day; may increase to total dosage >1.5 mg twice a day at 1 week or greater	Mild or moderate impairment (CrCl ≥30 mL/minute): reduce dose Severe impairment (CrCl <30 mL/minute): initial 0.5 mg twice a day, increase by no more than 0.5 mg twice a day; may increase to dosage >1.5 mg twice a day at 1 week or greater

TABLE 4. Antipsychotic medications: pharmacokinetics/pharmacodynamics of oral and short-acting intramuscular formulations *(continued)*

	Trade name	Oral bio-availability	Time to peak level	Protein binding	Metabolic enzymes/ transporters	Metabolites	Elimination half-life in adults	Excretion	Hepatic impairment[a]	Renal impairment
Second-generation antipsychotics *(continued)*										
Ziprasidone	Geodon	Oral with food: 60% IM:100%	Oral: 6–8 hours IM: 60 minutes	>99%	CYP1A2 (minor), CYP3A4 (minor) substrate, glutathione, aldehyde oxidase	Active: benziso-thiazole sulfox-ide (major), benzisothi-azole sulfone (major), ziprasidone sulfoxide, S-methyl-dihydro-ziprasidone	Oral: 7 hours IM: 2–5 hours	66% fecal, 20% renal	Use with caution	No oral dose adjustments noted IM formula-tion con-tains a renally cleared ex-cipient, cy-clodextrin; use with caution

[a]As described by Pugh et al. (1973). Child-Pugh class A corresponds to a Child-Pugh score of 5–6, class B corresponds to a Child-Pugh score of 7–9, and class C corresponds to a Child-Pugh score of 10–15.

Abbreviations. CrCl = creatinine clearance; CYP = cytochrome P450; MDD = major depressive disorder; UGT = uridine 5'-diphospho-glucuronosyltransferase.

Source. Hiemke et al. 2018; Koytchev et al. 1996; Lexicomp 2019; Micromedex 2019; Mountjoy et al. 1999; Procyshyn et al. 2019; Vermeir et al. 2008.

TABLE 5. Antipsychotic receptor binding properties

	Trade name	D$_1$	D$_2$	D$_3$	D$_4$	D$_5$	5-HT$_{1A}$	5-HT$_{2A}$	5-HT$_{2C}$	5-HT$_7$	H$_1$	Musc M$_1$	α$_1$	α$_2$	Comments
First-generation antipsychotics															
Chlorpromazine	Thorazine	+	+++	+++	++	+	0	+++	++	++	+++	++	+++	+	
Fluphenazine	Prolixin	++	++++	+++++	++	++	+	++	+	+++	++	0	+++	0	
Haloperidol	Haldol	+	+++	+++	+++	+	0	++	0	+	0	0	++	0	
Loxapine	Loxitane	++	++	++	+++	++	0	+++	++	++	+++	+	++	0	
Molindone	Moban	0	++	++	0	0	0	0	0	0	0	0	0	+	
Perphenazine	Trilafon	++	++++	+++++	++	+	0	+	++	++	+++	0	++	+	
Pimozide	Orap	0	++++	+++	++	+	+	++	0	++++	+	+	+	+	Moderate activity at dopamine transporter
Thioridazine	Mellaril	++	++	+++	++	+	+	++	++	++	++	+++	+++	+	
Thiothixene	Navane	+	++++	+++++	+	+	+	++	0	++	+++	0	++	0	
Trifluoperazine	Stelazine	+	+++	++++	++	+	+	+	+	+	++	+	++	0	
Second-generation antipsychotics															
Aripiprazole	Abilify	+	////	+++	+	0	///	+++	++	++	++	0	++	+	
Asenapine	Saphris, Secuado	+++	+++	+++++	+++	++	+++	++++	++++	++++	+++	0	+++	+++	
Brexpiprazole	Rexulti	+	///	+++	++++		////	++++	++	+++	++	0	+++	++++	
Cariprazine	Vraylar		///	++++			///	++	+	+	+	0	+		
Clozapine	Clozaril, FazaClo, Versacloz	+	+	+	++	+	/	+++	++	++	+++	///	+++	+	
Iloperidone	Fanapt	+	++	++	++	+	//	++++	++	++	+	0	+++	+++	
Lurasidone	Latuda	+	+++	++	++	+	/	++++	+	++++	0	0	++	++	
Olanzapine	Zyprexa	++	++	++	++	++	0	+++	+++	+	+++	+++	++	+	
Paliperidone	Invega	+	+++	+++	++	++	+	++++	++	+++	+++	0	+++	++	
Quetiapine	Seroquel	0	+	+	0	0	/	+	0	+	+++	+	++	0	
Risperidone	Risperdal	+	+++	+++	+++	+	+	++++	++	+++	++	0	+++	+++	
Ziprasidone	Geodon	+	+++	+++	++	+	///	++++	+++	+++	++	0	+++	+	Weak activity at norepinephrine and serotonin transporter

Note. ++++=very strong binding (K$_i$ <1 nM); +++=strong binding (1 nM ≤K$_i$ <10 nM); ++=moderate binding (10 nM ≤K$_i$ <100 nM); +=weak binding (100 nM ≤K$_i$ <1,000 nM); 0=very weak or negligible binding (K$_i$ ≥1,000 nM). For partial agonists, / is used instead of + to denote relative binding values.

Source. Latuda 2018; Lexicomp 2019; Maeda et al. 2014; Micromedex 2019; Olten and Bloch 2018; PDSP 2019; Procyshyn et al. 2019; Rexulti 2019; Roth et al. 2000; Saphris 2017; Vraylar 2019.

TABLE 6. Antipsychotic medications: relative side effects of oral formulations

	Trade name	Akathisia	Parkinsonism	Dystonia	Tardive dyskinesia	Hyperprolactinemia[a]	Anticholinergic	Sedation
First-generation antipsychotics								
Chlorpromazine	Thorazine	++	++	++	+++	+	+++	+++
Fluphenazine	Prolixin	+++	+++	+++	+++	+++	+	+
Haloperidol	Haldol	+++	+++	+++	+++	+++	+	+
Loxapine	Loxitane	++	++	++	++	++	++	++
Molindone	Moban	++	++	++	++	++	+	++
Perphenazine	Trilafon	++	++	++	++	++	++	++
Pimozide	Orap	+++	+++	++	+++	+++	+	+
Thioridazine	Mellaril	+	+	+	+	++	+++	+++
Thiothixene	Navane	+++	+++	+++	+++	+++	+	+
Trifluoperazine	Stelazine	++	++	++	++	++	++	+
Second-generation antipsychotics								
Aripiprazole	Abilify	++	+	+	+	+	+	+
Asenapine	Saphris	++	+	++	++	++	+	++
Brexpiprazole	Rexulti	++	+	+	+	+	+	++
Cariprazine	Vraylar	++	+	+	+	+	++	++
Clozapine	Clozaril, FazaClo, Versacloz	+	+	+	+	+	+++	+++
Iloperidone	Fanapt	+	+	+	+	++	+	++
Lurasidone	Latuda	++	++	++	++	+	+	++
Olanzapine	Zyprexa	++	++	+	+	++	++	+++
Paliperidone	Invega	++	++	++	++	+++	+	+
Quetiapine	Seroquel	+	+	+	+	+	++	+++
Risperidone	Risperdal	++	++	++	++	+++	+	++
Ziprasidone	Geodon	++	+	+	+	++	+	++

TABLE 6. Antipsychotic medications: relative side effects of oral formulations *(continued)*

	Trade name	Seizures	Orthostasis	QT prolongation	Weight gain	Hyperlipidemia	Glucose abnormalities	Comments
First-generation antipsychotics								
Chlorpromazine	Thorazine	++	+++	+++	++	+	++	
Fluphenazine	Prolixin	+	+	++	++	+	+	
Haloperidol	Haldol	+	+	++	++	+	+	
Loxapine	Loxitane	+	++	++	+	+	+	
Molindone	Moban	+	+	++	+	+	+	
Perphenazine	Trilafon	+	++	++	++	+	+	
Pimozide	Orap	+++	+	+++	+	+	+	
Thioridazine	Mellaril	++	+++	+++	++	+	+	Pigmentary retinopathy; high rates of sexual dysfunction; avoid use if QTc interval is >450 msec or with concomitant use of drugs that prolong the QTc interval or inhibit CYP2D6
Thiothixene	Navane	+++	+	++	+	+	+	
Trifluoperazine	Stelazine	+	+	++	++	+	+	
Second-generation antipsychotics								
Aripiprazole	Abilify	+	+	+	+	+	+	FDA safety alert for impulse control disorders (e.g., gambling, binge eating); may reduce hyperprolactinemia with other antipsychotics
Asenapine	Saphris	+	++	++	++	++	++	Oral hypoesthesia
Brexpiprazole	Rexulti	+	+	++	+	++	+	
Cariprazine	Vraylar	+	+	++	++	+	+	

TABLE 6. Antipsychotic medications: relative side effects of oral formulations *(continued)*

	Trade name	Seizures	Orthostasis	QT prolongation	Weight gain	Hyperlipidemia	Glucose abnormalities	Comments
Second-generation antipsychotics *(continued)*								
Clozapine	Clozaril, FazaClo, Versacloz	+++	+++	++	+++	+++	+++	Increased salivation common; high rate of sexual dysfunction; severe constipation and paralytic ileus possible; fever can occur with initiation; myocarditis is infrequent; cardiomyopathy and severe neutropenia are rare
Iloperidone	Fanapt	+	+++	+++	++	+	++	
Lurasidone	Latuda	+	+	+	+	++	++	Dose-related creatinine increase in some patients
Olanzapine	Zyprexa	++	++	++	+++	+++	+++	
Paliperidone	Invega	+	++	++	++	++	+	
Quetiapine	Seroquel	++	++	++	++	+++	++	
Risperidone	Risperdal	+	++	++	++	+	++	Intraoperative floppy iris syndrome reported
Ziprasidone	Geodon	+	++	+++	+	+	+	

[a]In general, rates of sexual dysfunction parallel rates of hyperprolactinemia except where noted in comments.

Note.   +=seldom; ++=sometimes; +++=often. CYP=cytochrome P450.

Source.   Credible Meds 2019; Hirsch et al. 2017; La Torre et al. 2013; Lexicomp 2019; Micromedex 2019; Pisani et al. 2002; Procyshyn et al. 2019; van Dijk et al. 2018.

TABLE 7. Long-acting injectable antipsychotic medications: availability and injection-related considerations[a]

	Trade name	Available strengths[b] (mg, unless otherwise noted)	How supplied	Injection site and technique[c]	Reactions at injection site[d]	Comments
First-generation antipsychotics						
Fluphenazine	Prolixin Decanoate	25/mL (5 mL)	Vial, sesame oil vehicle with 1.2% benzyl alcohol	Deep IM gluteal or deltoid injection; use of Z-track technique recommended[e]	Skin reactions reported	Monitor for hypotension. In sesame oil, be alert for allergy. For detailed instructions on needle size and product handling, refer to labeling.
Haloperidol	Haldol Decanoate	50/mL (1 mL, 5 mL), 100/mL (1 mL, 5 mL)	Vial, sesame oil vehicle with 1.2% benzyl alcohol	Deep IM gluteal or deltoid injection; use of Z-track technique recommended[e]	Inflammation and nodules reported, especially with dose >100 mg/mL	Do not administer more than 3 mL per injection site. In sesame oil, be alert for allergy. For detailed instructions on needle size, refer to labeling.
Second-generation antipsychotics						
Aripiprazole monohydrate	Abilify Maintena	300, 400	Kit with either prefilled syringe or single-use vial	Slow IM injection into gluteal or deltoid muscle	Occasional redness, swelling, induration (mild to moderate)	Rotate injection sites. Do not massage muscle after injection. For detailed instructions on needle size and product reconstitution, refer to labeling.
Aripiprazole lauroxil	Aristada Initio	675/2.4 mL	Kit with prefilled syringe	IM deltoid or gluteal muscle	Common: pain Infrequent: induration, swelling, redness	Only to be used as a single dose to initiate Aristada treatment or to reinitiate treatment following a missed dose of Aristada. Not for repeat dosing. Not interchangeable with Aristada. Avoid concomitant injection of Aristada Initio and Aristada into the same deltoid or gluteal muscle. Refer to labeling for detailed instructions on injection site, needle length, and instructions to ensure a uniform suspension.
Aripiprazole lauroxil	Aristada	441/1.6 mL, 662/2.4 mL, 882/3.2 mL, 1,064/3.9 mL	Kit with prefilled syringe	IM deltoid or gluteal muscle for 441 mg IM gluteal muscle for 662 mg, 882 mg, or 1,064 mg	Common: pain Infrequent: induration, swelling, redness	Not interchangeable with Aristada Initio. Avoid concomitant injection of Aristada Initio and Aristada into the same deltoid or gluteal muscle. Refer to labeling for detailed instructions on injection site, needle length, and instructions to ensure a uniform suspension.

TABLE 7. Long-acting injectable antipsychotic medications: availability and injection-related considerations[a] *(continued)*

	Trade name	Available strengths[b] (mg, unless otherwise noted)	How supplied	Injection site and technique[c]	Reactions at injection site[d]	Comments
Second-generation antipsychotics *(continued)*						
Olanzapine	Zyprexa Relprevv	210, 300, 405	Kit with vial containing diluent and vial with powder for reconstituting suspension	Deep IM gluteal injection only; do not administer subcutaneously	Infrequent induration or mass at injection site	Because of risk of postinjection delirium/sedation syndrome, must be given in a registered health care facility with ready access to emergency response services, and patient must be observed for at least 3 hours postinjection and accompanied on discharge. Requires use of FDA REMS program (www.zyprexarelprevv program.com/public/Default.aspx). Do not massage muscle after injection. The combined effects of age, smoking, and biological sex may lead to significant pharmacokinetic differences. For detailed instructions on product handling and reconstitution, refer to labeling.
Paliperidone palmitate	Invega Sustenna	39/0.25 mL, 78/0.5 mL, 117/0.75 mL, 156/1 mL, 234/1.5 mL	Kit with prefilled syringe	IM only; slow, deep IM deltoid injection for first 2 doses, then deep deltoid or gluteal injection (upper outer quadrant) thereafter	Occasional redness, swelling, induration	The two initial deltoid IM injections help attain therapeutic concentrations rapidly. Alternate deltoid injections (right and left deltoid muscle). For detailed instructions on needle size and product reconstitution, refer to labeling.
Paliperidone palmitate	Invega Trinza	273/0.875 mL, 410/1.315 mL, 546/1.75 mL, 819/2.625 mL	Kit with prefilled syringe	IM only; slow, deep IM deltoid or gluteal injection	Infrequent redness or swelling	Shake prefilled syringe for 15 seconds within 5 minutes prior to administration. For detailed instructions on needle size, product handling, and reconstitution, refer to labeling.

TABLE 7. Long-acting injectable antipsychotic medications: availability and injection-related considerations[a] (continued)

	Trade name	Available strengths[b] (mg, unless otherwise noted)	How supplied	Injection site and technique[c]	Reactions at injection site[d]	Comments
Second-generation antipsychotics (continued)						
Risperidone	Risperdal Consta	12.5, 25, 37.5, 50	Kit with prefilled syringe and vial for reconstitution	Deep IM injection into the deltoid or gluteal (upper outer quadrant)	Occasional redness, swelling, induration	Alternate injection sites. Refrigerate and store at 2°C–8°C and protect from light. Vial should come to room temperature for at least 30 minutes before reconstituting. May be stored at 25°C for up to 7 days prior to administration. For detailed instructions on product handling and reconstitution, refer to labeling.
Risperidone	Perseris	90/0.6 mL, 120/0.8 mL	Kit with prefilled syringes containing powder and diluent	Abdominal subcutaneous injection only	Lump at injection site may persist for several weeks	Alternate injection sites. Inject only in area without skin conditions, irritation, reddening, bruising, infection, or scarring; do not rub or massage injection sites. Store at 2°C–8°C and protect from light. Allow package to come to room temperature for at least 15 minutes before injection. For detailed instructions on product handling and reconstitution, refer to labeling.

[a]This table and the subsequent table on long-acting injectable antipsychotic medications include information compiled from multiple sources. It is recommended that readers consult product labeling information for authoritative information on these medications. Detailed information on issues such as dose regimen, dose adjustments, medication administration procedures, appropriate needle size based on injection site and patient weight, product reconstitution, handling precautions, and storage can also be found in product labeling.

[b]Available strengths are based on U.S. products; strengths and products available in other countries may differ.

[c]Each injection must be administered only by a health care professional. Long-acting injectable antipsychotic medications should never be administered intravenously.

[d]Pain at injection site noted for all products.

[e]*Source.* Government of South Australia Health: Injection Sites. Available at: www.sahealth.sa.gov.au/wps/wcm/connect/public+content/sa+health+internet/clinical+resources/clinical+programs+and+practice+guidelines/medicines+and+drugs/injection+techniques#Z%20track. Accessed July 21, 2020. Northumberland, Tyne and Wear NHS Foundation Trust: Standard for the Assessment and Management of Physical Health. Appendix 2: Injection Sites. Available at: www.ntw.nhs.uk/content/uploads/2015/06/AMPH-PGN-10-IMI-App2-Injection-Sites-V01-iss-Sep7.pdf. Accessed January 20, 2019.

Abbreviations. REMS=risk evaluation and mitigation strategy.

Source. Abilify Maintena 2018; Andorn et al. 2019; Aristada 2019; Aristada Initio 2019; Invega Sustenna 2018a, 2018b; Invega Trinza 2018a, 2018b; Lexicomp 2019; Micromedex 2019; Perseris 2018; Procyshyn et al. 2019; Risperdal Consta 2019; Zyprexa Relprevv 2018.

The APA Practice Guideline for the Treatment of Patients With Schizophrenia

TABLE 8. Long-acting injectable antipsychotic medications: dosing

	Trade name	Dose conversions	Initial dose (mg)	Typical dose (mg)	Maximum dose (mg)	Dosing frequency	Need for initial oral supplementation	Comments
First-generation antipsychotics								
Fluphenazine	Prolixin Decanoate	For each 10 mg/day oral, give 12.5 mg decanoate every 3 weeks	6.25–25 every 2 weeks	6.25–25 every 2–4 weeks	100	2–4 weeks	Decrease oral dose by half after first injection, then discontinue with second injection	Increase in 12.5 mg increments if doses >50 mg are needed.
Haloperidol	Haldol Decanoate	For each 5 mg/day oral, give 50–75 mg decanoate every 4 weeks	Determined by oral dose and/or risk of relapse up to a maximum of 100 mg	50–200 (10–15 times previous oral dose)	450/month	4 weeks	Taper and discontinue after two to three injections	If initial dose is >100 mg, split into two injections separated by 3–7 days.
Second-generation antipsychotics								
Aripiprazole monohydrate	Abilify Maintena	Not applicable	400	400	400/month	Monthly	Continue oral for 14 days after initial injection	Follow labeling if scheduled injections are missed. Dose adjust for poor CYP2D6 metabolizers, for those taking CYP2D6 and/or CYP3A4 inhibitors, or because of adverse effects. Avoid use with CYP3A4 inducers.
Aripiprazole lauroxil	Aristada Initio	Not applicable	675	675	675	Single dose to initiate Aristada treatment or reinitiate treatment after a missed Aristada dose. Not for repeated dosing.	Must be administered in conjunction with one 30 mg dose of oral aripiprazole	For patients who have never taken aripiprazole, establish tolerability with oral aripiprazole before use. Aristada Initio and Aristada are not interchangeable. See labeling for dose adjustments.

TABLE 8. Long-acting injectable antipsychotic medications: dosing *(continued)*

Second-generation antipsychotics *(continued)*

	Trade name	Dose conversions	Initial dose (mg)	Typical dose (mg)	Maximum dose (mg)	Dosing frequency	Need for initial oral supplementation	Comments
Aripiprazole lauroxil	Aristada	10 mg/day orally, give 441 mg IM/month 15 mg/day orally, give 662 mg/month IM, 882 mg IM every 6 weeks, or 1,064 mg IM every 2 months 20 mg/day or greater orally, give 882 mg/month IM	Monthly: 441, 662, 882 Every 6 weeks: 882 Every 2 months: 1,064	Monthly: 441, 662, 882 Every 6 weeks: 882 Every 2 months: 1,064	882/month	Monthly: 441, 662, 882 Every 6 weeks: 882 Every 2 months: 1,064	There are two ways to initiate treatment: 1. Give one IM injection of Aristada Initio 675 mg and one dose of oral aripiprazole 30 mg or 2. Give 21 days of oral aripiprazole in conjunction with the first Aristada injection	Aristada Initio and Aristada are not interchangeable. The first Aristada injection may be given on the same day as Aristada Initio or up to 10 days thereafter.
Olanzapine	Zyprexa Relprevv	10 mg/day orally, 210 mg every 2 weeks for four doses or 405 mg every 4 weeks 15 mg/day orally, 300 mg every 2 weeks for four doses 20 mg/day orally, 300 mg every 2 weeks	Determined by oral dose	150 mg, 210 mg, or 300 mg every 2 weeks or 300 mg or 405 mg every 4 weeks	300 mg every 2 weeks or 405 mg every 4 weeks	2–4 weeks	Not required	Give 150 mg every 4 weeks in patients who may have sensitivity to side effects or slower metabolism. Smokers may require a greater daily dose than nonsmokers, and women may need lower daily doses than expected.

	Trade name	Dose conversions	Initial dose (mg)	Typical dose (mg)	Maximum dose (mg)	Dosing frequency	Need for initial oral supplementation	Comments
Second-generation antipsychotics *(continued)*								
Paliperidone palmitate	Invega Sustenna	3 mg oral paliperidone, give 39–78 mg IM 6 mg oral, give 117 mg IM 9 mg oral, give 156 mg IM 12 mg oral, give 234 mg IM	234 mg IM on day 1 and 156 mg IM 1 week later, both administered in the deltoid muscle	78–234 mg monthly beginning at week 5	234 mg/month	Monthly	Not required	Contains range of particle sizes for rapid and delayed absorption. For changes to oral or other LAI to Sustenna, see labeling. Doses are expressed as amount of paliperidone palmitate rather than as paliperidone. Avoid using with a strong inducer of CYP3A4 and/or P-glycoprotein.
Paliperidone palmitate	Invega Trinza	Conversion from monthly Invega Sustenna to every 3-month injections of Invega Trinza: 78 mg, give 273 mg 117 mg, give 410 mg 156 mg, give 546 mg 234 mg, give 819 mg	Dependent on last dose of monthly paliperidone	273–819	819/3 months	Every 3 months	Not applicable	Change to Trinza after at least four Invega Sustenna doses (with two doses at same strength). For changes from IM Trinza to oral or to IM Sustenna, see labeling. Doses are expressed as amount of paliperidone palmitate rather than as paliperidone. Avoid using with a strong inducer of CYP3A4 and/or P-glycoprotein.

TABLE 8. Long-acting injectable antipsychotic medications: dosing *(continued)*

	Trade name	Dose conversions	Initial dose (mg)	Typical dose (mg)	Maximum dose (mg)	Dosing frequency	Need for initial oral supplementation	Comments
Second-generation antipsychotics *(continued)*								
Risperidone	Risperdal Consta	Oral risperidone to Risperdal Consta IM: ≤3 mg/day, give 25 mg/2 weeks >3 to ≤5 mg/day, give 37.5 mg/ 2 weeks >5 mg/day, give 50 mg/2 weeks	25 every 2 weeks	25–50 every 2 weeks	50 every 2 weeks	2 weeks	Continue oral for 3 weeks (21 days)	Upward dose adjustment should not be made more frequently than every 4 weeks.
Risperidone	Perseris	Oral risperidone to subcutaneous risperidone extended release: 3 mg/day, give 90 mg/month 4 mg/day, give 120 mg/month	Determined by oral dose	90–120 monthly	120/month	Monthly	Neither a loading dose nor oral overlap is needed	May not be appropriate for patients taking less than 3 mg or more than 4 mg of oral risperidone daily. Adjust dose with concomitant CYP2D6 inhibitors or CYP3A4 inducers.

Abbreviations. CYP=cytochrome P450; LAI=long-acting injectable.

Source. Abilify Maintena 2018; Aristada 2019; Aristada Initio 2019; Bai et al. 2007; Hamann et al. 1990; Invega Sustenna 2018a, 2018b; Invega Trinza 2018a, 2018b; Kreyenbuhl et al. 2010; Lexicomp 2019; Micromedex 2019; Nasser et al. 2016; Perseris 2018; Procyshyn et al. 2019; Risperdal Consta 2019; Zyprexa Relprevv 2018.

TABLE 9. Long-acting injectable antipsychotic medications: pharmacological characteristics

	Trade name	Time to peak plasma level	Time to steady state	Elimination half-life	Comments[a]
First-generation antipsychotics					
Fluphenazine	Prolixin Decanoate	8–10 hours	2 months	6–9 days for single injection and 14–26 days for multiple doses	Major CYP2D6 substrate
Haloperidol	Haldol Decanoate	6 days	3–4 months	21 days	Major CYP2D6 and CYP3A4 substrate
Second-generation antipsychotics					
Aripiprazole monohydrate	Abilify Maintena	4 days (deltoid); 5–7 days (gluteal)	By fourth dose	300 mg: 29.9 days 400 mg: 46.5 days (400 mg) with gluteal injection	Give no sooner than 26 days between injections. Major CYP2D6 and CYP3A4 substrate
Aripiprazole lauroxil	Aristada Initio	16–35 days (median 27 days)	Not applicable	15–18 days	Not interchangeable with Aristada because of differing pharmacokinetic profiles CYP2D6 and CYP3A4 substrate
Aripiprazole lauroxil	Aristada	Not available	4 months	53.9–57.2 days	Not interchangeable with Aristada Initio because of differing pharmacokinetic profiles CYP2D6 and CYP3A4 substrate
Olanzapine	Zyprexa Relprevv	7 days	~3 months	30 days	Major CYP1A2 substrate
Paliperidone palmitate	Invega Sustenna	13 days	2–3 months	25–49 days; increased in renal disease	CrCl 50–79 mL/minute: initiate at 156 mg on day 1, followed by 117 mg 1 week later, both administered in the deltoid muscle. Maintenance dose of 78 mg. Use not recommended in patients with CrCl <50 mL/minute. Substrate of P-glycoprotein/ABCB1
Paliperidone palmitate	Invega Trinza	30–33 days	Not applicable	84–95 days with deltoid injection; 118–139 days with gluteal injection; increased in renal disease	Do not use in patients with CrCl <50 mL/minute. Substrate of P-glycoprotein/ABCB1

TABLE 9. Long-acting injectable antipsychotic medications: pharmacological characteristics *(continued)*

	Trade name	Time to peak plasma level	Time to steady state	Elimination half-life	Comments[a]
Second-generation antipsychotics *(continued)*					
Risperidone	Risperdal Consta	29–31 days	2 months	3–6 days; increased in renal or hepatic disease	For renal/hepatic impairment: initiate with oral dosing (0.5 mg twice a day for 1 week, then 1 mg twice a day or 2 mg daily for 1 week); if tolerated, begin 25 mg IM every 2 weeks and continue oral dosing for 21 days. An initial IM dose of 12.5 mg may also be considered. Major substrate of CYP2D6 and minor substrate of CYP3A4 (minor) substrate; weak CYP2D6 inhibitor
Risperidone	Perseris	Two peaks: 4–6 hours and 10–14 days	2 months	9–11 days	For renal/hepatic impairment: use with caution with renal impairment; has not been studied. If oral risperidone is tolerated and effective at doses up to 3 mg/day, 90 mg/month can be considered. Major CYP2D6 substrate and minor CYP3A4 substrate; weak CYP2D6 inhibitor

[a]If a dose of a long-acting injectable antipsychotic medication is missed, refer to product labeling for information on adjustments to medication dose or administration frequency.

Abbreviations. CrCl=creatinine clearance; CYP=cytochrome P450.

Source. Abilify Maintena 2018; Aristada 2019; Aristada Initio 2019; Invega Sustenna 2018a, 2018b; Invega Trinza 2018a, 2018b; Jann et al. 1985; Lexicomp 2019; Lindenmayer 2010; Micromedex 2019; Perseris 2018; Procyshyn et al. 2019; Risperdal Consta 2019; Risperdal Consta 2019; Saklad 2018; Zyprexa Relprevv 2018.

Factors Influencing Choice of an Antipsychotic Medication

Available Drug Formulations

Medication choice may be influenced by available formulations of specific medications, such as oral concentrates or rapidly dissolving tablets for patients who have difficulty swallowing pills or who are ambivalent about medications and inconsistent in swallowing them. Use of ingestible sensors with associated monitoring technology may assist in evaluating ingestion, although the FDA notes that improvements in adherence have not yet been shown (U.S. Food and Drug Administration 2017). LAI formulations may be preferred by some patients (Heres et al. 2007; Patel et al. 2009; Walburn et al. 2001) and may be particularly useful for patients with a history of poor or uncertain adherence (see Statement 10). Short-acting parenteral formulations of antipsychotic agents are available for short-term use in individuals who are unable to take oral medications or for emergency administration in acutely agitated patients.

Drug-Drug Interactions and Metabolism

Careful attention must be paid to the potential for interactions of antipsychotic agents with other prescribed medications. For example, when multiple medications are prescribed, side effects (e.g., sedation, anticholinergic effects) can be additive. In addition, drug interactions can influence the amount of free drug in the blood that is available to act at receptors. Because most antipsychotic medications are highly bound to plasma proteins, the addition of other protein-bound medications will displace drug molecules from proteins, resulting in a greater proportion of unbound drug in the blood. Another common cause of drug-drug interactions relates to interactions at metabolic enzymes such as cytochrome P450 (CYP) enzymes, UDP-glucuronosyltransferases, and flavin-containing monooxygenases (Ouzzine et al. 2014; Phillips and Shephard 2017; Rowland et al. 2013; Zanger and Schwab 2013). In particular, hepatic metabolism of antipsychotic medications via CYP enzymes has been widely studied (see Lexicomp 2019; Micromedex 2019). Medications may compete with each other for the same CYP enzyme, or they may induce or inhibit the activity of CYP enzymes, altering levels of drugs that are metabolized through that route. For antipsychotic medications that have active metabolites, shifts in CYP enzyme activity can influence the relative amounts of the active metabolite. Consequently, when a patient is taking multiple medications, it is useful to check for possible drug-drug interactions using electronic drug interaction software (e.g., Web-based software, drug interaction checking embedded in electronic health record software).

In addition to drug-drug interactions, a number of other factors can influence CYP enzymes and thereby affect antipsychotic medication levels in blood. For example, smoking tobacco or marijuana induces CYP1A2, resulting in a corresponding reduction of levels of drugs that are metabolized through that enzyme, including clozapine and olanzapine (Anderson and Chan 2016; Kroon 2007; Scherf-Clavel et al. 2019). Conversely, with cessation of smoking (either intentionally or with admission to a smoke-free facility), there will be corresponding increases in the levels of drugs metabolized via CYP1A2. These shifts in blood levels can be quite significant and contribute to shifts in medication effectiveness or toxicity. Several of the main phytocannabinoids in marijuana (e.g., Δ^9-tetrahydrocannabinol, cannabidiol) are metabolized via CYP3A4, and cannabidiol may also inhibit CYP2C19 (Anderson and Chan 2016).

Furthermore, levels of antipsychotic medications, the relative proportions of active metabolites, and other pharmacokinetic properties such as medication or active metabolite half-life can be influenced by genetic differences in metabolic enzyme activity. Polymorphisms of CYP2D6 have been subjected to the most study (Eum et al. 2016; Zhou 2009), show substantial variation in their occurrence in the population by ethnicity (Bertilsson 2007; Gaedigk et al. 2017), and are likely to have the greatest potential for impact on antipsychotic medication metabolism. Polymorphisms of the ATP-binding cassette subfamily B member 1 (ABCB1) gene, which affects P-glycoprotein membrane transport, may influence brain concentrations of drugs, including antipsychotic agents (Moons et al. 2011). Although the applicability of gene polymorphism testing to the clinical choice of an antipsychotic medication is still being explored (Bousman and Dunlop 2018; Koopmans et al. 2018; Lagishetty et al. 2016), the FDA has incorporated testing for CYP2D6 polymorphisms into its labeling recommendations for dosing of pimozide on the basis of the increased risk of electrocardiographic changes in poor metabolizers at doses higher than 4 mg/day (0.05 mg/kg/day in children) (Rogers et al. 2012; U.S. Food and Drug Administration 2011b). In addition, product labeling for a number of other antipsychotic medications refers to a need for dose adjustments based on metabolizer status (U.S. Food and Drug Administration 2019). Additional information on the clinical pharmacogenomics of antipsychotic medications is available through the Clinical Pharmacogenetics Implementation Consortium (https://cpicpgx.org; Relling and Klein 2011), the Pharmacogene Variation Consortium (www.pharmvar.org; Gaedigk et al. 2018), and the Pharmacogenomics Knowledgebase (www.pharmgkb.org; Whirl-Carrillo et al. 2012).

Pharmacokinetic Properties

The absorption of some antipsychotic medications is affected by the presence of food in the stomach (see Statement 4, Tables 3 and 4). Some individuals may have difficulty in adhering to appropriate meal size or content, which could influence choice of these medications.

The half-life of an antipsychotic medication is another pharmacokinetic property that may be useful to consider in choosing among antipsychotic agents. Antipsychotic agents with a short half-life (see Statement 4, Tables 3 and 4) are more likely to require divided dosing in contrast to antipsychotic medications with a half-life that is closer to 24 hours. An oral antipsychotic medication with a longer half-life or an LAI may be preferable for patients who are prone to forget doses or who are intermittently nonadherent to treatment. Nevertheless, if an antipsychotic medication (or active metabolite) half-life is significantly longer than 24 hours, it is important to be aware that steady state may not be reached for some time. This can complicate interpreting the patient's response to adjustments in doses in terms of therapeutic benefits and side effects. Additional caution may be needed when an antipsychotic medication with a long half-life is chosen for older individuals, for an individual who is taking other medications that may affect drug metabolism, or for individuals with renal or hepatic impairment.

Older individuals often exhibit additional physiological changes relative to younger persons, including a reduced cardiac output (and concomitant reduction in renal and hepatic blood flow), reduced glomerular filtration rate, possible reduction in hepatic metabolism, and increased fat content. These changes may alter the absorption, distribution, metabolism, and excretion of medications and may also result in prolonged drug effects and greater sensitivity to medications, in terms of both therapeutic response and side effects (Kaiser 2015).

Side-Effect Profile

The side-effect profile of an antipsychotic agent is a significant factor in the choice of a specific medication (see Statement 4, Table 6). Often, a patient will express concerns about a particular side effect of medication (e.g., weight gain). A specific side effect (e.g., akathisia, weight gain, sedation, orthostatic hypotension, sexual dysfunction) may also have limited a patient's treatment adherence or ability to function in the past. If a patient has a concomitant physical condition (e.g., diabetes, cardiac conduction abnormalities, a seizure disorder), choice of medication will need to consider the likelihood of exacerbating an existing health condition. Older individuals may be more sensitive to some medication side effects, such as tardive dyskinesia, orthostatic hypotension, or anticholinergic effects of medications. Thus, a medication that has a lower likelihood of these side effects might be preferred. In contrast, there may be circumstances in which a medication side effect may be helpful. For example, in a patient who is not sleeping well, a more sedating antipsychotic might be chosen and administered at bedtime. Regardless of the initial side effect–related considerations in the choice of an antipsychotic medication, it is important to continue to monitor for side effects as treatment proceeds and to have additional discussions with the patient about side effects as they relate to treatment preferences.

Initiation of Treatment With an Antipsychotic Medication

The initial goal of acute treatment with an antipsychotic medication is to reduce acute symptoms, with the aim of returning the individual to his or her baseline level of functioning. Later, maintenance treatment will aim to prevent recurrence of symptoms and maximize functioning and quality of life.

The initial dose of medication will depend on such factors as the medication formulation, the characteristics of the patient, and whether a prior trial of antipsychotic medication has occurred. With the exception of clozapine, the dose of most antipsychotic medications can be increased relatively quickly to a typical therapeutic dose once an initial dose has been tolerated. For patients who have previously been treated with an oral or LAI antipsychotic medication, more rapid resumption of an effective medication dose is often appropriate. Although as-needed or emergency administration of antipsychotic medication may, at times, be useful in individuals with acute agitation, it can also reduce tolerability and contribute to a perception that premature dose increases are needed.

Younger individuals who are experiencing a first episode of psychosis may be more likely to gain weight or develop adverse metabolic effects of antipsychotic medications (Correll et al. 2014; Jensen et al. 2019). This can influence selection of an initial medication. In such individuals, a lower initial medication dose may help in minimizing acute side effects of antipsychotic medication and may improve a patient's willingness to continue with treatment (Czobor et al. 2015; Gaebel et al. 2010). Because a first episode of psychosis may respond more rapidly and may require a lower medication dose than later episodes do, use of a lower initial medication dose is also reasonable (Takeuchi et al. 2019). In older individuals, particularly those with concomitant physical health issues who are receiving multiple medications, recommended starting doses of medication are one-quarter to one-half of the usual adult starting dose on the basis of pharmacokinetic considerations (Howard et al. 2000).

Determining the optimal dose of antipsychotic medication during acute treatment is complicated by the fact that there is usually a delay between initiation of treatment and full therapeutic response. Patients may take between 2 and 4 weeks to show an initial response and longer periods of time to show full or optimal response. Once a therapeutic dose of the antipsychotic medication is reached, overly rapid or premature escalation of medication doses can affect tolerability. Premature dose increases can also create the false impression of enhanced efficacy due to a higher dose when the observed response is actually related to elapsed time at a steady state level of medication. Available evidence suggests that patients who have not exhibited at least a 20% reduction in symptoms (or minimal improvement) by about 2 weeks on a therapeutic dose are unlikely to be much improved at 4–6 weeks as reflected by at least a 50% reduction in symptoms (Samara et al. 2015). Consequently, monitoring of the patient's clinical status for 2–4 weeks is warranted on a therapeutic dose unless the patient is having uncomfortable side effects.

Initiation of treatment with clozapine is a notable exception to this general approach because it requires a slow dose titration to minimize the risks of seizure, orthostatic hypotension, and excessive sedation (Clozaril 2019). Large, rapid increases in clozapine dosage have led to cardiovascular collapse and death, particularly in patients taking respiratory depressant medications such as benzodiazepines. From a starting dose of 12.5 mg once or twice daily, the daily clozapine dosage can be increased by, at most, 25–50 mg/day to a target dose of 300–450 mg/day (Clozaril 2019). Subsequent dose increases, if needed, should be of 100 mg or less, once or twice weekly. A slower rate of titration may be needed for patients with an initial episode of schizophrenia and in those who are older, severely debilitated, or sensitive to side effects. Those with a preexisting central nervous system condition, including individuals with 22q11.2 deletion syndrome, also warrant a slower rate of titration and may have an increased risk of seizures at usual doses. Use of divided doses can be helpful in reducing side effects during initial dose titration, although many patients are ultimately treated with a single dose at bedtime to minimize daytime sedation and facilitate adherence (Takeuchi et al. 2016). Although efficacy is often seen at a dosage of 300–450 mg/day, some individuals may need higher dosages of clozapine, to a maximum daily dose of 900 mg, for full response. Blood levels of clozapine can be helpful to obtain if making adjustments to clozapine doses (see Statement 7).

With clozapine, safety monitoring during treatment is important in order to minimize the risk of adverse events. The U.S. Clozapine Risk Evaluation and Mitigation Strategy (REMS) Program (www.clozapinerems.com)[1] includes required training that must be completed by prescribers (Clozapine REMS Program 2019a), resource materials (Clozapine REMS Program 2019b), and a shared patient registry for all clozapine manufacturers' products that permits tracking of absolute neutrophil counts (ANCs) and documentation of decisions about continued treatment. The Clozapine REMS site provides instructions about threshold values for ANCs in hematologically normal individuals and in those with benign ethnic neutropenia, which is most common in individuals of African descent and is associated with normal ANCs that are lower than standard reference ranges (Clozapine REMS Program 2014). The site also describes the required frequencies for ANC monitoring, which vary with ANC values. Because the highest risk of severe neutropenia (ANC<500/μL) occurs within the initial 6 months of clozapine treatment (Alvir et al. 1993; Clozapine REMS Program 2019c; Myles et al. 2018), the frequency of ANC monitoring is also reduced with longer treatment duration. In patients who have stopped or interrupted treatment with clozapine for 30 days or more, the initial dose titration for clozapine and the monitoring frequency for treatment initiation should be followed.

With clozapine as well as with other antipsychotic medications, some common early side effects such as sedation, postural hypotension, or nausea may improve or resolve after the first several days or weeks of treatment, and patients can be encouraged to tolerate or temporarily manage these short-term effects. Other side effects, notably parkinsonism and akathisia, are likely to persist with long-term treatment, and additional approaches to management may be needed (see Statements 12 and 13).

If treatment with an LAI antipsychotic medication is planned, a trial of the oral formulation of the same medication is usually given to assure tolerability. The conversion from an oral dose of medication to a corresponding dose of an LAI antipsychotic depends on the specific medication (Meyer 2017), and product labeling for each medication describes approximate conversion ratios and whether a period of concomitant oral and LAI medication is needed.

Strategies to Address Initial Nonresponse or Partial Response to Antipsychotic Treatment

If a patient is showing response within several weeks of treatment initiation, continuing with the same medication and monitoring for continued improvement is appropriate. However, if there is no significant improvement after several weeks of treatment (e.g., <20% improvement in symptoms) or if improvement plateaus before substantial improvement is achieved (e.g., >50% improvement in symptoms, minimal impairment in functioning), it is important to consider whether factors are present that are influencing treatment response. Such factors may include concomitant substance use, rapid medication metabolism, poor medication absorption, interactions with other medications, and other effects on drug metabolism (e.g., smoking) that could affect blood levels of medication.

Difficulties with adherence are a common contributor to reduced response. (For a detailed discussion of adherence, see Statement 3.) When adherence is poor or uncertain, use of an LAI formulation of an antipsychotic may improve adherence as well as response. Determination of the blood concentration of the drug may also be helpful if the patient is being treated with a medication (e.g., clozapine) for which blood level has some correlation with clinical response. For other antipsychotic medications, a blood level can help to determine if poor adherence or subtherapeutic levels may be contributing to poor response (Bishara et al. 2013; de Oliveira et al. 1996; Hiemke et al. 2004; Lopez and Kane 2013; McCutcheon et al. 2018; Melkote et al. 2018; Sparshatt et al. 2010; Uchida et al. 2011b; Van Putten et al. 1991). Depending on the patient's symptoms, the possibility of another concomitant disorder should be considered. For example, in a patient with negative symptoms, an untreated major depressive disorder may also be present.

---

[1]For Canadian prescribers, use the appropriate Canadian clozapine registry, not the U.S. Clozapine REMS Program.

If no factors that would affect treatment response have been identified, raising the dose for a finite period, such as 2–4 weeks, can be tried. Although the incremental efficacy of higher doses has not been established (Samara et al. 2018), some patients may show benefit if they are able to tolerate a higher dose of antipsychotic medication without significant side effects. If dose adjustment does not result in an adequate response, a different antipsychotic medication should be considered. Tables 5 and 6 in Statement 4 can be consulted to identify antipsychotic medications with other receptor binding profiles or different side effects. Because each patient responds differently to antipsychotic medications in terms of therapeutic effects and side effects, adequate trials of multiple antipsychotic medications may be needed before antipsychotic treatment is optimized, and it can be helpful to advise patients of this possibility.

If a patient has had minimal or no response to two trials of antipsychotic medication of 2–4 weeks' duration at an adequate dose (Howes et al. 2017; Samara et al. 2015), a trial of clozapine is recommended (see Statement 7). A trial of clozapine is also recommended for a patient with a persistent risk of suicide that has not responded to other treatments and is suggested for a patient with a persistent risk of aggressive behavior that has not responded to other treatments (see Statements 8 and 9). A trial of clozapine may also be appropriate in individuals who show a response to treatment (i.e., have more than a 20% reduction in symptoms) yet still have significant symptoms or impairments in functioning (Howes et al. 2017). In fact, clozapine is often underused (Carruthers et al. 2016; Latimer et al. 2013; Olfson et al. 2016; Stroup et al. 2014; Tang et al. 2017), and many patients would benefit from earlier consideration of clozapine initiation.

For individuals with treatment-resistant schizophrenia who are unable to tolerate clozapine or are not interested in pursuing a trial of clozapine, the limited available evidence suggests no benefit from high doses of antipsychotic medication, and treatment-related side effects are likely to be increased (Dold et al. 2015). However, a trial of a different antipsychotic medication may be helpful, particularly if there is no response or only a partial response to the most recently used medication.

Augmentation treatment can also be considered, although a trial of clozapine should not be delayed by multiple attempts at augmentation therapy. Particularly for patients with negative symptoms or depression, augmentation of antipsychotic therapy with an antidepressant medication may also be helpful (Helfer et al. 2016; Stroup et al. 2019). Use of a benzodiazepine, such as lorazepam, is also suggested in patients who exhibit catatonia (Bush et al. 1996b; Fink 2013; Pelzer et al. 2018; Unal et al. 2017). Other augmentation approaches (e.g., antipsychotics, anticonvulsants, benzodiazepines, lithium) have also been studied, although evidence is mixed and primarily from small, short-term open-label studies (Correll et al. 2017b; Galling et al. 2017; Ortiz-Orendain et al. 2017). For combination therapy with two antipsychotic medications, data from a large nationwide cohort study suggest that emergency visits and rehospitalization rates may be reduced in individuals receiving polypharmacy as compared with monotherapy (Tiihonen et al. 2019). In addition, there is no evidence that combining drugs is any more harmful than using a single medication, beyond the common side effects from each drug. Nevertheless, if multiple drugs are used, monitoring for benefits and side effects is important, and it is preferable to limit changes in dose to one drug at a time. In addition, if a patient experiences an exacerbation of symptoms while on a stable dose of medication, a reconsideration of the treatment plan is warranted rather than simply adding medications to the existing regimen.

Monitoring During Treatment With an Antipsychotic Medication

During treatment with an antipsychotic medication, it is important to monitor medication adherence, therapeutic benefits of treatment, and treatment-related side effects. The patient's clinical status can also be affected by changes in physical health, adjustments to other psychotropic and nonpsychotropic medications, and other factors, such as cessation or resumption of smoking.

Adherence to antipsychotic treatment is a common problem that affects treatment outcomes. There are many barriers to treatment adherence as well as facilitators and motivators of adherence, each of which will differ for an individual patient (Hatch et al. 2017; Kane et al. 2013; Pyne et al. 2014). Thus, it is important to take a patient-centered approach in inquiring in a nonjudgmental way whether the individual has experienced difficulties with taking medication since the last visit. (For a detailed discussion of factors related to adherence, see Statement 3.)

Monitoring of treatment response is also essential for identifying whether there are reductions in the severity of functional impairments or target symptoms, including positive symptoms, negative symptoms, and other symptoms that are a focus of treatment. Use of a quantitative measure (see Statement 2) can assist in determining whether the antipsychotic medication is producing therapeutic benefits, including reductions in symptom severity and improvements in functioning. If a lack of response or a partial response is noted, additional assessment will be needed to identify and address possible contributors as described in the subsection "Strategies to Address Initial Nonresponse or Partial Response to Antipsychotic Treatment." If an antipsychotic medication dose is being decreased, monitoring can help detect a return of symptoms prior to a more serious relapse.

Monitoring for the presence of side effects is also important throughout the course of antipsychotic treatment. Some side effects (e.g., sedation, nausea) are prominent with treatment initiation but dissipate, at least to some extent, with continued treatment. Other side effects (e.g., hypotension, akathisia) may be present initially and increase in severity with titration of the medication dose. Still other side effects emerge only after longer periods of treatment (e.g., tardive dyskinesia) or become more noticeable to patients as their acute symptoms are better controlled (e.g., sexual dysfunction). Table 2 in Statement 1 gives suggestions for baseline assessments and monitoring frequencies for some side effects, clinical measurements, and laboratory studies. Specific attention may need to be given to clinical workflow to assure that indicated monitoring is conducted because rates of follow-up testing and screening for metabolic side effects of treatment appear to be low (Morrato et al. 2009). Patients should also be asked about other common side effects of antipsychotic medications, which may vary with the specific medication that is prescribed (see Statement 4, Table 6).

Use of rating scales can help assure that patients are asked about side effects in a systematic fashion. Although the clinician-rated Udvalg for Kliniske Undersogelser (UKU) Side Effect Rating Scale (Lingjaerde et al. 1987) is often used to assess side effects of antipsychotic medications in clinical trials (van Strien et al. 2015), it can be time-consuming to administer. However, a self-rated version of the UKU Side Effect Rating Scale (Lindström et al. 2001) is also available (http://scnp.org/fileadmin/SCNP/SCNP/UKU/UKU-Pat-%20English%20.pdf). Another self-rating scale, the Glasgow Antipsychotic Side-effect Scale, has two versions: one for use in patients treated with clozapine (www.sussexpartnership.nhs.uk/sites/default/files/documents/gass_for_clozapine.pdf) (Hynes et al. 2015) and one for patients treated with other antipsychotic medications (www.southernhealth.nhs.uk/_resources/assets/inline/full/0/38222.pdf) (Waddell and Taylor 2008). Other rating scales are aimed at identifying and assessing the severity of a specific type of side effect. For example, the clinician-administered Abnormal Involuntary Movement Scale (AIMS; www.aacap.org/App_Themes/AACAP/docs/member_resources/toolbox_for_clinical_practice_and_outcomes/monitoring/AIMS.pdf) (Guy 1976) or the Dyskinesia Identification System: Condensed User Scale (DISCUS; https://portal.ct.gov/-/media/DDS/Health/hcsma20002b.pdf) (Kalachnik and Sprague 1993) can complement clinical assessment in identifying and monitoring tardive dyskinesia and other abnormal movements. Another example, the self-rated Changes in Sexual Functioning Questionnaire (www.dbsalliance.org/wp-content/uploads/2019/02/Restoring_Intimacy_CSFQ_Handout.pdf) (Clayton et al. 1997a, 1997b; Depression and Bipolar Support Alliance 2019; Keller et al. 2006), can help to identify sexual side effects of antipsychotic treatment, which is an issue that patients may find difficult to discuss yet can lead them to discontinue treatment.

Treatment-Emergent Side Effects of Antipsychotic Medications

As with most medications, antipsychotic medications have been associated with a number of side effects that can develop as treatment proceeds. Table 6 in Statement 4 shows the relative tendencies for antipsychotic medications to be associated with specific side effects. In addition, each of these side effects is described in further detail below.

Early in the course of treatment, common side effects include sedation; orthostatic changes in blood pressure; and anticholinergic side effects such as dry mouth, constipation, and difficulty with urination.

Of the side effects related to dopamine D_2 receptor antagonist effects of antipsychotics, acute dystonia also appears early in treatment. It is particularly common with high-potency antipsychotic medications (e.g., haloperidol, fluphenazine) and can be life-threatening if associated with laryngospasm. Neuroleptic malignant syndrome (NMS) can also be life-threatening because of associated hyperthermia and autonomic instability. It typically occurs within the first month of antipsychotic treatment, with resumption of treatment, or with an increase in the dose of antipsychotic medication. Akathisia and medication-induced parkinsonism can also occur in the initial weeks of treatment or after increases in medication doses. Hyperprolactinemia, related to D_2 receptor antagonism in the hypothalamic-pituitary axis, can lead to breast enlargement, galactorrhea, sexual dysfunction, and, in women, menstrual disturbances. These elevations in prolactin also occur in the initial weeks to months of treatment. On the other hand, tardive syndromes, including tardive dyskinesia, develop later, often months or even years after treatment initiation.

Side effects related to metabolic syndrome are common. Generally, they are observed in the initial months of treatment, but they can also occur later in treatment. These side effects include weight gain; hyperlipidemia; and glucose dysregulation, including development of diabetes mellitus.

Clozapine treatment is associated with a number of side effects that are less commonly seen with other antipsychotic medications. Severe neutropenia is most often seen early in treatment and is potentially life-threatening; however, with current regulatory requirements for monitoring ANC levels during treatment, it is rare. When seizures occur with clozapine, it is typically with very high doses or blood levels of clozapine, rapid increases in clozapine dose, or shifts in medication levels (related to drug-drug interactions or effects of smoking on drug metabolism). Myocarditis is infrequent and generally occurs early in treatment. Cardiomyopathy is rare and generally occurs later in the treatment course. Gastrointestinal effects of clozapine can also be significant, and in some patients it is associated with fecal impaction or paralytic ileus. Sialorrhea and tachycardia are each commonly observed during treatment with clozapine but can generally be managed conservatively.

Allergic and Dermatological Side Effects

Cutaneous allergic reactions occur infrequently with antipsychotic medications, but hypersensitivity can manifest as maculopapular erythematous rashes, typically of the trunk, face, neck, and extremities. Medication discontinuation or administration of an antihistamine is usually effective in reversing these symptoms.

In terms of other dermatological side effects, on rare occasions, thioridazine treatment is noted to be associated with hyperpigmentation of the skin. Dermatological reactions, including hyperpigmentation and cutaneous reactions, have also been reported with risperidone, clozapine, olanzapine, quetiapine, and haloperidol (Bliss and Warnock 2013). Photosensitivity reactions, resulting in severe sunburn, are also most commonly observed with low-potency phenothiazine medications. A blue-gray discoloration of the skin in body areas exposed to sunlight has been reported in patients receiving long-term chlorpromazine treatment. Consequently, patients who are taking these medications should be instructed to avoid excessive sunlight and use sunscreen.

Cardiovascular Effects

Hyperlipidemia

There is some evidence that certain antipsychotic medications, particularly clozapine and olanzapine, may increase the risk for hyperlipidemias (Buhagiar and Jabbar 2019; Bushe and Paton 2005; Meyer and Koro 2004; Mitchell et al. 2013a). However, there is also a suggestion that some patients may have a dyslipidemia prior to starting on antipsychotic treatment (Misiak et al. 2017; Pillinger et al. 2017b; Yan et al. 2013). Some patients develop an elevation of triglyceride levels in association with antipsychotic treatment that rarely is sufficiently high as to be associated with development of pancreatitis (Alastal et al. 2016). It is unclear whether triglyceridemia with antipsychotic treatment is a direct result of the medication or an indirect result of increased triglycerides in the blood with concomitant diabetes (Yan et al. 2013). In any patient with hyperlipidemia, it is also important to assess for other contributors to metabolic syndrome (Mitchell et al. 2012, 2013b) and ensure that the patient is receiving treatment with a lipid-lowering agent, as clinically indicated.

Myocarditis and Cardiomyopathy

Myocarditis and cardiomyopathy have been reported in some patients treated with clozapine and have resulted in death in some individuals. The etiology of these cardiac effects is unclear, although an immune-mediated mechanism has been suggested (Røge et al. 2012). For myocarditis, the reported incidence has varied from 0.015% to 8.5% (Bellissima et al. 2018). For reasons that are unclear, the highest rates have been reported in Australia (Ronaldson et al. 2015); rates elsewhere appear to be much lower. For example, an early study using the U.S. Clozaril National Registry found 17 confirmed cases of myocarditis in a total of 189,405 individuals who had received clozapine (La Grenade et al. 2001). A recent national registry study of outpatients in Denmark found 1 of 3,262 (0.03%) clozapine-treated patients developed myocarditis in the initial 2 months of treatment (Rohde et al. 2018). These authors estimated that a maximum of 0.28% of patients treated with clozapine would experience fatality due to clozapine-associated myocarditis, which is comparable to rates of cardiac adverse effects with other antipsychotic medications. For cardiomyopathy, the reported incidence is even less clear but appears to be considerably lower than rates of clozapine-associated myocarditis (Higgins et al. 2019; Khan et al. 2017; Rohde et al. 2018; Ronaldson et al. 2015).

Although cardiomyopathy has been reported throughout the course of clozapine treatment, the onset of myocarditis typically occurs during the first month of treatment and is heralded by shortness of breath, tachycardia, and fever (Bellissima et al. 2018; Ronaldson et al. 2015). Other features can include fatigue, chest pain, palpitations, and peripheral edema. Diagnosis can be challenging because of the nonspecific nature of these symptoms. For example, primary tachycardia is common with clozapine treatment without signifying underlying cardiac disease. Fever can also occur with clozapine initiation yet often resolves quickly and without evidence of myocarditis (Bruno et al. 2015; Lowe et al. 2007; Pui-yin Chung et al. 2008).

Recommendations for monitoring have varied, but there is no evidence or consensus that preemptive screening is necessary or helpful. However, if myocarditis or cardiomyopathy is suspected, a recent systematic review suggests seeking cardiology consultation as well as monitoring C-reactive protein and troponin (I and T subtypes) and obtaining an electrocardiogram as indicated (Knoph et al. 2018). Cardiac magnetic resonance imaging may also be indicated in some individuals.

In patients who do develop myocarditis or cardiomyopathy in conjunction with clozapine treatment, clozapine is typically discontinued. Subsequent decisions about resuming clozapine are individualized and should be based on the benefits and risks of treatment as compared with other therapeutic alternatives.

Orthostatic Hypotension

Orthostatic hypotension, a drop in blood pressure when changing from lying down or sitting to standing, is dose-related and due to the α-receptor-blocking effects of antipsychotic medications. When severe, orthostatic hypotension can cause syncope, dizziness, or falls. Older or severely debilitated patients, patients in the dose-titration phase of clozapine therapy, and patients with peripheral vascular disease or a compromised cardiovascular status may be at particular risk. Patients who experience orthostatic hypotension must be cautioned to sit on the edge of the bed for a minute before standing up, to move slowly when going from lying down or sitting to standing, and to seek assistance when needed. Management strategies for orthostatic hypotension include using supportive measures (e.g., use of support stockings, increased dietary salt and fluid intake); reducing the speed of antipsychotic dose titration; decreasing or dividing doses of antipsychotic medication; switching to an antipsychotic medication without antiadrenergic effects; and, as a last resort, administration of the salt/fluid-retaining corticosteroid fludrocortisone to increase intravascular volume (Mar and Raj 2018; Shen et al. 2017). For patients who are receiving concomitant antihypertensive treatment, adjustments to the dose of these medications may be needed.

QTc Prolongation

The QT interval on the electrocardiogram reflects the length of time required for ventricular repolarization and varies with heart rate (Funk et al. 2018). Several approaches exist for calculating a QT interval corrected for heart rate (QTc). Although the Bazett formula remains the one most widely used for drug monitoring and research, alternative correction formulas, such as the Fridericia and Framingham formulas, have been shown to most accurately correct for rate and improve prediction of mortality. In order to accurately predict risk, clinicians should be familiar with an alternative correction formula (Aytemir et al. 1999; Rautaharju et al. 2009; Vandenberk et al. 2016). Significant prolongation of the QTc interval is associated with increased risk for a ventricular tachyarrhythmia, torsades de pointes (TdP), which can lead to life-threatening consequences (e.g., ventricular fibrillation, sudden death). When the QTc interval is prolonged, a decision about the antipsychotic medication choice or changes requires a comprehensive risk-benefit assessment. A QTc interval >500 msec is sometimes viewed as a threshold for concern; however, "there is no absolute QTc interval at which a psychotropic should not be used" (Funk et al. 2018, p. 2).

Studies that have examined the risks of QTc prolongation with antipsychotic treatment have varied in study quality, sample sizes, and the physical health of study subjects. Sources are available that categorize medications on the basis of their level of risk for QTc prolongation and TdP (Woosley et al. 2009), but the quality of data that informs such categorizations is also variable (Funk et al. 2018). Nevertheless, among the FGAs, chlorpromazine, droperidol, thioridazine, and pimozide appear to be associated with the greatest risk of QTc prolongation. The FDA recommends that thioridazine be used only when patients have not had a clinically acceptable response to other available antipsychotics (U.S. National Library of Medicine 2018b). Pimozide labeling also includes specific instructions related to medication dosing and QTc interval prolongation (U.S. National Library of Medicine 2018a). Orally administered haloperidol has been associated with only a mild increase in QTc interval length in healthy individuals; however, the risk of QTc interval prolongation and TdP appears to be greater with intravenous administration in medically ill individuals (Funk et al. 2018). Most SGAs have also been associated with some QTc interval prolongation, with ziprasidone and iloperidone appearing to have the greatest likelihood of QTc prolongation. The FDA has required that a warning about QTc prolongation be included with product labeling for ziprasidone (Geodon 2018), quetiapine (Quetiapine 2011; Seroquel XR 2019), iloperidone (Fanapt 2017), and paliperidone (Invega 2018, 2019; Invega Sustenna 2018a, 2018b; Invega Trinza 2018a, 2018b).

Factors to consider when making a determination about selecting or changing antipsychotic medications include whether the patient is taking other medications that are known to prolong QTc intervals; whether the patient has factors that would influence drug metabolism, leading to higher blood levels of a drug (e.g., poor metabolizer status, pharmacokinetic drug-drug interactions, hepatic or renal disease, drug toxicity); whether the patient is known to have a significant cardiac risk factor (e.g., congenital long QT syndrome, structural or functional cardiac disease, bradycardia, family history of sudden cardiac death); and other factors associated with an increased risk of TdP (e.g., female sex; advanced age; personal history of drug-induced QTc prolongation; severe acute illness; starvation; risk or presence of hypokalemia, hypomagnesemia, or hypocalcemia) (Funk et al. 2018). For individuals with these risk factors, antipsychotic medications with a regulatory warning or those with a known risk of QTc prolongation are not recommended for use if safer medication alternatives are available. Input from cardiology consultants should be considered when significant cardiac disease or other risk factors for QTc prolongation are present, although routine cardiology consultation is not indicated for patients without cardiac risk factors (Funk et al. 2018).

Tachycardia

Tachycardia can be primary (e.g., with clozapine), a reflex response to orthostatic hypotension, or a result of anticholinergic effects. It appears to be particularly common in individuals who are treated with clozapine (Lally et al. 2016a), but it may also be seen in individuals treated with other antipsychotic medications, particularly low-potency phenothiazines. Although healthy patients may be able to tolerate some increase in resting pulse rate, this may not be the case for patients with preexisting heart disease. In patients with significant tachycardia (heart rates above 110–120 bpm), ECG is warranted, as is an assessment for other potential causes of tachycardia (e.g., fever, anemia, smoking, hyperthyroidism, respiratory disease, cardiovascular disorders, caffeine and other stimulants, side effects of other medications). Early in treatment with clozapine, the possibility of myocarditis should be considered. Management strategies for tachycardia with antipsychotic medications include reducing the dose of medication, discontinuing medications with anticholinergic or stimulant properties, and using the strategies described above to reduce any contributing orthostatic hypotension. Case reports have discussed the use of medications such as β-blocking agents for persistent and significant tachycardia with clozapine. Nevertheless, treatment is not indicated unless the patient is symptomatic or the patient's heart rate is substantially greater than 120 bpm because data from more rigorous studies are not available and these medications can contribute to other side effects, such as orthostatic hypotension (Lally et al. 2016a). If tachycardia is accompanied by pain, shortness of breath, fever, or signs of a myocardial infarction or heart rhythm problem, emergency assessment is essential.

Endocrine Side Effects

Glucose Dysregulation and Diabetes Mellitus

Evidence from meta-analyses of RCTs, population-based studies, and case-control studies suggests that some antipsychotic medications, clozapine and olanzapine in particular, are associated with an increased risk of hyperglycemia and diabetes (Hirsch et al. 2017; Ward and Druss 2015; Whicher et al. 2018; Zhang et al. 2017). Complicating the evaluation of antipsychotic-related risk of diabetes is that some patients with first-episode psychosis seem to have abnormal glucose regulation that precedes antipsychotic treatment (Greenhalgh et al. 2017; Perry et al. 2016; Pillinger et al. 2017a). In addition, obesity and treatment-related weight gain may contribute to diabetes risk. Nevertheless, there are some patients without other known risk factors who develop insulin resistance early in the course of antipsychotic treatment. In some individuals, diabetic ketoacidosis and nonketotic hyperosmolar coma have been reported in the absence of a known diagnosis of diabetes (Guenette et al. 2013; Kato et al. 2015; Liao and Phan 2014; Polcwiartek et al. 2016; Vuk et al. 2017). Given the rare occurrence of extreme hyperglycemia, ketoacidosis, hyperosmolar coma, or death and the suggestion from epidemiological studies of an increased risk of treatment-emergent adverse events with SGAs, the FDA has requested that all manufacturers of SGA medications include a warning in their product labeling regarding hyperglycemia and diabetes mellitus (Rostack 2003). When individuals with schizophrenia do develop diabetes, management principles should follow current guidelines for any patient with diabetes (Holt and Mitchell 2015; Scott et al. 2012). Given the existence of frequent health disparities for individuals with serious mental illness (Mangurian et al. 2016; Scott et al. 2012), clinicians can also help in ensuring that patients are obtaining appropriate diabetes care and encourage patients to engage in lifestyle interventions to improve diabetes self-management (Cimo et al. 2012). In any patient with diabetes, it is also important to assess for other contributors to metabolic syndrome (Mitchell et al. 2012, 2013b).

Hyperprolactinemia

Prolactin elevation is frequent in patients treated with antipsychotics (Ajmal et al. 2014; Cookson et al. 2012; Kinon et al. 2003; Lally et al. 2017a; Leucht et al. 2013; Rubio-Abadal et al. 2016), which increase prolactin secretion by blocking the inhibitory actions of dopamine on lactotrophic cells in the anterior pituitary. Consequently, hyperprolactinemia is observed more frequently with the use of antipsychotics that are more potent at blocking dopamine receptors (Tsuboi et al. 2013).

In both men and women, prolactin-related disruption of the hypothalamic-pituitary-gonadal axis can lead to decreased sexual interest and impaired sexual function (Kirino 2017; Rubio-Abadal et al. 2016). Other effects of hyperprolactinemia may include breast tenderness, breast enlargement, and lactation (Ajmal et al. 2014; Cookson et al. 2012). Because prolactin also regulates gonadal function, hyperprolactinemia can lead to decreased production of gonadal hormones, including estrogen and testosterone, resulting in disruption or elimination of menstrual cycles in women. In addition, in lactating mothers, suppression of prolactin may be detrimental, and the potential for this effect should be considered.

The long-term clinical consequences of chronic elevation of prolactin are poorly understood. Chronic hypogonadal states may increase the risk of osteopenia/osteoporosis and fractures may be increased in individuals with schizophrenia, but a direct link to antipsychotic-induced hyperprolactinemia has not been established (Bolton et al. 2017; Stubbs et al. 2014, 2015; Tseng et al. 2015; Weaver et al. 2019). In addition, some concern has been expressed about potential effects of hyperprolactinemia on the risk of breast or endometrial cancer; however, the available evidence suggests that such risks, if they exist, are likely to be small (De Hert et al. 2016; Froes Brandao et al. 2016; Klil-Drori et al. 2017; Pottegård et al. 2018; Wang et al. 2002).

If a patient is experiencing clinical symptoms of prolactin elevation, the dose of antipsychotic medication may be reduced, or the medication regimen may be switched to an antipsychotic with less effect on prolactin such as one with partial agonist activity at dopamine receptors (Ajmal et al. 2014; Grigg et al. 2017; Yoon et al. 2016). Administration of a dopamine agonist such as bromocriptine may also be considered.

Sexual Function Disturbances

A majority of patients with schizophrenia report some difficulties with sexual function. Although multiple factors are likely to contribute and rates vary widely depending on the study, it is clear that antipsychotic treatment contributes to sexual dysfunction (de Boer et al. 2015; La Torre et al. 2013; Marques et al. 2012; Serretti and Chiesa 2011; van Dijk et al. 2018). Effects of antipsychotic agents on sexual function may be mediated directly via drug actions on adrenergic and serotonergic receptors or indirectly through effects on prolactin and gonadal hormones (Kirino 2017; Knegtering et al. 2008; Rubio-Abadal et al. 2016). Loss of libido and anorgasmia can occur in men and in women; erectile dysfunction and ejaculatory disturbances also occur in men (La Torre et al. 2013; Marques et al. 2012; Serretti and Chiesa 2011; van Dijk et al. 2018). Retrograde ejaculation has also been reported with specific antipsychotic medications (e.g., thioridazine, risperidone) (Chouinard et al. 1993; de Boer et al. 2015; Kotin et al. 1976). In addition, it is important to note that priapism can also occur in association with antipsychotic treatment, particularly in individuals with other underlying risk factors such as sickle cell disease (Burnett and Bivalacqua 2011; Sood et al. 2008).

Despite the high rates of occurrence of sexual dysfunction with antipsychotic medication, many patients will not spontaneously report such difficulties. Thus, it is important to ask patients specifically about these side effects. Structured rating scales also exist to assess sexual side effects during antipsychotic treatment, and these can be used to supplement information obtained via interview (Clayton et al. 1997a, 1997b; de Boer et al. 2014; Depression and Bipolar Support Alliance 2019; Keller et al. 2006). Education about sexual side effects of medication can also be provided to the patient to communicate that these symptoms may occur but can be addressed (de Boer et al. 2015).

When sexual side effects of antipsychotic therapy are of significant concern to the patient, a reduction in medication dose or change in medication may be considered in addition to an assessment of other potential contributing factors (e.g., hyperprolactinemia, other medications, psychological factors) (de Boer et al. 2015; La Torre et al. 2013). Priapism, if it occurs, requires urgent urological consultation.

Gastrointestinal Side Effects

The most common gastrointestinal side effects of antipsychotic medications are related to anticholinergic side effects and include dry mouth and constipation, as noted in the subsection "Treatment-Emergent Side Effects of Antipsychotic Medications." Patients and families should be educated about monitoring for constipation, and, if present, constipation should be reported promptly to clinicians. With clozapine in particular, gastrointestinal hypomotility can be severe and can result in fecal impaction or paralytic ileus (Every-Palmer and Ellis 2017; Leung et al. 2017; Palmer et al. 2008). Thus, if constipation is severe or does not resolve, the patient should obtain urgent medical care.

To prevent development of constipation in patients at increased risk (e.g., older patients, patients treated with clozapine), it is useful to minimize the doses and number of contributory medications such as other anticholinergic medications and opioids. A stool softener (e.g., docusate [Colace]) can be started. Activity and exercise should be encouraged to stimulate motility.

If constipation does develop, initial treatment can include stool softeners (e.g., docusate [Colace]) or osmotic laxatives (e.g., lactulose [Enulose], polyethylene glycol [Miralax], bisacodyl [Dulcolax]). Second-line treatments include stimulant laxatives (e.g., senna [Senokot], senna tea, cascara, sodium picosulfate). If constipation persists, an enema (e.g., Fleet) should be considered. A combination of treatments may be needed to treat constipation and then to prevent its recurrence.

Hepatic effects have also been reported with antipsychotic medications, including elevation of liver enzyme levels and cholestatic jaundice (U.S. Department of Health and Human Services and U.S. National Library of Medicine 2017b). Cholestatic jaundice is rare and has been reported primarily with chlorpromazine (U.S. Department of Health and Human Services and U.S. National Library of Medicine 2017a). It usually occurs within the first month after the initiation of treatment and generally requires discontinuation of treatment. However, given the relative infrequency of antipsychotic-induced jaundice, other etiologies for jaundice should be evaluated before the cause is judged to be antipsychotic medication.

Hematological Effects

Hematological effects are of greatest concern with clozapine; however, they have also been reported with other antipsychotic agents and may include inhibition of leukopoiesis, purpura, hemolytic anemia, and pancytopenia (Balon and Berchou 1986; Myles et al. 2019; Pisciotta 1969). For example, with chlorpromazine, transient benign leukopenia (white blood cell count <3,500/mm^3) is common, and severe neutropenia has been reported in 0.08% of patients, typically within the first few months of treatment (Pisciotta 1969).

There is no clear etiology of severe neutropenia or agranulocytosis with antipsychotic medications. With clozapine, a complex polygenic trait appears likely, perhaps involving the human leukocyte antigen locus or a group of hepatic transporter genes (de With et al. 2017; Legge et al. 2017). Initial estimates suggested that severe neutropenia would develop in 1%–2% of patients treated with clozapine, with fatal agranulocytosis in approximately 15% of those individuals (Alvir et al. 1993; Honigfeld et al. 1998). However, data from the initial 5 years of monitoring through clozapine registries showed a rate of severe neutropenia of 0.38%, with death occurring in only 3.1% of those cases (Honigfeld et al. 1998). A recent meta-analysis suggested an incidence of severe neutropenia in 0.9% of clozapine-treated patients, with a case fatality rate for individuals with severe neutropenia of 2.1% (Myles et al. 2018). For clozapine-treated patients as a group, the incidence of death due to severe neutropenia was 0.013% (Myles et al. 2018), suggesting that clozapine is quite safe with appropriate monitoring. Nevertheless, patients who are receiving clozapine should be advised to report any sign of infection (e.g., sore throat, fever, weakness, lethargy) immediately so that a decision can be made about obtaining additional evaluation.

If severe neutropenia does develop, it is usually reversible if clozapine is discontinued immediately and secondary complications (e.g., sepsis) are given intensive treatment. Granulocyte colony–

stimulating factor has been used to accelerate granulopoietic function and shorten recovery time (Lally et al. 2017c; Myles et al. 2017).

Although there have been reports of successful resumption of clozapine after severe neutropenia, the risk of recurrence remains high (Lally et al. 2017b; Manu et al. 2018). For patients with a good clinical response to clozapine after multiple unsuccessful trials of other antipsychotic medications, the benefits and risks of rechallenge require thorough consideration and discussion with the patient and involved family members. Under such circumstances, case reports have suggested using granulocyte colony–stimulating factor to reduce the risk of recurrence, although evidence is limited (Lally et al. 2017b).

Neurological Side Effects

Acute Dystonia

Medication-induced acute dystonia is defined in DSM-5 as

> [a]bnormal and prolonged contraction of the muscles of the eyes (oculogyric crisis), head, neck (torticollis or retrocollis), limbs, or trunk developing within a few days of starting or raising the dosage of a medication (such as a neuroleptic) or after reducing the dosage of a medication used to treat extrapyramidal symptoms. (American Psychiatric Association 2013a, p. 711)

A dystonic spasm of the axial muscles along the spinal cord can result in opisthotonos, in which the head, neck, and spinal column are hyperextended in an arched position. Rarely, acute dystonia can also present as life-threatening laryngospasm, which results in an inability to breathe (Ganesh et al. 2015; Koek and Pi 1989). Acute dystonia is sudden in onset and painful and can cause patients great distress. Because of the dramatic appearance of acute dystonia, health professionals who are unfamiliar with the condition may incorrectly attribute these reactions to catatonic signs or unusual behavior on the part of patients, and oculogyric crises can sometimes be misinterpreted as indicative of seizure activity.

In individuals treated with FGAs, it is estimated that up to 10% of patients may experience an acute dystonic episode, and with SGAs, rates of acute dystonia may be less than 2% (Martino et al. 2018; Miller et al. 2008; Satterthwaite et al. 2008). Additional factors that increase the risk of acute dystonia with antipsychotic medication include young age, male sex, ethnicity, recent cocaine use, high medication dose, and intramuscular route of medication administration (Gray and Pi 1998; Spina et al. 1993; van Harten et al. 1999). For further discussion of acute dystonia, including its treatment, see Statement 11.

Akathisia

Medication-induced acute akathisia is defined in DSM-5 as

> [s]ubjective complaints of restlessness, often accompanied by observed excessive movements (e.g., fidgety movements of the legs, rocking from foot to foot, pacing, inability to sit or stand still), developing within a few weeks of starting or raising the dosage of a medication (such as a neuroleptic) or after reducing the dosage of a medication used to treat extrapyramidal symptoms. (American Psychiatric Association 2013a, p. 711)

Akathisia is sometimes difficult to distinguish from psychomotor agitation associated with psychosis, leading to a cycle of increasing doses of antipsychotic medication that lead to further increases in akathisia. Even in mild forms in which the patient is able to control most movements, akathisia is often extremely distressing to patients and is a frequent cause of nonadherence with antipsychotic treatment. If allowed to persist, akathisia can contribute to feelings of dysphoria and, in some instances, suicidal behaviors. The reported rates of akathisia vary from 10%–15% to as many as one-third of patients treated with antipsychotic medication, even when SGAs are used (Juncal-Ruiz et al. 2017; Martino et al. 2018; Mentzel et al. 2017; Miller et al. 2008). For further discussion of akathisia, including its treatment, see Statement 13.

Parkinsonism

Medication-induced parkinsonism, which is termed neuroleptic-induced parkinsonism and other medication-induced parkinsonism in DSM-5, is defined as

> [p]arkinsonian tremor, muscular rigidity, akinesia (i.e., loss of movement or difficulty initiating movement), or bradykinesia (i.e., slowing movement) developing within a few weeks of starting or raising the dosage of a medication (e.g., a neuroleptic) or after reducing the dosage of a medication used to treat extrapyramidal symptoms. (American Psychiatric Association 2013a, p. 709)

These symptoms of medication-induced parkinsonism are dose-dependent and generally resolve with discontinuation of antipsychotic medication. It is important to appreciate that medication-induced parkinsonism can affect emotional and cognitive function, at times in the absence of detectable motor symptoms. As a result, it can be difficult to distinguish the negative symptoms of schizophrenia or concomitant depression from medication-induced parkinsonism. In addition, emotional and cognitive features of medication-induced parkinsonism can be subjectively unpleasant and can contribute to poor medication adherence (Acosta et al. 2012; Ascher-Svanum et al. 2006). For further discussion of medication-induced parkinsonism, including its treatment, see Statement 12.

Neuroleptic Malignant Syndrome

NMS is characterized by a classic triad of rigidity, hyperthermia (>100.4°F/38.0°C on at least two occasions, measured orally), and sympathetic nervous system lability, including hypertension and tachycardia, in the context of exposure to a dopamine antagonist (or withdrawal of a dopamine agonist), typically within 72 hours of symptom development (American Psychiatric Association 2013a; Gurrera et al. 2011, 2017). In addition, NMS is associated with an elevated level of serum creatine kinase (typically, at least four times the upper limit of normal), tachypnea, change in mental status (e.g., delirium, stupor), and lack of another identified etiology for the symptoms. Notably, however, the onset and clinical features of NMS can vary and may make recognition more difficult. If misdiagnosed and mistreated, NMS can be fatal (Berman 2011; Rosebush and Stewart 1989; Strawn et al. 2007).

Other diagnostic considerations in patients presenting with possible NMS include malignant catatonia, malignant hyperthermia (in association with anesthetic administration), heat stroke (for which patients treated with antipsychotics have a heightened susceptibility), serotonin syndrome (in patients also taking serotonergic drugs such as selective serotonin reuptake inhibitors), benign elevations in the level of serum creatine kinase, fever in association with clozapine treatment, alcohol or sedative withdrawal, anticholinergic syndrome, hyperthermia associated with use of stimulants and hallucinogens, central nervous system infections, limbic encephalitis, and inflammatory or autoimmune conditions (American Psychiatric Association 2013a; Berman 2011; Rosebush and Stewart 1989; Strawn et al. 2007).

NMS has been reported with almost all medications that block dopamine receptors, but a greater risk of occurrence appears to be associated with high-potency FGAs (Schneider et al. 2018; Stübner et al. 2004). Risk also may be increased by use of short-acting intramuscular formulations of antipsychotic medications, use of higher total drug dosages, or rapid increases in the dosage of the antipsychotic medication (Keck et al. 1989; Sachdev et al. 1997; Viejo et al. 2003). Additional risk factors for NMS include acute agitation, dehydration, exhaustion, iron deficiency, physical illness, preexisting neurological disability, and a prior episode of NMS (American Psychiatric Association 2013a; Keck et al. 1989; Sachdev et al. 1997; Strawn et al. 2007).

Because NMS is rare, with an estimated incidence of 0.01%–0.02% among individuals treated with antipsychotics (Schneider et al. 2018; Stübner et al. 2004), most evidence regarding NMS treatment comes from single case reports or case series. Antipsychotic medications should always be discontinued, and supportive treatment to maintain hydration and to treat the fever and cardiovascular, renal, or other symptoms should be provided (American Psychiatric Association 2013a; Berman 2011; Strawn et al. 2007). NMS is usually self-limited, with resolution within a week of medication discontinuation in the majority of patients; however, prolonged symptoms of NMS do occur and may be associated with use of LAI antipsychotic medications (Caroff and Mann 1988; Caroff et al. 2000).

In addition to antipsychotic discontinuation and supportive care, a number of approaches have been used to treat NMS, although evidence is limited to case reports and case series (Pileggi and Cook 2016; Strawn et al. 2007). Benzodiazepines, such as lorazepam, have been used because of their benefits in treating catatonia and the parallels between malignant catatonia and NMS. As a postsynaptic D_2 receptor agonist, bromocriptine has been used to counteract the dopamine antagonist effects of the antipsychotic medication. Dantrolene, a direct-acting skeletal muscle relaxant, has also been used, particularly in severe cases of NMS, because of its benefits in treating malignant hyperthermia. When NMS has not responded to these interventions or when catatonic symptoms persist after the resolution of NMS, case reports suggest that ECT can be beneficial (Caroff et al. 2000; Pileggi and Cook 2016; Strawn et al. 2007; Wittenauer Welsh et al. 2016). Assistance with emergency management of NMS is recommended and can be obtained through NMSContact (www.mhaus.org/nmsis/nmscontact).

Once NMS has resolved, caution is needed when resuming an antipsychotic medication because recurrence has been reported (Rosebush and Stewart 1989; Strawn et al. 2007; Susman and Addonizio 1988). Generally, when treatment is resumed, doses are increased gradually, and a medication other than the precipitating agent is used, typically one with a lower potency at blocking dopamine D_2 receptors.

Seizures

Among the antipsychotic medications, clozapine is associated with the greatest likelihood of a seizure, and patients with a history of an idiopathic or medication-induced seizure may have a higher risk (Alldredge 1999; Devinsky and Pacia 1994; Wong and Delva 2007). Although generalized tonic-clonic seizures are most frequent, other types of seizures may occur. Seizures may also be preceded by myoclonus or drop attacks.

The seizure risk with clozapine is increased by rapid increases in dose as well as at high blood levels or doses of the drug. The overall seizure rate is 2.8%; with low-dose treatment (<300 mg/day) the risk is 1%, with medium doses (300–599 mg/day) the risk is 2.7%, and with high doses (>599 mg/day) the risk is 4.4% (Devinsky et al. 1991). Therefore, a slow initial titration of clozapine dose is essential, and patients should be cautioned not to drive or engage in other potentially hazardous activities while clozapine is being titrated. In individuals at high risk of seizure, prophylactic treatment with an anticonvulsant medication can be considered. FGAs can also lower the seizure threshold in a dose-related manner and result in the development of generalized tonic-clonic seizures (Alldredge 1999). Nevertheless, at usual dose ranges, seizure rates are below 1% for all FGAs.

In patients who do experience a seizure while taking clozapine or another antipsychotic medication, neurological consultation will be important for delineating the risks of a further seizure, determining whether anticonvulsant therapy (e.g., valproate) is indicated, and collaborating with the clinician in determining whether changes to the patient's antipsychotic regimen are indicated (Alldredge 1999; Wong and Delva 2007).

Tardive Syndromes, Including Tardive Dyskinesia

Tardive syndromes are persistent abnormal involuntary movement disorders caused by sustained exposure to antipsychotic medication, the most common of which are tardive dyskinesia, tardive dystonia, and tardive akathisia (Frei et al. 2018). They begin later in treatment than acute dystonia, akathisia, or medication-induced parkinsonism, and they persist and may even increase, despite reduction in dose or discontinuation of the antipsychotic medication. Typically, tardive dyskinesia presents as "[i]nvoluntary athetoid or choreiform movements (lasting at least a few weeks) generally of the tongue, lower face and jaw, and extremities (but sometimes involving the pharyngeal, diaphragmatic, or trunk muscles)" (American Psychiatric Association 2013a, p. 712), whereas tardive dystonia and tardive akathisia resemble their acute counterparts in phenomenology.

Tardive dyskinesia has been reported after exposure to any of the available antipsychotic medications (Carbon et al. 2017, 2018). It occurs at a rate of approximately 4%–8% per year in adult patients treated with FGAs (Carbon et al. 2018; Woods et al. 2010), a risk that appears to be at least three times that observed with SGAs (Carbon et al. 2018; O'Brien 2016; Woods et al. 2010). Various factors are associated with greater vulnerability to tardive dyskinesia, including age greater than 55 years; female sex; white or African race/ethnicity; presence of a mood disorder, intellectual disability, or central nervous system injury; and past or current akathisia, clinically significant parkinsonism, or acute dystonic reactions (Patterson-Lomba et al. 2019; Solmi et al. 2018a).

Although the majority of patients who develop tardive dyskinesia have mild symptoms, a small proportion will develop symptoms of moderate or severe degree. Tardive dyskinesia can have significant effects on quality of life and can be associated with social withdrawal (McEvoy et al. 2019). Although the impact appears to be influenced by the severity of tardive dyskinesia, individuals with mild symptoms can also experience negative effects on quality of life.

Evaluation of the risk of tardive dyskinesia is complicated by the fact that dyskinetic movements may be observed with a reduction in antipsychotic medication dose, which is termed a withdrawal-emergent dyskinesia (American Psychiatric Association 2013a). Fluctuations in symptoms are also common and may be influenced by such factors as psychosocial stressors. Furthermore, spontaneous dyskinesias, which are clinically indistinguishable from tardive dyskinesia, have been described in elderly patients before the advent of antipsychotic medications and in up to 20% of never-medicated patients with chronic schizophrenia (Blanchet et al. 2004; Crow et al. 1982; Fenton et al. 1997; Saltz et al. 1991). In longer-term studies, findings are often confounded by the sequential or concomitant use of more than one antipsychotic medication and the lack of systematic prospective assessments for the presence of a movement disorder (Tarsy and Baldessarini 2006). Nevertheless, evaluation for the presence of tardive syndromes is important in order to identify them, minimize worsening, and institute clinically indicated treatment. For further discussion of tardive syndromes, including their treatment, see Statement 14.

Ophthalmological Effects

The most common ophthalmological effects of antipsychotic medications are related to the anticholinergic effects of these agents and include blurred vision and exacerbation of open-angle glaucoma. Pigmentary retinopathies and corneal opacities can occur with chronic administration of the low-potency medications thioridazine and chlorpromazine, particularly at high doses (e.g., more than 800 mg/day of thioridazine) (Matsuo et al. 2016). With SGAs, including quetiapine, evidence does not suggest any increase in the likelihood of cataract development (Laties et al. 2015; Pakzad-Vaezi et al. 2013). If patients do undergo cataract surgery, however, there have been case reports of intraoperative floppy-iris syndrome in individuals treated with antipsychotic medications, a complication that has been associated with use of medications that block α_1-adrenergic receptors (Chatziralli and Sergentanis 2011). Although adverse ophthalmological effects of antipsychotic medications are infrequent, encouraging regular eye care is important to maintaining good vision for individuals with schizophrenia (Viertiö et al. 2007), particularly because of high rates of diabetes and other health conditions that can affect sight.

Other Side Effects

Anticholinergic Effects

The anticholinergic effects of some antipsychotic medications (along with the anticholinergic effects of antiparkinsonian medications, if concurrently administered) can produce a variety of peripheral side effects, including dry mouth, blurred vision, constipation, tachycardia, urinary retention, and effects on thermoregulation (e.g., hyperthermia in hot weather) (Nasrallah and Tandon 2017; Ozbilen and Adams 2009). Central anticholinergic effects can include impaired learning and memory and slowed cognition (Ang et al. 2017; Vinogradov et al. 2009).

Because most anticholinergic side effects are mild and tolerable, they are often overlooked. Nevertheless, they can have multiple implications for patients, including impaired quality of life and significant health complications (Salahudeen et al. 2015). For example, dry mouth is associated with an increased risk for multiple dental complications (Singh and Papas 2014), and drinking high-calorie fluids in response to dry mouth can contribute to weight gain. The muscarinic receptor antagonist properties of antipsychotic drugs can be particularly problematic in older individuals and can contribute to problems such as urinary retention, confusion, fecal impaction, and anticholinergic toxicity (with delirium, somnolence, and hallucinations) (Nasrallah and Tandon 2017). Anticholinergic properties of antipsychotic or antiparkinsonian medications can also precipitate acute angle-closure glaucoma (Lachkar and Bouassida 2007), although patients with treated glaucoma seem to be able to tolerate these medications with careful monitoring (Bower et al. 2018).

The propensity of an antipsychotic medication to cause anticholinergic effects should be considered when choosing an antipsychotic agent initially, particularly in older individuals or those with physical conditions that may confer a greater risk of anticholinergic complications. In selecting a medication, it is also important to keep in mind the total anticholinergic burden from antipsychotic medications, antiparkinsonian medications, urological medications (e.g., oxybutynin), nonselective antihistamines (e.g., hydroxyzine, diphenhydramine), and other medications with anticholinergic side effects. For this reason, antiparkinsonian medications with anticholinergic properties are not typically administered on a prophylactic basis. When anticholinergic side effects do occur, they are often dose-related and thus may improve with lowering of the dose or administering the medications that have anticholinergic properties in divided doses. For additional discussion of anticholinergic properties of antiparkisonian medications, see Statement 12.

Fever

Fever (>38°C) should prompt assessment for possible etiologies, including NMS or infection. In hot weather, the possibility of heat stroke should be considered in patients who do not have access to air-conditioned environments due to the increased risk of heat-related events in individuals with psychiatric illness (Bouchama et al. 2007) and the effects of some antipsychotics and anticholinergic agents on thermoregulation (Martin-Latry et al. 2007). In patients who are treated with clozapine, a brief self-limiting fever may occur during the first few weeks of treatment and responds to supportive measures (Bruno et al. 2015; Lowe et al. 2007; Pui-yin Chung et al. 2008). However, it is also essential to assess for the presence of potentially life-threatening complications, including NMS, severe neutropenia, and myocarditis.

Sedation

Sedation is a very common side effect of antipsychotic medications (Citrome 2017a; Leucht et al. 2013). This effect may be related to antagonist effects of those drugs on histamine, adrenergic, and dopamine receptors (Michl et al. 2014). Sedation is most pronounced in the initial phases of treatment, and many patients develop some tolerance to the sedating effects with continued administration. For agitated patients, the sedating effects of these medications in the initial phase of treatment can have therapeutic benefits. Bedtime sedation can also be desirable for patients who are having difficulty sleeping. However, persistent sedation, including daytime drowsiness, increased sleep time, and reduced cognitive acuity, can interfere with social, recreational, and vocational function.

Lowering of the daily dose, consolidation of divided doses into one evening dose, or changing to a less sedating antipsychotic medication may be effective in reducing the severity of sedation. Coffee or other caffeine can be helpful in the morning but can also interact with medications (e.g., contribute to tachycardia; raise blood levels of medications, including clozapine). Adding a stimulant medication is not typically helpful and can lead to additional side effects. If sedation or the risk of sedation is significant (e.g., during initial clozapine titration), patients should be cautioned not to drive or engage in potentially hazardous activities.

Sialorrhea

Sialorrhea (or hypersalivation) is a frequent side effect of clozapine (Maher et al. 2016) but can also be observed with other antipsychotic medications (Essali et al. 2013). The etiology of sialorrhea is unclear but may relate to decreased saliva clearance, although actions on muscarinic or α-adrenergic receptors have also been postulated (Ekström et al. 2010). Sialorrhea can contribute to reductions in quality of life and can also be associated with complications such as aspiration pneumonia (Dzahini et al. 2018; Kaplan et al. 2018; Stoecker et al. 2017).

During the day, patients can be encouraged to chew sugarless gum, which stimulates the swallowing reflex. Because sialorrhea may be more bothersome at night, patients may be advised to place a towel on their pillow and change to a clean towel in the middle of the night to minimize discomfort. Pharmacological approaches to address sialorrhea come from small studies and case reports and include use of low-dose or topical anticholinergic medications, such as glycopyrrolate or sublingual ophthalmic atropine 1% drops (Bird et al. 2011; Liang et al. 2010; Man et al. 2017). Diphenhydramine has also been studied (Chen et al. 2019); however, because clozapine and other antipsychotics can have significant anticholinergic properties themselves and anticholinergics have small effects on sialorrhea, the use of agents with added anticholinergic effects should be approached cautiously. Terazosin and, in severe refractory cases, botulinum toxin have also been used (Bird et al. 2011; Liang et al. 2010; Man et al. 2017).

Weight Gain

Weight gain occurs with most antipsychotic agents and appears to relate to actions of these medications as histamine H_1 receptor antagonists, although actions on serotonin and muscarinic receptors may also play a role (He et al. 2013; Kroeze et al. 2003; Michl et al. 2014; Olten and Bloch 2018). Reviews and meta-analyses have compared average weight gains with antipsychotic treatment and the proportion of patients who gain 7% or more of body weight (Bak et al. 2014; Leucht et al. 2013; Zhang et al. 2013). Nevertheless, there is substantial variability in the amount of weight gain that will occur in an individual patient who is treated with a specific antipsychotic medication. Typically, weight gain is progressive over the first 6 months of treatment, although some patients continue to gain weight indefinitely (Alvarez-Jimenez et al. 2008). In addition, younger individuals who are experiencing a first episode of psychosis may be more likely than older individuals to gain weight with antipsychotic medication (Correll et al. 2014; Jensen et al. 2019). In identifying individuals with schizophrenia who experience weight gain with antipsychotic treatment, self-reported awareness may be less effective than objective measurement (Gao et al. 2016).

Obesity, in general, can contribute to an increase in risk for mortality and morbidity, including increased rates of cardiovascular disease, hypertension, cancers, diabetes, osteoarthritis, and sleep apnea (Aune et al. 2016; Bellou et al. 2018; Jehan et al. 2018; Lauby-Secretan et al. 2016; Stringhini et al. 2017). Consequently, weight gain with antipsychotic medications is also likely to contribute to an increase in physical health conditions and mortality. Prevention of weight gain should, thus, be a high priority because weight loss is difficult for most patients. Efforts should be made to intervene proactively with weight gain of 5–10 pounds because people who are obese rarely lose more than 10% of body weight with weight loss regimens.

A number of studies have evaluated the effectiveness of specific interventions to prevent or treat antipsychotic-induced weight gain (Caemmerer et al. 2012; Das et al. 2012; de Silva et al. 2016; Gierisch et al. 2014; Mahmood et al. 2013; Manu et al. 2015; Mizuno et al. 2014; Mukundan et al. 2010; Vancampfort et al. 2019; Zheng et al. 2015). Nutritional interventions have shown small but consistent benefits (Bonfioli et al. 2012), although patients who are willing to enroll in and are able to adhere to such studies may not be representative. Nevertheless, nutritional approaches may be suggested for their benefits for overall health as well as for weight. Such approaches include specialized behavioral health interventions, in-person community interventions (e.g., Weight Watchers), services that include meal delivery (e.g., Jenny Craig), and Internet-based interventions (e.g., Omada Health). In addition, some programs have begun to integrate dietitians into the treatment team, given the nutritional challenges that exist for many individuals with serious mental illness (Teasdale et al. 2017). Other nonpharmacological approaches that have been studied include exercise and cognitive-behavioral therapy approaches (Bonfioli et al. 2012; Caemmerer et al. 2012; Das et al. 2012).

In collaboration with the patient's primary care clinician, medication strategies for weight loss can be considered. Of the pharmacological treatments that have been assessed, metformin has been studied most often. It has been shown to be safe in individuals without hyperglycemia, shows modest benefits on weight (with average weight loss of 3–4 kg), and can reverse metabolic abnormalities in patients with obesity or other metabolic problems (Das et al. 2012; de Silva et al. 2016; McGinty et al. 2016; Mizuno et al. 2014; Siskind et al. 2016a; Vancampfort et al. 2019; Zheng et al. 2015; Zhuo et al. 2018). However, most studies have been small, and follow-up periods have not been longer than 6 months. Modest benefit has also been seen in several studies of glucagon-like peptide-1 receptor agonists (Siskind et al. 2019) and small studies of topiramate (Mahmood et al. 2013; Mizuno et al. 2014; Vancampfort et al. 2019; Zhuo et al. 2018). Other medications have been examined in small trials or case series, with less consistent findings (Mizuno et al. 2014). This limited evidence and the modest benefit of these pharmacological treatments need to be considered in light of potential adverse effects.

Another consideration for a patient who has experienced significant weight gain with antipsychotic treatment is to change or augment treatment with a medication with lower weight-gain liability (Vancampfort et al. 2019). When possible, other medications that can cause weight gain (e.g., valproate) should be tapered and discontinued. Such decisions need to consider the extent of the patient's response to the current medication regimen, the risks to the patient if relapse occurs with a medication change, and the likelihood that a medication change will be beneficial in terms of weight loss or other side effects (Manu et al. 2015; Mukundan et al. 2010; Newcomer et al. 2013; Vancampfort et al. 2019). In any patient with weight gain, it is also important to assess for other contributors to metabolic syndrome (Mitchell et al. 2012, 2013b).

The benefits of exercise appear to be small in terms of weight loss in individuals with schizophrenia (Firth et al. 2015; Pearsall et al. 2014; Vancampfort et al. 2017, 2019). Nevertheless, many individuals with schizophrenia do not engage in physical activity (Stubbs et al. 2016a; Vancampfort et al. 2016b), and exercise can be suggested for its benefits to overall health, improved cardiorespiratory fitness, and other aspects of functioning (Dauwan et al. 2016; Firth et al. 2015, 2017; Vancampfort et al. 2017, 2019). Health promotion coaching interventions focused on individuals with mental illness, such as the In SHAPE program, can also be pursued and may be associated with weight loss and reduced cardiovascular risk (Bartels et al. 2015; Naslund et al. 2016; Van Citters et al. 2010; Verhaeghe et al. 2013).

Balancing of Potential Benefits and Harms in Rating the Strength of the Guideline Statement

Benefits

Use of an antipsychotic medication in the treatment of schizophrenia can improve positive and negative symptoms of psychosis (high strength of research evidence) and can also lead to reductions in depression and improvements in quality of life and functioning (moderate strength of research evidence). A meta-analysis of double-blind, randomized, placebo-controlled trials showed a medium effect size for overall efficacy (Leucht et al. 2017), with the greatest effect on positive symptoms. The rates of achieving any response or a good response were also significantly greater in patients who received an antipsychotic medication. In addition, the proportion of individuals who dropped out of treatment for any reason and for lack of efficacy was significantly less in those who were treated with an antipsychotic medication. Research evidence from head-to-head comparison studies and network meta-analysis (McDonagh et al. 2017) showed no consistent evidence that favored a specific antipsychotic medication, with the possible exception of clozapine.

Harms

The harms of using an antipsychotic medication in the treatment of schizophrenia include sedation, side effects mediated through dopamine receptor blockade (e.g., acute dystonia, akathisia, parkinsonism, tardive syndromes, NMS, hyperprolactinemia), disturbances in sexual function, anticholinergic effects, weight gain, glucose abnormalities, hyperlipidemia, orthostatic hypotension, tachycardia, and QTc prolongation. Clozapine has additional harms associated with its use, including sialorrhea, seizures, neutropenia (which can be severe and life-threatening), myocarditis, and cardiomyopathy. Among the antipsychotic medications, there is variability in the rates at which each of these effects occurs, and no specific medication appears to be devoid of possible side effects.

Patient Preferences

Clinical experience suggests that many patients are cooperative with and accepting of antipsychotic medications as part of a treatment plan. A survey of patient preferences reported that patients viewed an ability to think more clearly and an ability to stop hallucinations or paranoia as important efficacy-related reasons to take an antipsychotic medication (Achtyes et al. 2018). However, patients also reported concerns about side effects, particularly weight gain, sedation, and restlessness, as reasons that they might not wish to take antipsychotic medications. Some patients might also choose not to take an antipsychotic medication when they are feeling well or if they do not view themselves as having a condition that requires treatment. Some patients may also prefer one medication over another medication on the basis of prior treatment experiences or other factors.

Balancing of Benefits and Harms

The potential benefits of this guideline statement were viewed as far outweighing the potential harms. Although harms of antipsychotic medications can be significant, the impact of schizophrenia on patients' lives is also substantial, and consistent benefits of antipsychotic treatment were found. Harms of treatment can be mitigated by selecting medications on the basis of individual characteristics and preferences of patients as well as by choosing a medication on the basis of its side-effect profile, pharmacological characteristics, and other factors. For clozapine, the additional benefits of treatment were viewed as outweighing the additional rare but serious harms and the need for ANC monitoring to reduce the likelihood of severe neutropenia. For additional discussion of the research evidence, see Appendix C, Statement 4.

Differences of Opinion Among Writing Group Members

There were no differences of opinion. The writing group voted unanimously in favor of this recommendation.

Review of Available Guidelines From Other Organizations

Information from other guidelines is consistent with this guideline statement. Other guidelines on the treatment of schizophrenia (BAP, Canadian Schizophrenia Guidelines [CSG], NICE, PORT, RANZCP, SIGN, WFSBP) all recommend use of an antipsychotic medication in the treatment of schizophrenia, with the selection of a specific medication on an individualized basis with consideration of medication characteristics, patient characteristics, and patient preferences (Addington et al. 2017a, 2017b; Barnes et al. 2011; Buchanan et al. 2010; Crockford and Addington 2017; Galletly et al. 2016; Hasan et al. 2012; National Institute for Health and Care Excellence 2014; Pringsheim et al. 2017; Remington et al. 2017; Scottish Intercollegiate Guidelines Network 2013). Each guideline also recommends monitoring during the course of treatment to assess therapeutic response and treatment-related side effects.

Quality Measurement Considerations

In clinical practice, almost all individuals with schizophrenia are offered an antipsychotic medication. Thus, a quality measure is unlikely to enhance outcomes if it examines only whether an individual with schizophrenia is offered or receives an initial prescription for antipsychotic treatment. An existing National Quality Forum–endorsed measure, "Adherence to Antipsychotic Medications for Individuals with Schizophrenia" (NQF #1879, www.qualityforum.org/QPS/1879), is aimed at assessing whether an antipsychotic medication is continued once it is begun. For individuals who are at least 18 years old and who have a diagnosis of schizophrenia or schizoaffective disorder, this measure assesses the percentage who have been dispensed an antipsychotic medication (as reflected by at least two such prescriptions being filled) and who had a proportion of covered days of at least 0.8 during a 12 consecutive month measurement period. By requiring ongoing prescribing of antipsychotic medication, this measure is more likely to be associated with improvements in outcomes for patients. Nevertheless, this measure does have several limitations. It uses pharmacy claims data or electronic prescription orders to examine whether a medication has been prescribed, but such measures do not guarantee treatment adherence. For instance, a prescriber could submit an antipsychotic medication prescription and the patient could fill the prescription at the pharmacy, but the patient might not actually take the medication. This measure also does not determine the adequacy of the medication or the medication dose and could be met through continuous prescriptions of a subtherapeutic dose or clinically ineffective antipsychotic. Another limitation is the difficulty in determining the proportion of covered days in a 12 consecutive month period, particularly when patients have transitions in care between settings or treating clinicians.

Quality measures, quality improvement initiatives, or electronic decision supports may be appropriate for monitoring side effects of antipsychotic treatment. Evidence suggests that rates of guideline concordant monitoring are low for metabolic risk factors, including lipids, diabetes, and weight (Mitchell et al. 2012; Morrato et al. 2009). Several measures endorsed by NQF address such monitoring. NQF #1932, "Diabetes Screening for People With Schizophrenia or Bipolar Disorder Who Are Using Antipsychotic Medications" (www.qualityforum.org/QPS/1932) measures the percentage of patients ages 18–64 years with schizophrenia or bipolar disorder "who were dispensed an antipsychotic medication and had a diabetes screening test during the measurement year." Because this measure is focused on screening, it excludes monitoring of individuals who had diabetes in the measurement year or in the preceding year.

NQF #1927, "Cardiovascular Health Screening for People With Schizophrenia or Bipolar Disorder Who Are Prescribed Antipsychotic Medications" (www.qualityforum.org/QPS/1927) measures the percentage of individuals ages 25–64 years with schizophrenia or bipolar disorder "who were prescribed any antipsychotic medication and who received a cardiovascular health screening during the measurement year," where cardiovascular health screening consists of "one or more LDL-C screenings performed during the measurement year." Individuals are excluded from this screening measure for having evidence of preexisting cardiovascular disease as defined by precise criteria in the measure text. Presently, the specific elements of these criteria can often be challenging to determine from unstructured electronic health records.

Two additional NQF-approved measures, NQF #1933 (www.qualityforum.org/QPS/1933) and NQF #1934 (www.qualityforum.org/QPS/1934) address cardiovascular and diabetes monitoring, respectively, for individuals with preexisting cardiovascular disease or diabetes. Each of these measures is limited to individuals who are ages 18–64 years. The cardiovascular monitoring measure requires that individuals receive "an LDL-C test performed during the measurement year," whereas the diabetes monitoring measure requires "[o]ne or more HbA1c tests and one or more LDL-C tests performed during the measurement year." These measures have been tested for feasibility, usability, reliability, and validity at the health plan, integrated delivery system, and population levels; however, before holding individual clinicians or facilities accountable for the delivered quality of care, the measures would need additional testing at these levels.

STATEMENT 5: Continuing Medications

APA *recommends* **(1A)** that patients with schizophrenia whose symptoms have improved with an antipsychotic medication continue to be treated with an antipsychotic medication.*

Implementation

For individuals with a diagnosis of schizophrenia whose symptoms have improved with an antipsychotic medication, there are a number of benefits to maintenance treatment, including reduced risks of relapse (Bowtell et al. 2018; Goff et al. 2017; Hui et al. 2018; Kishi et al. 2019; Leucht et al. 2012; Thompson et al. 2018), rehospitalization (Tiihonen et al. 2018), and death (Tiihonen et al. 2018; Vermeulen et al. 2017). When administered on a long-term basis, however, antipsychotic medications are also associated with a greater incidence of weight gain, sedation, and movement disorders (Leucht et al. 2012). In addition, some studies have raised questions about whether long-term antipsychotic treatment might be associated with other adverse effects on functioning or health, including loss of brain volume (Davidson 2018; Goff et al. 2017). These data are heterogeneous, and when compared with withholding treatment, there was minimal evidence to suggest negative effects of maintenance treatments on outcomes (Goff et al. 2017; Huhtaniska et al. 2017). In addition, it may be possible to mitigate these risks by preventive interventions (e.g., early intervention for weight gain, screening for lipid and glucose abnormalities) and careful monitoring for side effects of medication. Nevertheless, as treatment proceeds, the pluses and minuses of continuing treatment with an antipsychotic medication should be reviewed with the patient in the context of shared decision-making. It will typically be beneficial to include family members or other persons of support in such discussions (Hamann and Heres 2019).

Despite the benefits of continued antipsychotic treatment for the majority of patients, maintaining adherence to an antipsychotic medication can be difficult (Acosta et al. 2012; Shafrin et al. 2016; Valenstein et al. 2006). Barriers to, facilitators of, and motivators of treatment adherence will differ for each patient. Engaging family members or other persons of support can be helpful in fostering adherence (Mueser et al. 2015). Other approaches to assessing and enhancing adherence are described in detail in Statement 3.

For some patients, the formulation of the antipsychotic medication may influence adherence (see Statement 4, Table 3). For example, rapidly dissolving tablets or oral concentrates may be preferable for patients who have difficulty swallowing pills or who are ambivalent about medications and inconsistent in swallowing them. LAI formulations may be preferred by some patients (Heres et al. 2007; Patel et al. 2009; Walburn et al. 2001) and may be particularly useful for patients with a history of poor or uncertain adherence (see Statement 10).

It is also important to assess the ongoing benefits and side effects of treatment that may indicate a need for adjustments to medication doses or changes in medications. The use of quantitative measures can be helpful in systematically assessing each of these realms (see Statement 2). The optimal dose of medication is one that provides the best medication benefits yet is tolerable in terms of medication side effects. For some patients, adjustments in dose will be required during the course of treatment to maintain this balance (Essock et al. 2006). Such factors as addition or discontinuation of interacting medications, changes in smoking status, changes in patient body mass, changes in renal or hepatic status, or changes in drug absorption (e.g., with bariatric surgery) may influence medication pharmacokinetics and require increases or decreases in medication dose. In order to minimize the risk of extended side effects, when medications with a long half-life are used and particularly when LAI antipsychotic medications are used, considerations about changes in dose need to consider the extended actions of these medications.

---

*This guideline statement should be implemented in the context of a person-centered treatment plan that includes evidence-based nonpharmacological and pharmacological treatments for schizophrenia.

Evidence on the rationale and approach to planned reductions of medication doses is limited. Unless a medication requires emergent discontinuation, gradual reductions in doses are preferable, with close monitoring for recurrent symptoms.

Shared decision-making discussions with the patient should consider the patient's recovery goals, the potential benefits of medication changes or dose reductions in terms of changes or diminution of side effects, and the potential harms of medication changes or dose reductions (Davidson 2018). The longitudinal course of the patient's episode and the certainty of the diagnosis should also be considered. There may be some individuals with a brief episode of psychosis or uncertain psychotic diagnosis (e.g., possible substance-induced psychosis or mood-related psychosis) who may not require continuing antipsychotic treatment. On the other hand, individuals with chronic symptoms, repeated relapses, and clear diagnostic features of schizophrenia will likely have poorer outcomes if medications are stopped. In addition to symptom recurrence and relapse, medication cessation may be associated with hospitalization, legal difficulties, reduced likelihood of response with reinstatement of treatment, or poorer psychosocial outcomes (Correll et al. 2018; Hui et al. 2018; Takeuchi et al. 2019; Wilper et al. 2009). It will typically be beneficial to include family members or other persons of support in discussions of medication changes or dose reductions.

Balancing of Potential Benefits and Harms in Rating the Strength of the Guideline Statement

Benefits

Use of an antipsychotic medication that has already been associated with symptom response can maintain improvements in symptoms as well as promote enhanced functioning and quality of life (high strength of research evidence). Long-term treatment with an antipsychotic medication has also been associated with a reduction in mortality as compared with no antipsychotic treatment in individuals with schizophrenia. In contrast, discontinuation of antipsychotic treatment can be associated with increases in symptoms and risk of hospitalization and poorer long-term outcomes, including greater mortality in the long term (low strength of research evidence).

Harms

The harms of continuing use of an antipsychotic medication can vary depending on whether the patient is experiencing any significant side effects from the medication that would have long-term untoward effects. For patients whose medications are well tolerated, long-term risks include tardive syndromes from antipsychotic medications. For other patients, long-term risks will vary according to the specific side effect, with metabolic effects of antipsychotic medication serving as a possible contributor to long-term health risks. Some studies have raised concerns about changes in brain region volumes with antipsychotic treatment, but these findings are heterogeneous and inconsistent.

Patient Preferences

Clinical experience suggests that many patients are cooperative with and accepting of antipsychotic medications as part of a treatment plan. This is particularly true when the medication has been associated with a response in symptoms. Indeed, a survey of patient preferences reported that patients viewed an ability to think more clearly and an ability to stop hallucinations or paranoia as important efficacy-related reasons to take an antipsychotic medication (Achtyes et al. 2018). Patients are also likely to value the long-term benefits that have been shown with continued antipsychotic treatment, including reductions in relapses, hospitalizations, and mortality. However, patients also report concerns about side effects, particularly weight gain, sedation, and restlessness, that can make them reluctant to take antipsychotic medications on a long-term basis. In addition, some patients may choose not to take an antipsychotic medication when they are feeling well or if they do not view themselves as having a condition that requires treatment.

Balancing of Benefits and Harms

The potential benefits of this guideline statement were viewed as far outweighing the potential harms. Although harms of antipsychotic medications can be significant and the long-term effects of antipsychotic medications are not well studied, the impact of schizophrenia on patients' lives is also substantial, and consistent benefits of continued antipsychotic treatment were found. Overall, rates of mortality appear to be reduced by ongoing treatment with an antipsychotic medication as compared with no treatment. In addition, harms of treatment can be mitigated by using the lowest effective dose; by selecting medications on the basis of individual characteristics and preferences of patients; and by choosing a medication on the basis of its side-effect profile, pharmacological characteristics, and other factors. For additional discussion of the research evidence, see Appendix C, Statement 5.

Differences of Opinion Among Writing Group Members

There were no differences of opinion. The writing group voted unanimously in favor of this recommendation.

Review of Available Guidelines From Other Organizations

Information from other guidelines is consistent with this guideline statement. Other guidelines on the treatment of schizophrenia (BAP, NICE, PORT, SIGN, WFSBP) recommend continued use of an antipsychotic medication in the treatment of schizophrenia once symptom response has been achieved (Barnes et al. 2011; Buchanan et al. 2010; Hasan et al. 2013; National Institute for Health and Care Excellence 2014; Scottish Intercollegiate Guidelines Network 2013). Other guidelines (RANZCP, BAP, SIGN, NICE) also suggest the use of LAI antipsychotic medications on the basis of patient preference or when adherence has been poor or uncertain (Barnes et al. 2011; Galletly et al. 2016; National Institute for Health and Care Excellence 2014; Scottish Intercollegiate Guidelines Network 2013). Use of a gradual reduction in dose, including a gradual cross-taper when changing medications, is noted by several guidelines (BAP, NICE, SIGN) along with an emphasis on close monitoring for signs of relapse (Barnes et al. 2011; National Institute for Health and Care Excellence 2014; Scottish Intercollegiate Guidelines Network 2013).

Quality Measurement Considerations

See Statement 4 for a discussion of quality measures related to initiation and ongoing use of an antipsychotic medication.

STATEMENT 6: Continuing the Same Medications

APA *suggests* **(2B)** that patients with schizophrenia whose symptoms have improved with an antipsychotic medication continue to be treated with the same antipsychotic medication.*

Implementation

As noted in Statement 5, it is important for treatment with an antipsychotic medication to be maintained once symptoms have improved. Specifically, for individuals with a diagnosis of schizophrenia,

---

*This guideline statement should be implemented in the context of a person-centered treatment plan that includes evidence-based nonpharmacological and pharmacological treatments for schizophrenia.

there are a number of benefits to continued treatment with an antipsychotic medication, including reduced risks of relapse (Bowtell et al. 2018; Goff et al. 2017; Hui et al. 2018; Kishi et al. 2019; Leucht et al. 2012; Thompson et al. 2018), rehospitalization (Tiihonen et al. 2018), and death (Tiihonen et al. 2018; Vermeulen et al. 2017). Implicitly, continued treatment with an effective and tolerable medication would be preferable to potential destabilization or treatment discontinuation. This inference is also consistent with clinical observations that individualizing choice of an antipsychotic medication is important. In clinical trials, a change to a different medication has been associated with earlier discontinuation of treatment as compared with continuation of the same antipsychotic medication (Essock et al. 2006; Stroup et al. 2011).

For these reasons, it will be optimal to continue on the same medication for most patients. Nevertheless, under some circumstances, it may be necessary to consider a change from one antipsychotic medication to another one. For example, a patient may have experienced some degree of response to initial treatment but may still have significant symptoms or difficulties in functioning that would warrant a trial of a different medication. Another reason to change medications would be to initiate treatment with an LAI antipsychotic if the current oral medication is unavailable in an LAI formulation (see Statement 10). A medication change may also be considered because of patient preferences, medication availability, or side effects. Given the long-term health risks of metabolic syndrome and obesity, weight gain and development of diabetes or metabolic syndrome are common reasons that a change to a different medication may be discussed.

In a randomized study that examined the effects of switching from olanzapine, quetiapine, or risperidone to aripiprazole to reduce metabolic risk, a change to aripiprazole was associated with improvements in non-HDL cholesterol, serum triglycerides, and weight as well as a small reduction in 10-year risk of coronary heart disease but no difference in the odds of having metabolic syndrome (Stroup et al. 2011, 2013). Individuals who switched to aripiprazole, as compared with those who remained on their initial medication, had a higher rate of discontinuing treatment but showed no significant increases in symptoms or hospitalizations. In addition, the Clinical Antipsychotic Trials of Intervention Effectiveness (CATIE) showed that individuals who experienced issues with medication efficacy or tolerability in an early phase of the trial could still go on to do well with a different medication in a subsequent phase of the trial (McEvoy et al. 2006; Rosenheck et al. 2009; Stroup et al. 2007, 2009).

These findings suggest that a change in medication can be of benefit to patients under some circumstances but also suggest that the possible benefits and risks of a medication change should be reviewed with the patient in the context of shared decision-making. Such discussions with the patient should consider the patient's recovery goals, the potential benefits of medication changes or dose reductions in terms of changes in or diminution of side effects, and the potential harms of medication changes or dose reductions (Davidson 2018). It will typically be beneficial to include family members or other persons of support in such discussions.

Only a limited amount of research has explored the optimal approach for changing antipsychotic medications when warranted. The typical approach is a gradual cross-taper in which the second antipsychotic medication is begun and gradually increased in dose as the initial antipsychotic medication is gradually tapered. However, the few studies that are available do not suggest differences between gradual discontinuation as compared with immediate discontinuation of the first medication (Takeuchi et al. 2017a). In addition, no differences have been seen between starting the second antipsychotic and discontinuing the first antipsychotic at the same time as compared with starting the second antipsychotic and waiting before discontinuing the first antipsychotic agent (Takeuchi et al. 2017b). Regardless of the approach that is taken, careful monitoring is essential to avoid the risks of reduced adherence and clinical destabilization if a change in medications is undertaken. Depending on the pharmacological properties of the medications, including pharmacokinetic and receptor binding profiles (see Statement 4, Tables 4 and 5), side effects of medications may also emerge (e.g., insomnia with a shift to a less sedating medication, withdrawal dyskinesia with a shift to a medication with less prominent dopamine D_2 receptor blockade) (Cerovecki et al. 2013).

Balancing of Potential Benefits and Harms in Rating the Strength of the Guideline Statement

Benefits

Use of an antipsychotic medication that has already been associated with symptom response can maintain improvements in symptoms as well as promote enhanced functioning and quality of life. In contrast, changes in antipsychotic treatment can be associated with early treatment discontinuation, increases in symptoms, clinical destabilization, and worsening of treatment tolerability.

Harms

The harms of continuing use of the same antipsychotic medication can vary depending on whether the patient is experiencing any significant side effects from the medication that would have long-term untoward effects. Continuing the same medication could lead to greater long-term risks such as metabolic effects or tardive syndromes from antipsychotic medications, but this would depend on the side-effect profile of the medication. In some instances, changing to a different medication could worsen long-term side-effect risk rather than reduce such risks.

Patient Preferences

Clinical experience suggests that most patients prefer to continue to take an antipsychotic medication that has led to a response in symptoms. Once they have found a medication that is effective and well tolerated, many individuals experience anxiety if they are unable to continue with that medication because of realistic concerns about a possible return of symptoms, reductions in functioning, risk of hospitalization, and other potential consequences of medication changes. However, other patients may not wish to remain on a given antipsychotic medication because of concerns about side effects or other factors that make continued treatment difficult.

Balancing of Benefits and Harms

The potential benefits of this guideline statement were viewed as likely to outweigh the potential harms. Although most patients prefer to continue taking the same medication once their symptoms have responded, there are reasons that a change in medication may be indicated, and factors such as medication side-effect profiles, medication availability, and patient preferences for specific medications also may play a role in decisions to continue with the same medication. For additional discussion of the research evidence, see Appendix C, Statement 6.

Differences of Opinion Among Writing Group Members

There were no differences of opinion. The writing group voted unanimously in favor of this suggestion.

Review of Available Guidelines From Other Organizations

Information from other guidelines is consistent with this guideline statement. Other guidelines on the treatment of schizophrenia (SIGN, WFSBP) note that treatment should usually continue with the same antipsychotic medication that led to the best response and had the best individual side-effect profile, given the risk of destabilization with switching an antipsychotic regimen (Hasan et al. 2013; Scottish Intercollegiate Guidelines Network 2013).

Quality Measurement Considerations

As a suggestion, this guideline statement is not appropriate for use as a quality measure or for electronic decision support. However, health plans may wish to implement internal process measures to assess and reduce rates at which changes to stable medication regimens are made on the basis of nonclinical factors such as pre-authorization requirements or formulary changes.

STATEMENT 7: Clozapine in Treatment-Resistant Schizophrenia

APA *recommends* **(1B)** that patients with treatment-resistant schizophrenia be treated with clozapine.*

Implementation

Identification of Treatment-Resistant Schizophrenia

Clozapine is recommended for individuals with treatment-resistant schizophrenia, but there is considerable variation in definitions of treatment-resistant schizophrenia in clinical trials and in practice (Howes et al. 2017). For the purpose of future research trials, the Treatment Response and Resistance in Psychosis (TRRIP) Working Group conducted a detailed systematic review of clinical trials in treatment-resistant schizophrenia and used a consensus-based approach to establish minimum and optimum criteria for identifying treatment-resistant schizophrenia (Howes et al. 2017). In addition to a diagnosis of schizophrenia, the identification of treatment-resistant schizophrenia rests on the persistence of significant symptoms despite adequate pharmacological treatment (Howes et al. 2017). More specifically, the TRRIP Working Group recommended that symptoms be of at least 12 weeks' duration in total, be of at least moderate severity, and be associated with at least moderate functional impairment as determined by validated rating scales (e.g., PANSS, BPRS, or SANS and SAPS for symptoms and a score <60 on the SOFAS as a measure of functioning). If a prospective medication trial of at least 6 weeks at adequate dose has not led to symptom reduction of more than 20%, this provides additional evidence of treatment resistance. It is helpful to note whether the persistent symptoms include positive, negative, or cognitive symptoms because responses to these symptom domains may differ.

In terms of treatment adequacy, the TRRIP Working Group recommended that at least two antipsychotic trials should be conducted with different antipsychotic medications with at least 6 weeks at a therapeutic dosage of medication for each and with adherence of at least 80% of prescribed dosages (Howes et al. 2017). A therapeutic dosage of medication was defined as the midpoint of the target range for acute treatment of schizophrenia according to the manufacturer's product labeling or the equivalent of at least 600 mg of chlorpromazine per day (Howes et al. 2017). (For tables of dose equivalents, see College of Psychiatric and Neurologic Pharmacists 2019; Leucht et al. 2014, 2015; Rothe et al. 2018.) The consensus criteria include at least one antipsychotic blood level to assess adherence, obtaining information on adherence from at least two sources (e.g., pill counts, dispensing chart reviews, patient/carer reports), and obtaining information on past treatment response from patient/carer reports and other sources.

For clinical purposes, a common definition is that a patient's symptoms have shown no response or partial and suboptimal response to two antipsychotic medication trials of at least 6 weeks each at an adequate dosage of medication, and some definitions specify using medications from different classes (e.g., SGA vs. FGA). However, if there is no significant improvement after several weeks of treatment (e.g., <20% improvement in symptoms), the likelihood of substantial improvement (e.g., >50% improvement in symptoms) is small (Howes et al. 2017; Samara et al. 2015), and a longer trial of the medication may not be warranted. It should also be noted that a medication trial cannot be viewed as adequate if truncated in terms of duration or dosage because of poor tolerability or if limited by poor adherence. Accordingly, some experts suggest a trial of an LAI antipsychotic medication before deciding that a patient's symptoms are treatment-resistant.

---

*This guideline statement should be implemented in the context of a person-centered treatment plan that includes evidence-based nonpharmacological and pharmacological treatments for schizophrenia.

Initiation of Treatment With Clozapine

After a patient is identified as having treatment-resistant schizophrenia, the clinician should engage the patient in discussion about clozapine treatment. A trial of clozapine may also be appropriate in individuals who show a response to treatment (i.e., have at least a 20% reduction in symptoms) yet still have significant symptoms or impairments in functioning (Howes et al. 2017). In fact, clozapine is often underused (Carruthers et al. 2016; Latimer et al. 2013; Olfson et al. 2016; Stroup et al. 2014; Tang et al. 2017), and many patients would benefit from earlier consideration of clozapine initiation.

Discussion of clozapine should emphasize principles of shared decision-making; including family members or other persons of support in such discussions is often beneficial. In terms of a patient's recovery goals, most individuals value an ability to think more clearly and stop hallucinations or delusions when deciding about medication changes (Achtyes et al. 2018). In addition, most patients who receive clozapine view it positively. For example, one large survey of individuals with schizophrenia or schizoaffective disorder who were taking an antipsychotic medication found that the vast majority of those taking clozapine adhered to treatment and found it helpful, whereas only approximately 5% found it not helpful (Siskind et al. 2017a). In contrast, most other antipsychotic medications were viewed less positively (Siskind et al. 2017a). Nevertheless, it is important to identify patient concerns about clozapine and address them insofar as is possible. For example, patients may express concerns about the burdens of required blood work and may encounter logistical barriers such as access to transportation (Farooq et al. 2019; Gee et al. 2017; Verdoux et al. 2018). However, they may be willing to consider clozapine if logistical barriers can be overcome or if given the information that blood monitoring requirements become less frequent over time. Concerns about other side effects, such as weight gain or somnolence, may also contribute to a reluctance to switch to clozapine (Achtyes et al. 2018). It can be helpful to have an open discussion of these side effects and a well-defined plan for monitoring as treatment proceeds. Peer-run support groups that directly address living with side effects can help patients develop strategies for coping with side effects.

Clinicians may also have concerns about clozapine that can serve as a barrier to treatment. For example, many clinicians have limited experience in using clozapine and sometimes express concerns about paperwork burdens, patient adherence with monitoring, and side effects (Daod et al. 2019; Farooq et al. 2019; Gee et al. 2017; Kelly and Love 2019; Kelly et al. 2018; Leung et al. 2019; Verdoux et al. 2018; Warnez and Alessi-Severini 2014). Many clinicians overestimate the likelihood of severe neutropenia and are reluctant to begin clozapine on an outpatient basis (Farooq et al. 2019). Education about the use of clozapine and its side effects can be useful in addressing clinician-related prescribing barriers.

When initiating treatment with clozapine, a slow dose titration is essential to minimize the risks of seizure, orthostatic hypotension, and excessive sedation (Clozaril 2019). Large, rapid increases in clozapine dosage have led to cardiovascular collapse and death, particularly in patients taking respiratory depressant medications such as benzodiazepines. From a starting dosage of 12.5 mg once or twice daily, the dosage of clozapine can be increased by, at most, 25–50 mg/day to a target dosage of 300–450 mg/day (Clozaril 2019). Subsequent dose increases, if needed, should be of 100 mg or less, once or twice weekly. Although efficacy is often seen at a dosage of 300–450 mg/day, some individuals may need higher dosages of clozapine, to a maximum daily dose of 900 mg, for full response. A slower rate of titration may be needed for patients with an initial episode of schizophrenia and in those who are older, severely debilitated, or sensitive to side effects. Those with a preexisting central nervous system condition, including individuals with 22q11.2 deletion syndrome, also warrant a slower rate of titration and may have an increased risk of seizures at usual doses. Use of divided doses can be helpful in reducing side effects during initial dose titration, although many patients are ultimately treated with a single dose at bedtime to minimize daytime sedation and facilitate adherence (Takeuchi et al. 2016).

Monitoring for therapeutic benefits and side effects of clozapine should occur throughout the dose titration phase (see Statement 4). Because titration of clozapine proceeds slowly, the therapeutic benefits may not be noticed immediately, and side effects may be more prominent than benefits. Thus, it can be helpful to provide patients with education and reassurance about the expected timetable of therapeutic effects of clozapine.

If clozapine is being resumed after a gap in treatment of 48 hours or more, it should be restarted at 12.5 mg once or twice daily. If that dosage is well tolerated, the dose may be increased to a therapeutic range more quickly than recommended for initial treatment. If a decision is made to stop clozapine, it is best to taper the dose unless the medication is being stopped for medically urgent reasons (e.g., severe neutropenia, myocarditis, NMS).

Use of Clozapine Levels During Treatment With Clozapine

While the dose of clozapine is being titrated, it is useful to obtain blood levels of clozapine and its major active metabolite, norclozapine (N-desmethylclozapine) (Couchman et al. 2010). Blood levels can also be helpful if there are questions about medication adherence, less efficacy or more side effects than expected, potential medication interactions, or other factors that may be influencing clozapine levels. Although there is substantial variation between individuals, clozapine levels on a specific dosage will generally be greater in nonsmokers than in smokers, in heavy caffeine users than in nonusers, in women than in men, and in older individuals than in younger individuals (Carrillo et al. 1998; Ismail et al. 2012). In addition, changing between different generic forms of clozapine can lead to a 5%–10% difference in blood levels. Levels of clozapine should be drawn at steady state (3 days or more after a dose change) and at a trough in medication levels (about 12 hours after the last dose). Typically, patients will receive a bedtime dose of clozapine and then have a level drawn the following morning before receiving an additional dose. There is not an absolute level of clozapine that is associated with either efficacy or toxicity (Remington et al. 2013; Spina et al. 2000; Stark and Scott 2012; Suzuki et al. 2011; VanderZwaag et al. 1996). In most patients, efficacy will be highest at levels greater than 350 ng/mL of clozapine, but some patients will show response or prevention of relapse at levels as low as 200 ng/mL. The risk of developing seizures increases with the blood level of clozapine.

As with the results of any laboratory test, interpretation of clozapine levels should consider the clinical context. For example, if a clozapine level is much higher than expected, assess for dose-related side effects and clinical evidence of toxicity. If the patient's clinical status does not suggest signs of clozapine toxicity, then determine the timing of the level (e.g., peak vs. trough) and identify any potential for drug interactions, changes in smoking status, or incorrect specimen labeling. If levels are much lower than expected, such factors as poor adherence, rapid metabolism, drug interactions, or changes in smoking status may also be relevant.

Typically, the level of norclozapine will be reported along with the blood level of clozapine. Norclozapine is the major active metabolite of clozapine and appears to differ from clozapine in efficacy and side effects. Nevertheless, the value of norclozapine levels in guiding clinical decisions is unclear. Because the half-life of norclozapine is greater than the half-life of clozapine, a clozapine:norclozapine ratio less than 0.5 can suggest poor adherence over the previous day or rapid metabolism of clozapine (e.g., via CYP1A2 induction). A clozapine:norclozapine ratio greater than 3.0 could suggest that metabolic pathways are saturated or inhibited by a concomitant medication. Shifts in the ratio of clozapine to norclozapine can also result from other drug-drug interactions or if nontrough levels are obtained (Couchman et al. 2010; Ellison and Dufresne 2015).

Monitoring for Side Effects During Treatment With Clozapine

With clozapine, safety monitoring during treatment is important to minimize the risk of adverse events. The Clozapine REMS Program (www.clozapinerems.com)[1] is required for prescribing of clozapine in the United States. The REMS program includes required training that must be completed by prescribers (Clozapine REMS Program 2019a), resource materials (Clozapine REMS Program 2019b), and a shared patient registry for all clozapine manufacturers' products that permits tracking of ANCs and documentation of decisions about continued treatment. The Clozapine REMS site provides instructions about threshold values for ANCs in hematologically normal individuals and in those with benign ethnic neutropenia, which is most common in individuals of African descent and is associated with ANCs that are lower than standard reference ranges (Clozapine REMS Program 2014). It also describes the required frequencies for ANC monitoring, which vary with ANC values. In patients who have stopped or interrupted treatment with clozapine for 30 days or more, the initial dose titration for clozapine and the monitoring frequency for treatment initiation should be followed.

Because the highest risk of severe neutropenia (ANC <500/μL) occurs within the initial 6 months of clozapine treatment (Alvir et al. 1993; Clozapine REMS Program 2019c; Myles et al. 2018), ANC monitoring is more frequent early in treatment and is required less often with longer treatment duration. The need for ANC monitoring can be a common practical issue for patients because of the time and transportation needed to obtain blood tests at a laboratory. The availability of point-of-care testing for white blood cell counts may mitigate these barriers for patients and facilitate treatment with clozapine.

In addition to neutropenia, clozapine treatment can be associated with several other important side effects. Potentially serious cardiac complications of clozapine treatment include myocarditis and cardiomyopathy. Myocarditis is infrequent and generally occurs during the first month of treatment, whereas cardiomyopathy is rare and generally occurs later in the treatment course (Bellissima et al. 2018; Ronaldson et al. 2015). Myocarditis usually is heralded by shortness of breath, tachycardia, and fever, but diagnosis can be challenging because of the nonspecific nature of other symptoms, which can include fatigue, chest pain, palpitations, peripheral edema, and hypereosinophilia. In patients who do develop myocarditis or cardiomyopathy in conjunction with clozapine treatment, clozapine is typically discontinued. Subsequent decisions about resuming clozapine are individualized and are based on the benefits and risks of treatment as compared with other therapeutic alternatives.

In patients who are treated with clozapine, a brief self-limiting fever (>38°C) may also occur during the first few weeks of clozapine treatment; this fever responds to supportive measures (Bruno et al. 2015; Lowe et al. 2007; Pui-yin Chung et al. 2008). However, in a febrile patient, it is essential to assess for the presence of potentially life-threatening complications, including NMS, severe neutropenia, infection, and myocarditis.

Other potentially serious side effects of clozapine treatment include seizures, orthostatic hypotension, and gastrointestinal effects. When seizures occur with clozapine, they typically occur with very high doses of clozapine, rapid increases in clozapine dose, or shifts in medication levels (related to drug-drug interactions or effects of smoking on drug metabolism) (Devinsky et al. 1991). Therefore, a slow initial titration of clozapine dose is essential, and patients should be cautioned not to drive or engage in other potentially hazardous activities while clozapine is being titrated. If a seizure does occur with clozapine, dose adjustment may be needed, or adjunctive anticonvulsant medication (e.g., valproate) may be considered in conjunction with neurological consultation (Alldredge 1999; Wong and Delva 2007).

Orthostatic hypotension can also occur with clozapine and is most common with treatment initiation. Older patients and patients with peripheral vascular disease or a compromised cardiovascular status may be at particular risk. When severe, orthostatic hypotension can cause syncope, dizziness, or falls. Patients who experience orthostatic hypotension must be cautioned to sit on the edge of the bed for a minute before standing up, move slowly when going from lying down or sitting to standing, and seek assistance when needed. Management strategies for orthostatic hypotension include supportive measures (e.g., use of support stockings, increased dietary salt and fluid intake), reducing the speed of clozapine dose titration, and decreasing or dividing doses of clozapine. As a last re-

---

[1]For Canadian prescribers, use the appropriate Canadian clozapine registry, not the U.S. Clozapine REMS Program.

sort, administration of the salt/fluid-retaining corticosteroid fludrocortisone can be considered to increase intravascular volume, but it is important to be mindful of the potential for immunosuppressive effects and development of diabetes with this medication (Mar and Raj 2018; Shen et al. 2017). For patients who are receiving concomitant antihypertensive treatment, adjustments to the dose of these medications may be needed.

Gastrointestinal effects of clozapine can also be significant and in some patients are associated with fecal impaction or paralytic ileus (Every-Palmer and Ellis 2017; Leung et al. 2017). Thus, the patient should obtain urgent medical care if experiencing constipation that is severe or does not resolve. To prevent development of constipation, it is useful to minimize the doses and number of contributory medications such as other anticholinergic medications and opioids. Activity and exercise should be encouraged to stimulate motility. A stool softener (e.g., docusate [Colace]) can be started for patients at increased risk (e.g., older patients). If constipation does develop, initial treatment can include stool softeners (e.g., docusate [Colace]) or osmotic laxatives (e.g., lactulose [Enulose], polyethylene glycol [Miralax], bisacody, [Dulcolax]). Second-line treatments include stimulant laxatives (e.g., senna [Senokot], senna tea, cascara, sodium picosulfate). If constipation persists, an enema (e.g., Fleet) should be considered. A combination of treatments may be needed to treat constipation and then to prevent its recurrence.

Side effects related to metabolic syndrome are common and generally are observed in the initial months of treatment but can also occur later in treatment. These side effects include weight gain (Alvarez-Jimenez et al. 2008; Leucht et al. 2013; Zhang et al. 2013); hyperlipidemia (Buhagiar and Jabbar 2019; Bushe and Paton 2005; Meyer and Koro 2004; Mitchell et al. 2013a); and glucose dysregulation, including development of diabetes mellitus (Hirsch et al. 2017; Ward and Druss 2015; Whicher et al. 2018; Zhang et al. 2017). Monitoring of body mass index, hemoglobin A1c, and lipid levels is important during clozapine treatment, as outlined in Statement 1, Table 2. If diabetes or hyperlipidemia is identified, it should be treated, typically by the patient's primary care clinician. When weight gain occurs, it is usually progressive over the first 6 months of treatment, although some patients continue to gain weight indefinitely (Alvarez-Jimenez et al. 2008). Prevention of weight gain should, thus, be a high priority because weight loss is difficult for most patients. Efforts should be made to intervene proactively with weight gain of 5–10 pounds, and other medications that can cause weight gain (e.g., valproate) should be tapered and discontinued when possible. Dietary interventions, such as specialized behavioral health interventions, in-person community interventions (e.g., Weight Watchers), services that include meal delivery (e.g., Jenny Craig), or Internet-based interventions (e.g., Omada Health), should be suggested (Bonfioli et al. 2012).

In collaboration with the patient's primary care clinician, metformin or nonstimulant medications for weight loss can be considered. Metformin has been shown to be safe in individuals without hyperglycemia and can reduce body weight and reverse metabolic abnormalities in patients with obesity or other metabolic problems (Das et al. 2012; de Silva et al. 2016; McGinty et al. 2016; Mizuno et al. 2014; Siskind et al. 2016a; Vancampfort et al. 2019; Zheng et al. 2015; Zhuo et al. 2018). Fewer studies have been done with glucagon-like peptide-1 agonist medications, but the available data suggest that body weight and metabolic risk factors are reduced by these medications as compared with placebo (Siskind et al. 2019). The benefits of exercise appear to be small in terms of weight loss in individuals with schizophrenia (Firth et al. 2015; Pearsall et al. 2014; Vancampfort et al. 2017, 2019). Nevertheless, many individuals with schizophrenia do not engage in physical activity (Stubbs et al. 2016a; Vancampfort et al. 2016b), and exercise can be suggested for its benefits for overall health, improved cardiorespiratory fitness, and other aspects of functioning (Dauwan et al. 2016; Firth et al. 2015, 2017; Vancampfort et al. 2017, 2019).

Sedation, sialorrhea, and tachycardia are each commonly observed during treatment with clozapine but can generally be managed conservatively. Sedation is most pronounced in the initial phases of treatment with clozapine, and many patients develop some tolerance to the sedating effects with continued administration. However, persistent sedation, including daytime drowsiness and increased sleep time, can interfere with social, recreational, and vocational function. Lowering of the daily dose, consolidating divided doses into one evening dose, or changing to a less sedating antipsychotic medication may be effective in reducing the severity of sedation. Coffee or other forms of caffeine can be helpful in the morning but can also interact with medications (e.g., contribute to tachycardia; raise blood levels of medications, including clozapine). Adding a stimulant medication is not typically helpful and can lead to additional side effects. If sedation or the risk of sedation is significant (e.g., during initial clozapine titration), patients should be cautioned not to drive or engage in potentially hazardous activities.

Sialorrhea (or hypersalivation) is also a frequent side effect of clozapine that can contribute to reductions in quality of life and complications such as aspiration pneumonia (Dzahini et al. 2018; Kaplan et al. 2018; Stoecker et al. 2017). Because sialorrhea may be more bothersome at night, patients may be advised to place a towel on their pillow and change to a clean towel in the middle of the night to minimize discomfort. During the day, patients can be encouraged to chew sugarless gum, which stimulates the swallowing reflex. Pharmacological approaches to address sialorrhea come from small studies and case reports and include use of low-dose or topical anticholinergic medications, such as glycopyrrolate or sublingual ophthalmic atropine 1% drops (Bird et al. 2011; Liang et al. 2010; Man et al. 2017). Diphenhydramine has also been studied (Chen et al. 2019); however, because clozapine and other antipsychotics can have significant anticholinergic properties themselves and anticholinergics have small effects on sialorrhea, the use of agents with added anticholinergic effects should be approached cautiously. Terazosin and, in severe refractory cases, botulinum toxin have also been used (Bird et al. 2011; Liang et al. 2010; Man et al. 2017).

Healthy patients can usually tolerate some increase in resting pulse rate, although this may not be the case for patients with preexisting heart disease. In patients with significant tachycardia (heart rates above 110–120 bpm), an ECG is warranted, as is assessment for other potential causes of tachycardia (e.g., fever, anemia, smoking, hyperthyroidism, respiratory disease, cardiovascular disorders, caffeine, other stimulants, and side effects of other medications). Early in treatment with clozapine, the possibility of myocarditis should be considered. If tachycardia is accompanied by pain, shortness of breath, fever, or signs of a myocardial infarction or heart rhythm problem, emergency assessment is essential. Management strategies for tachycardia with any antipsychotic medication include reducing the dose of medication; discontinuing medications with anticholinergic or stimulant properties; and addressing orthostatic hypotension, if present. Case reports have discussed the use of medications such as β-blocking agents for persistent and significant tachycardia with clozapine. Nevertheless, treatment is not indicated unless the patient is symptomatic or the patient's heart rate is substantially greater than 120 bpm because data from more rigorous studies are not available and these medications can contribute to other side effects such as orthostatic hypotension (Lally et al. 2016a).

Side effects related to dopamine D_2 receptor antagonism (e.g., acute dystonia, akathisia, medication-induced parkinsonism, NMS, tardive syndromes, hyperprolactinemia) can occur but are less frequent with clozapine than with many other antipsychotic medications. For additional information on the recognition and management of these side effects, see Statement 4, subsection "Treatment-Emergent Side Effects of Antipsychotic Medications."

Other Approaches to Treatment-Resistant Schizophrenia

For all patients with treatment-resistant schizophrenia, it is important to conduct a review of the treatment plan at periodic intervals (see Statement 3). In addition to a review of prior medication trials, it is essential to review the psychosocial treatments that a patient has received and whether addition of one or more psychosocial interventions would be of benefit. For example, some patients may not have received cognitive-behavioral therapy for psychosis (CBTp) as recommended in Statement 16 or initial benefits of CBTp may have faded if CBTp was stopped. Under such circumstances, treatment with CBTp may be warranted (Burns et al. 2014; Morrison et al. 2018). Engaging families or persons of support in CBTp can also be helpful (Turkington and Spencer 2019). A similar review of potential additions to the treatment plan can occur with other psychosocial treatments.

Optimizing Treatment With Clozapine

Although studies suggest that at least one-third of individuals with treatment-resistant schizophrenia will respond to clozapine (Kahn et al. 2018; McEvoy et al. 2006), some patients will not have a complete response. Before concluding that a patient has not responded to clozapine, it is important to assure that an adequate target dose has been reached (typically 300–450 mg/day) and that steady state levels of clozapine and norclozapine appear sufficient to produce therapeutic benefit. Although no absolute level of clozapine is associated with efficacy (Remington et al. 2013; Spina et al. 2000; Suzuki et al. 2011; VanderZwaag et al. 1996), if no response is evident and clozapine is well tolerated, the clozapine dose should be increased to achieve a clozapine level of greater than 350 ng/mL. In general, this dose of medication should be continued for at least 8 weeks to determine response, although further increases in dose can also be made, as tolerated. If there continues to be no evidence of benefit, as for any patient treated with clozapine, the value of the medication should be assessed periodically in terms of the patient's response, the medication side effects, and the availability of any newer treatment options. Longitudinal use of a quantitative measure (see Statement 2) can be helpful in assessing functioning and overall response and identifying specific symptoms that have or have not responded to treatment.

Continuing Clozapine and Augmenting With Another Medication

For individuals who do not respond to clozapine alone, the evidence base for other treatments is limited, although a number of options have been tried. Augmentation of clozapine with another medication has shown no significant benefit in double-blind trials, although some benefit was noted in open-label trials and meta-analyses of trials that were generally of low quality (Barber et al. 2017; Correll et al. 2017b; Galling et al. 2017; Sinclair and Adams 2014; Siskind et al. 2018; Veerman et al. 2014; Wagner et al. 2019a). Studies have included augmentation with other antipsychotic medications (FGAs and SGAs), anticonvulsants, and other medications. If a trial of augmentation therapy is undertaken, it is important to consider the potential additive effects of the medications on side effects and the potential for drug-drug interactions. Periodic review of the patient's medication regimen is also important in order to identify and reduce or discontinue medications that are not effective, that are no longer necessary, or that are contributing to an inordinate burden of side effects. As noted in the previous subsection, longitudinal use of a quantitative measure can assist in making such determinations.

Augmenting Clozapine or Another Antipsychotic Medication With Electroconvulsive Therapy

There is also evidence for benefits of ECT in combination with clozapine as compared with clozapine alone in most (Ahmed et al. 2017; Grover et al. 2015; Lally et al. 2016b; Petrides et al. 2015; Pompili et al. 2013; G. Wang et al. 2018), but not all (Melzer-Ribeiro et al. 2017), studies. Rates of headache and reports of memory impairment were more frequent with clozapine plus ECT than with clozapine alone; however, symptomatic improvement and rates of remission at the end of treatment were significantly greater in the group that received adjunctive ECT. For this reason, ECT could be considered for clozapine-resistant schizophrenia, particularly in patients who also have catatonia or significant suicide risk or who require a rapid response because of the severity of their psychiatric or medical condition. For individuals who show a response to ECT, treatment with ECT on a maintenance basis could be considered as an adjunct to clozapine.

Some studies have shown evidence for benefits of ECT in combination with antipsychotic medications other than clozapine (Ahmed et al. 2017; Ali et al. 2019; Pompili et al. 2013; Sinclair et al. 2019; Zheng et al. 2016). Particularly in patients who also have catatonia or significant suicide risk or who require a rapid response due to the severity of their psychiatric or medical condition, ECT could be considered. For individuals who show a response to ECT, treatment with ECT on a maintenance basis could be considered.

Although studies have also been done with TMS for treatment of hallucinations and for treatment of negative symptoms, at present there is insufficient evidence of benefit to suggest use of TMS in individuals with schizophrenia (Dollfus et al. 2016; Dougall et al. 2015; He et al. 2017).

Balancing of Potential Benefits and Harms in Rating the Strength of the Guideline Statement

Benefits

Use of clozapine in individuals with treatment-resistant schizophrenia can be associated with reductions in psychotic symptoms, higher rates of treatment response, and lower rates of treatment discontinuation due to lack of efficacy (low to moderate strength of research evidence) as well as lower rates of self-harm, suicide attempts, or hospitalizations to prevent suicide (moderate strength of research evidence). Overall rates of hospitalization are also reduced during treatment with clozapine as compared with other oral antipsychotic medications (low strength of research evidence). All-cause mortality is also reduced in individuals treated with clozapine as compared with other individuals with treatment-resistant schizophrenia (moderate strength of research evidence).

Harms

Although overall rates of adverse events do not differ with clozapine as compared with risperidone (low strength of research evidence), clozapine does have a higher risk of study withdrawal due to adverse events than some other SGAs (low strength of research evidence). Specific harms of using clozapine include rare but serious effects, including severe neutropenia, myocarditis, cardiomyopathy, and NMS. These harms cannot be eliminated, but risks of severe neutropenia are lessened by required ANC monitoring. Early attention to and recognition of NMS and cardiac complications of clozapine use may also reduce risk. Seizures are also more frequent with clozapine than other antipsychotics but can be minimized by slow titration of the clozapine dose, avoidance of very high clozapine doses, and attention to pharmacokinetic factors that may lead to rapid shifts in clozapine levels. Constipation can also be significant with clozapine and in some patients is associated with fecal impaction or paralytic ileus. Other side effects that are more common with clozapine than other antipsychotic medications include sialorrhea, tachycardia, fever, dizziness, sedation, and weight gain. Rates of hyperglycemia and diabetes may also be increased.

Patient Preferences

Clinical experience suggests that many patients are cooperative with and accepting of clozapine as part of a treatment plan; however, other patients may express concerns about the burdens of required blood work, including logistical barriers such as access to transportation (Farooq et al. 2019; Gee et al. 2017; Verdoux et al. 2018). Concerns about other side effects, such as weight gain or somnolence, may also contribute to a reluctance to switch to clozapine (Achtyes et al. 2018). On the other hand, when deciding about medication changes, most patients value an ability to think more clearly and stop hallucinations or delusions (Achtyes et al. 2018; Kuhnigk et al. 2012; Levitan et al. 2015), and most patients who receive clozapine view it positively. For example, one large survey of individuals with schizophrenia or schizoaffective disorder who were taking an antipsychotic medication found that the vast majority of those taking clozapine adhered to treatment and found it helpful, whereas only approximately 5% found it not helpful (Siskind et al. 2017a). In contrast, most other antipsychotic medications were viewed less positively (Siskind et al. 2017a). In addition, in the CATIE study, clozapine and combination antipsychotic treatment regimens were frequently selected by patients who stopped a previous medication because of inadequate therapeutic effect and by those with relatively severe symptoms (Stroup et al. 2009).

Balancing of Benefits and Harms

The potential benefits of this guideline statement were viewed as far outweighing the potential harms. For individuals with treatment-resistant schizophrenia, the risks of inadequately treated illness are substantial in terms of reduced quality of life (Kennedy et al. 2014) and increased mortality (Cho et al. 2019; Vermeulen et al. 2019; Wimberley et al. 2017) as well as negative effects for informal caregivers (Brain et al. 2018). Even in individuals who have had an inadequate response to other antipsychotic medications, a substantial fraction shows a clinically relevant response to clozapine. With careful monitoring to minimize the risk of harms from clozapine, the benefits of clozapine in patients with treatment-resistant schizophrenia were viewed as significantly outweighing the harms of treatment. For additional discussion of the research evidence, see Appendix C, Statement 7.

Differences of Opinion Among Writing Group Members

There were no differences of opinion. The writing group voted unanimously in favor of this recommendation.

Review of Available Guidelines From Other Organizations

Practice guidelines (BAP, CSG, NICE, RANZCP, SIGN, WFSBP, PORT) are consistent in recommending clozapine for individuals with treatment-resistant schizophrenia (Barnes et al. 2011; Buchanan et al. 2010; Galletly et al. 2016; Hasan et al. 2012; National Institute for Health and Care Excellence 2014; Scottish Intercollegiate Guidelines Network 2013). In terms of other therapies for treatment-resistant schizophrenia, several guidelines (SIGN, WFSBP, BAP) recommend augmentation treatment with an antidepressant for treatment-resistant illness associated with negative symptoms (Barnes et al. 2011; Hasan et al. 2012; Scottish Intercollegiate Guidelines Network 2013). For individuals with catatonia, the WFSBP recommends benzodiazepines and ECT (Hasan et al. 2012). In addition, ECT is mentioned in several guidelines (e.g., SIGN, RANZCP, WFSBP) as being appropriate in individuals with treatment-resistant schizophrenia.

Quality Measurement Considerations

Studies suggest that clozapine is underused and that a significant proportion of individuals with treatment-resistant schizophrenia do not receive treatment with clozapine, although there is significant variation between and within countries (Addington et al. 2012; Bachmann et al. 2017; Carruthers et al. 2016; Keller et al. 2014; Olfson et al. 2016; Stroup et al. 2014; Tang et al. 2017). Thus, internal quality improvement programs may wish to focus on ways to increase use of clozapine in individuals with treatment-resistant schizophrenia and track rates of clozapine use in this patient population. Internal quality improvement programs could also focus on increasing use of quantitative measures (i.e., rating scales) to improve identification of individuals with treatment-resistant schizophrenia and facilitate systematic longitudinal tracking of functioning, symptoms, and side-effect burdens. If quality measures are considered for development at the provider, facility, health plan, integrated delivery system, or population level, testing of feasibility, usability, reliability, and validity would be essential prior to use for purposes of accountability.

Electronic decision support would be challenging to implement and would depend on accurate and consistent entry of structured information. Nevertheless, in combination with rating scale data and prior prescribing histories, electronic decision support could help identify individuals with treatment-resistant illness who would benefit from a trial of clozapine.

STATEMENT 8: Clozapine in Suicide Risk

APA *recommends* **(1B)** that patients with schizophrenia be treated with clozapine if the risk for suicide attempts or suicide remains substantial despite other treatments.*

Implementation

Treatment with clozapine can be effective in reducing suicidal behavior if risk remains substantial despite other treatments. In addition, treatment with clozapine can be effective in reducing rates of suicide attempts and suicide in individuals with schizophrenia, regardless of whether formal criteria for treatment resistance have been met. Risk factors for suicidal behavior in individuals with schizophrenia are described in Statement 1, subsection "Implementation." Although demographic and historical risk factors are static, a number of other risk factors are potentially modifiable and can serve as targets of intervention in constructing a plan of treatment (for additional details, see Statement 3). As in other circumstances in which patients do not appear to be responding fully to treatment, attention to adherence is crucial (for additional details, see Statement 3). For details of initiating and monitoring clozapine treatment, see Statement 7, subsections "Initiation of Treatment With Clozapine," "Use of Clozapine Levels During Treatment With Clozapine," and "Monitoring for Side Effects During Treatment With Clozapine."

Balancing of Potential Benefits and Harms in Rating the Strength of the Guideline Statement

Benefits

In individuals with schizophrenia who are at significant risk for suicide attempts or suicide, use of clozapine can be associated with lower rates of self-harm, suicide attempts, or hospitalization to prevent suicide (moderate strength of research evidence). Additional benefits of clozapine treatment include higher rates of treatment response (low to moderate strength of research evidence) and reductions in psychotic symptoms, all-cause mortality, overall hospitalization rates, and treatment discontinuation due to lack of efficacy (low to moderate strength of research evidence).

Harms

Although overall rates of adverse events do not differ with clozapine as compared with risperidone (low strength of research evidence), clozapine does have a higher risk of study withdrawal due to adverse events than some other SGAs (low strength of research evidence). Specific harms of using clozapine include rare but serious effects, including severe neutropenia, myocarditis, cardiomyopathy, and NMS. These harms cannot be eliminated, but risks of severe neutropenia are lessened by required ANC monitoring. Early attention to and recognition of NMS and cardiac complications of clozapine use may also reduce risk. Seizures are also more frequent with clozapine than other antipsychotics but can be minimized by slow titration of the clozapine dose, avoidance of very high clozapine doses, and attention to pharmacokinetic factors that may lead to rapid shifts in clozapine levels. Constipation can also be significant with clozapine and in some patients is associated with fecal impaction or paralytic ileus. Other side effects that are more common with clozapine than other antipsychotic medications include sialorrhea, tachycardia, fever, dizziness, sedation, and weight gain. Rates of hyperglycemia and diabetes may also be increased.

---

*This guideline statement should be implemented in the context of a person-centered treatment plan that includes evidence-based nonpharmacological and pharmacological treatments for schizophrenia.

Patient Preferences

Clinical experience suggests that many patients are cooperative with and accepting of clozapine as part of a treatment plan; however, other patients may express concerns about the burdens of required blood work, including logistical barriers such as access to transportation (Farooq et al. 2019; Gee et al. 2017; Verdoux et al. 2018). Concerns about other side effects, such as weight gain or somnolence, may also contribute to a reluctance to switch to clozapine (Achtyes et al. 2018). On the other hand, when deciding about medication changes, most patients value an ability to think more clearly and stop hallucinations or delusions (Achtyes et al. 2018; Kuhnigk et al. 2012; Levitan et al. 2015), and most patients who receive clozapine view it positively. For example, one large survey of individuals with schizophrenia or schizoaffective disorder who were taking an antipsychotic medication found that the vast majority of those taking clozapine adhered to treatment and found it helpful, whereas only approximately 5% found it not helpful (Siskind et al. 2017a). In contrast, most other antipsychotic medications were viewed less positively (Siskind et al. 2017a).

Balancing of Benefits and Harms

The potential benefits of this recommendation were viewed as far outweighing the potential harms. For individuals at significant risk for suicide attempts or suicide despite other treatments, the benefit of clozapine in reducing suicide-related risk is significant. With careful monitoring to minimize the risk of harms from clozapine, the benefit of clozapine in such patients was viewed as significantly outweighing the harms of treatment. For additional discussion of the research evidence, see Appendix C, Statement 8.

Differences of Opinion Among Writing Group Members

There were no differences of opinion. The writing group voted unanimously in favor of this recommendation.

Review of Available Guidelines From Other Organizations

Other guidelines do not specifically mention the use of clozapine for individuals with schizophrenia who are at substantial risk for suicide attempts or suicide despite other treatment. Guidelines (BAP, CSG, NICE, RANZCP, SIGN, WFSBP, PORT) are consistent, however, in recommending clozapine for individuals with treatment-resistant schizophrenia (Barnes et al. 2011; Buchanan et al. 2010; Galletly et al. 2016; Hasan et al. 2012; National Institute for Health and Care Excellence 2014; Scottish Intercollegiate Guidelines Network 2013).

Quality Measurement Considerations

Studies suggest that clozapine is underused and that a significant proportion of individuals with treatment-resistant schizophrenia do not receive treatment with clozapine, although there is significant variation between and within countries (Addington et al. 2012; Bachmann et al. 2017; Carruthers et al. 2016; Keller et al. 2014; Olfson et al. 2016; Stroup et al. 2014; Tang et al. 2017). Given low utilization of clozapine in general (Addington et al. 2012; Bachmann et al. 2017; Carruthers et al. 2016; Keller et al. 2014; Olfson et al. 2016; Stroup et al. 2014; Tang et al. 2017) and the high rates of suicidal ideas among individuals with treatment-resistant schizophrenia (Kennedy et al. 2014), it is likely that many individuals at significant suicide risk are not receiving treatment with clozapine. Thus, internal quality improvement programs may wish to focus on ways to increase and track use of clozapine in individuals with schizophrenia who have significant suicide risk that persists despite other treatments. Internal quality improvement programs could also focus on increasing the use of quantitative measures to improve identification and monitoring of individuals with risk factors for suicide.

If quality measures are considered for development at the provider, facility, health plan, integrated delivery system, or population level, testing of feasibility, usability, reliability, and validity would be essential prior to use for purposes of accountability. In particular, it is currently not possible to identify from most administrative data people at increased risk for suicide. Clinical assessment or patient self-report data are likely to be required.

Electronic decision support using passive alerts may be able to prompt clinicians to consider clozapine; however, such prompts would be challenging to implement because they would depend on accurate and consistent entry of structured information about diagnosis, suicidal ideation, and suicide attempts. Nevertheless, in combination with rating scale data, electronic decision support could help identify individuals with schizophrenia and significant suicide risk who would benefit from a trial of clozapine.

STATEMENT 9: Clozapine in Aggressive Behavior

APA *suggests* (2C) that patients with schizophrenia be treated with clozapine if the risk for aggressive behavior remains substantial despite other treatments.*

Implementation

Treatment with clozapine can be effective in reducing aggressive behavior if risk remains substantial despite other treatments. As in other circumstances in which patients do not appear to be responding fully to treatment, attention to adherence is crucial (for additional details, see Statement 3). Risk factors for aggressive behavior in individuals with schizophrenia are described in Statement 1, subsection "Implementation." Although demographic and historical risk factors are static, a number of other risk factors are potentially modifiable and can serve as targets of intervention in constructing a plan of treatment (for additional details, see Statement 3). For details of initiating and monitoring clozapine treatment, see Statement 7, subsections "Initiation of Treatment With Clozapine," "Use of Clozapine Levels During Treatment With Clozapine," and "Monitoring for Side Effects During Treatment With Clozapine."

Balancing of Potential Benefits and Harms in Rating the Strength of the Guideline Statement

Benefits

In individuals with schizophrenia who are at significant risk for aggressive behavior, use of clozapine may reduce the likelihood of aggressive behaviors (low strength of research evidence). Additional benefits of clozapine treatment include higher rates of treatment response (low to moderate strength of research evidence); reductions in psychotic symptoms, all-cause mortality, overall hospitalization rates, and treatment discontinuation due to lack of efficacy (low to moderate strength of research evidence); and lower rates of self-harm, suicide attempts, or hospitalizations to prevent suicide (moderate strength of research evidence).

Harms

Although overall rates of adverse events do not differ with clozapine as compared with risperidone (low strength of research evidence), clozapine does have a higher risk of study withdrawal due to adverse events than some other SGAs (low strength of research evidence). Specific harms of using clozapine include rare but serious effects, including severe neutropenia, myocarditis, cardiomyopa-

---

*This guideline statement should be implemented in the context of a person-centered treatment plan that includes evidence-based nonpharmacological and pharmacological treatments for schizophrenia.

thy, and NMS. These harms cannot be eliminated, but risks of severe neutropenia are lessened by required ANC monitoring. Early attention to and recognition of NMS and cardiac complications of clozapine use may also reduce risk. Seizures are also more frequent with clozapine than other antipsychotics but can be minimized by slow titration of the clozapine dose, avoidance of very high clozapine doses, and attention to pharmacokinetic factors that may lead to rapid shifts in clozapine levels. Constipation can also be significant with clozapine and in some patients is associated with fecal impaction or paralytic ileus. Other side effects that are more common with clozapine than other antipsychotic medications include sialorrhea, tachycardia, fever, dizziness, sedation, and weight gain. Rates of hyperglycemia and diabetes may also be increased.

Patient Preferences

Clinical experience suggests that many patients are cooperative with and accepting of clozapine as part of a treatment plan; however, other patients may express concerns about the burdens of required blood work, including logistical barriers such as access to transportation (Farooq et al. 2019; Gee et al. 2017; Verdoux et al. 2018). Concerns about other side effects, such as weight gain or somnolence, may also contribute to a reluctance to switch to clozapine (Achtyes et al. 2018). On the other hand, when deciding about medication changes, most patients value an ability to think more clearly and stop hallucinations or delusions (Achtyes et al. 2018; Kuhnigk et al. 2012; Levitan et al. 2015), and most patients who receive clozapine view it positively. For example, one large survey of individuals with schizophrenia or schizoaffective disorder who were taking an antipsychotic medication found that the vast majority of those taking clozapine adhered to treatment and found it helpful, whereas only approximately 5% found it not helpful (Siskind et al. 2017a). In contrast, most other antipsychotic medications were viewed less positively (Siskind et al. 2017a).

Balancing of Benefits and Harms

The potential benefits of this guideline statement were viewed as likely to outweigh the potential harms. For individuals at significant risk for aggressive behavior despite other treatments, there appears to be some benefit of clozapine in reducing aggression risk. In addition, clozapine may lead to indirect reductions in the risk of aggressive behavior by reducing other contributory risk factors for aggression such as hallucinations and delusions. Thus, with consideration of patient preferences and careful monitoring to minimize the risk of harms from clozapine, the benefit of clozapine in such patients was viewed as likely to outweigh the harms of treatment. For additional discussion of the research evidence, see Appendix C, Statement 9.

Differences of Opinion Among Writing Group Members

There were no differences of opinion. The writing group voted unanimously in favor of this suggestion.

Review of Available Guidelines From Other Organizations

Information from other guidelines is consistent with this guideline statement. The SIGN, RANZCP, BAP, and PORT guidelines all suggest consideration of clozapine for individuals with hostility or aggressive behaviors that do not respond to other interventions (Barnes et al. 2011; Buchanan et al. 2010; Galletly et al. 2016; Hasan et al. 2012; Scottish Intercollegiate Guidelines Network 2013). In addition, guidelines (BAP, CSG, NICE, RANZCP, SIGN, WFSBP, PORT) are consistent in recommending clozapine for individuals with treatment-resistant schizophrenia (Barnes et al. 2011; Buchanan et al. 2010; Galletly et al. 2016; Hasan et al. 2012; National Institute for Health and Care Excellence 2014; Scottish Intercollegiate Guidelines Network 2013).

Quality Measurement Considerations

As a suggestion, this guideline statement is not appropriate for use as a quality measure for purposes of accountability. Electronic decision support using passive alerts may be able to prompt clinicians to consider clozapine; however, such prompts would be challenging to implement because they would depend on accurate and consistent entry of structured information about diagnosis and risk factors for aggression. Nevertheless, in combination with rating scale data, electronic decision support could help identify individuals with schizophrenia and significant aggression risk who may benefit from a trial of clozapine.

STATEMENT 10: Long-Acting Injectable Antipsychotic Medications

APA *suggests* **(2B)** that patients receive treatment with a long-acting injectable antipsychotic medication if they prefer such treatment or if they have a history of poor or uncertain adherence.*

Implementation

LAI formulations of antipsychotic medications can provide a number of benefits for patients, families, and clinicians, yet they are often underutilized (Brown et al. 2014; Correll et al. 2016; Lawson et al. 2015; Sultana et al. 2019). Racial differences also exist in the proportion of individuals who are treated with LAI antipsychotic medications, with greater use of these formulations in Black patients than in white patients (Brown et al. 2014; Lawson et al. 2015).

With LAI antipsychotic medications, there is greater assurance that a patient will receive medication continuously because there are fewer opportunities to miss a medication dose and clinicians will be immediately aware of a missed visit or injection, yielding greater time for intervention before symptoms recur (Correll et al. 2016; Velligan et al. 2010; West et al. 2008). Presumably due to improved adherence, advantages of LAI antipsychotics include the potential for a decreased risk of mortality; reduced risk of hospitalization; and decreased rates of treatment discontinuation, including discontinuation due to inefficacy (see Appendix C, Statement 10). Other benefits for patients include a subjective sense of better symptom control, greater convenience as a result of needing to take fewer medications daily, and reduced conflict with family members or other persons of support related to medication-related reminders (Caroli et al. 2011; Correll et al. 2016; Iyer et al. 2013; Yeo et al. 2019). Although some patients may not wish to experience the discomfort associated with receiving injections of medications, this is not a major barrier for most patients. In addition, discomfort can often be minimized by using SGA LAIs rather than FGA LAIs, which have sesame oil–based vehicles, or by using an LAI with a small injection volume or lower administration frequency (Correll et al. 2016).

Consistent with principles of patient-centered care, it may be preferable to educate patients about the availability of LAI antipsychotic medications when discussing other aspects of antipsychotic treatment. Indeed, many patients will accept and may prefer LAIs if provided with information about the pluses and minuses of LAIs in the context of shared decision-making (Caroli et al. 2011; Heres et al. 2007; Kane et al. 2019; Waddell and Taylor 2009; Weiden et al. 2015; Yeo et al. 2019). Preference rates for LAIs are even higher among individuals who have personal experience in receiving an LAI formulation of an antipsychotic medication (Heres et al. 2007; Patel et al. 2009; Waddell and Taylor 2009).

---

*This guideline statement should be implemented in the context of a person-centered treatment plan that includes evidence-based nonpharmacological and pharmacological treatments for schizophrenia.

Discussions about LAI antipsychotic medications often occur with patients who have had difficulty in adhering to oral medications. However, such discussions can also take place at other junctures. For example, if an individual has not responded to treatment with an oral antipsychotic medication, a trial of an LAI may be warranted (Howes et al. 2017; see Statement 4, subsection "Strategies to Address Initial Nonresponse or Partial Response to Antipsychotic Treatment") because breaks in the continuity of oral medication therapy can be unrecognized (Lopez et al. 2017). An LAI formulation of an antipsychotic may also be considered when patients are transitioning between settings (e.g., at inpatient discharge, on release from a correctional facility), when future adherence is uncertain and the risk of reduced adherence may be increased. Although LAI antipsychotic medications have typically been used in individuals with multiple episodes of schizophrenia, some studies have used an LAI antipsychotic formulation earlier in the course of illness (Kane et al. 2019; Subotnik et al. 2015), when rates of poor adherence may be greater. Earlier discussion of an LAI may also be considered in individuals who are at increased risk of poor adherence due to a limited awareness of needing treatment or a co-occurring substance use disorder (García et al. 2016; Velligan et al. 2009).

If a decision is made to initiate treatment with an LAI, aspects of medication selection are similar to those for selection of an oral medication in terms of considering prior response, prior tolerability, pharmacological considerations, and side-effect profiles (see Statement 4). Patients may also have specific preferences and values related to the frequency of injection and the type and location of the injection (e.g., IM deltoid or gluteal sites, subcutaneous abdominal site; Heres et al. 2012). Because the oral and LAI formulations of a specific antipsychotic medication are comparable, a trial of the same oral antipsychotic will typically occur first to assure efficacy and tolerability (SMI Adviser 2019). Patients will experience medication side effects for a longer period of time after drug discontinuation with LAIs than with oral medications because of pharmacokinetic differences in the formulations, but this is not usually a problem if the oral formulation has first been well tolerated. Nevertheless, caution is warranted in a patient who has experienced NMS previously (Correll et al. 2016).

The conversion from an oral dose of medication to a corresponding dose of an LAI antipsychotic depends on the specific medication (see Statement 4, Tables 7, 8, and 9; Meyer 2013, 2017); product labeling for each medication describes approximate conversion ratios and whether a period of concomitant oral and LAI medication is needed. If the patient is taking an oral medication that lacks a corresponding LAI formulation, a change in antipsychotic medication may be needed if an LAI formulation is clinically indicated or preferred (see Statement 6).

When administering LAI antipsychotic injections, it is important to follow recommendations for safe injection practices (Centers for Disease Control and Prevention 2019a, 2019b) and infection control precautions (Centers for Disease Control and Prevention 2016, 2019b) as well as instructions from product labeling. Product labeling also contains important information on storage and reconstitution of LAI antipsychotic formulations as well as information on how to handle missed or late doses of medications (see Statement 4, Tables 7–9).

There are several barriers related to the use of LAI formulations of antipsychotic medications. For patients, there may be logistical barriers (e.g., access to transportation, childcare, school or work schedules) that depend on the frequency of appointments needed to receive an LAI antipsychotic medication. Other logistical barriers for patients may relate to such factors as cost or insurance authorizations for LAI antipsychotic agents. For clinicians, lack of knowledge and limited experience in using LAI antipsychotic medications contribute to underuse (Correll et al. 2016). Skill and experience in administering injections may be lacking, and nursing staff may not be available to give injections.

Additional barriers relate to the decision to suggest an LAI antipsychotic medication. Clinicians often do not consider LAI antipsychotic medications as a treatment option (Hamann et al. 2014; Heres et al. 2006; Kirschner et al. 2013; Weiden et al. 2015), even when such use is appropriate. Furthermore, clinicians may overestimate patients' adherence with oral medications when considering relative benefits of LAIs (Correll et al. 2016; Lopez et al. 2017) or underestimate the acceptability of

LAIs to patients (Hamann et al. 2010; Iyer et al. 2013; Patel et al. 2010a, 2010b; Weiden et al. 2015). At an organizational level, there may be a lack of resources, space, or trained personnel to administer injections (Correll et al. 2016; Velligan et al. 2011). Thus, workflows may need to be adjusted, partnerships may need to be developed with primary care clinicians to administer LAI antipsychotic injections, or other concerted efforts may be needed to address logistical and clinical barriers to LAI antipsychotic use.

Balancing of Potential Benefits and Harms in Rating the Strength of the Guideline Statement

Benefits

Use of an LAI antipsychotic medication in the treatment of schizophrenia may be associated with improved outcomes. Although meta-analyses of head-to-head RCTs comparing LAI with oral antipsychotics (McDonagh et al. 2017) and other meta-analyses of RCTs (Kishi et al. 2016a, 2016b; Kishimoto et al. 2014; Ostuzzi et al. 2017) do not show evidence of benefit from LAIs relative to oral antipsychotic medications, observational data from nationwide registry databases (Taipale et al. 2018a, 2018b; Tiihonen et al. 2011, 2017), cohort studies (Kishimoto et al. 2018), and "mirror image" studies (Kishimoto et al. 2013) suggest that use of LAI antipsychotic agents as compared with oral antipsychotic medications is associated with a decreased risk of mortality, reduced risk of hospitalization, and decreased rates of study discontinuation (including discontinuation due to inefficacy).

Harms

The harms of using an LAI antipsychotic medication in the treatment of schizophrenia are generally comparable to the harms of using an oral formulation of the same medication. For some patients, side effects with LAIs may be less problematic because peaks and troughs of medication levels will be less prominent than with oral medications because of the pharmacokinetic differences in the medication formulations. On the other hand, patients may experience medication side effects for a longer period of time with LAIs than with oral medications, again because of pharmacokinetic differences. In addition, patients may experience injection-related side effects, including pain, swelling, redness, or induration at the injection site, with LAI antipsychotic agents.

Patient Preferences

Clinical experience suggests that many patients are cooperative with and accepting of an LAI antipsychotic medication as part of a treatment plan, particularly when the option of an LAI and the pluses and minuses of an LAI antipsychotic are reviewed in the context of shared decision-making (Caroli et al. 2011; Heres et al. 2007; Kane et al. 2019; Waddell and Taylor 2009; Weiden et al. 2015; Yeo et al. 2019). Attitudes about LAIs are typically more positive among patients who have previously received or currently receive an LAI antipsychotic medication than in those who have never been treated with an LAI medication (Patel et al. 2009). Many patients prefer the convenience of receiving an infrequent injection rather than needing to remember to take oral medications. They also value the potential benefits of an LAI antipsychotic medication in terms of better subjective symptom reduction or improved long-term outcomes. On the other hand, some patients may not wish to experience the discomfort associated with receiving injections of medications.

Balancing of Benefits and Harms

The potential benefits of this guideline statement were viewed as likely to outweigh the potential harms. The outcomes associated with use of an LAI formulation of an antipsychotic medication are at least as good as using an oral formulation of the medication and may be better, particularly in terms of treatment discontinuation, rehospitalization, and mortality risk. Many experts infer that the relative benefits of LAI antipsychotic medications as compared with equivalent oral formulations are related to improved adherence (Velligan et al. 2010; West et al. 2008), although specific data to test this supposition are not available. Nevertheless, use of an LAI antipsychotic may have additional advantages in patients who have difficulty with adherence or in whom adherence is uncertain. The side effects of treatment with an LAI antipsychotic medication are also comparable to side effects with the corresponding oral medication. For additional discussion of the research evidence, see Appendix C, Statement 10.

Differences of Opinion Among Writing Group Members

There were no differences of opinion. The writing group voted unanimously in favor of this suggestion.

Review of Available Guidelines From Other Organizations

Information from other guidelines is consistent with this guideline statement (Barnes et al. 2011; Buchanan et al. 2010; Galletly et al. 2016; Hasan et al. 2012; National Institute for Health and Care Excellence 2014; Remington et al. 2017; Scottish Intercollegiate Guidelines Network 2013). Other guidelines on the treatment of schizophrenia suggest use of LAIs based on patient preference (BAP, CSG, NICE, PORT, RANZCP, SIGN) or in the context of poor or uncertain adherence (BAP, NICE, RANZCP, SIGN). The RANZCP and WFSBP guidelines also note that LAIs should be considered if there has been a poor response to oral medication, and the RANZCP guideline notes that LAIs should be offered to patients early in the clinical course of schizophrenia.

Quality Measurement Considerations

As a suggestion, this guideline statement is not appropriate for use as a quality measure. However, only a small proportion of individuals with schizophrenia receive an LAI antipsychotic medication in clinical practice (Brown et al. 2014; Correll et al. 2016; Lawson et al. 2015; Sultana et al. 2019). Because adherence is poor or uncertain in many individuals with schizophrenia, patients may benefit from or prefer to receive an LAI antipsychotic medication if one is offered. Consequently, electronic decision support could suggest that clinicians consider an LAI antipsychotic medication if poor adherence is documented or with repeated hospitalizations or emergency visits. In addition, health care organizations may wish to ensure that they will provide treatment with an LAI antipsychotic medication to patients when appropriate. Health care organizations and health plans may also wish to implement internal process measures to assess and increase rates at which LAI antipsychotics are used.

STATEMENT 11: Anticholinergic Medications for Acute Dystonia

APA *recommends* **(1C)** that patients who have acute dystonia associated with antipsychotic therapy be treated with an anticholinergic medication.

Implementation

Medication-induced acute dystonia is defined in DSM-5 as

> [a]bnormal and prolonged contraction of the muscles of the eyes (oculogyric crisis), head, neck (torticollis or retrocollis), limbs, or trunk developing within a few days of starting or raising the dosage of a medication (such as a neuroleptic) or after reducing the dosage of a medication used to treat extrapyramidal symptoms. (American Psychiatric Association 2013a, p. 711)

A dystonic spasm of the axial muscles along the spinal cord can result in opisthotonos, in which the head, neck, and spinal column are hyperextended in an arched position. Rarely, acute dystonia can also present as life-threatening laryngospasm, which results in an inability to breathe (Ganesh et al. 2015; Koek and Pi 1989). Acute dystonia is sudden in onset and painful and can cause patients great distress. Because of the dramatic appearance of acute dystonia, health professionals who are unfamiliar with the condition may incorrectly attribute these reactions to catatonic signs or unusual behavior on the part of patients, and oculogyric crises can sometimes be misinterpreted as indicative of seizure activity. In individuals treated with FGAs, it is estimated that up to 10% of patients may experience an acute dystonic episode, and with SGAs, rates of acute dystonia may be less than 2% (Martino et al. 2018; Miller et al. 2008; Satterthwaite et al. 2008). Additional factors that increase the risk of acute dystonia with antipsychotic medication include young age, male sex, ethnicity, recent cocaine use, high medication dose, and intramuscular route of medication administration (Gray and Pi 1998; Spina et al. 1993; van Harten et al. 1999).

There are a limited number of clinical studies of anticholinergic medications in acute dystonia associated with antipsychotic therapy. Nevertheless, a large amount of clinical experience suggests that acute dystonia can be reversed by administration of diphenhydramine, a histamine receptor antagonist with anticholinergic properties. Typically, it is administered intramuscularly to treat acute dystonia, but it can also be administered intravenously in emergent situations, as with acute dystonia associated with laryngospasm. Alternatively, benztropine can also be administered intramuscularly. Once the acute dystonia has resolved, it may be necessary to continue an oral anticholinergic medication to prevent recurrence, at least until other changes in medications can take place such as reducing the dose of medication or changing to an antipsychotic medication that is less likely to be associated with acute dystonia. Typically, a medication such as benztropine or trihexyphenidyl is used for this purpose because of the shorter half-life of oral diphenhydramine and a need for more frequent dosing. For additional details of dosing and use of these medications, see Statement 12, Table 10. Regardless of the anticholinergic medication that is chosen, it is important to use the lowest dose that is able to treat acute dystonia and continue the anticholinergic medication for the shortest time needed to prevent dystonia from recurring. After several weeks to months, anticholinergic medications can sometimes be reduced or withdrawn without recurrence of dystonia or worsening of other antipsychotic-induced neurological symptoms (Desmarais et al. 2012). Medications with anticholinergic effects can result in multiple difficulties for patients, including impaired quality of life, impaired cognition, and significant health complications (Salahudeen et al. 2015). Dry mouth due to anticholinergic effects is associated with an increased risk for multiple dental complications (Singh and Papas 2014), and drinking high-calorie fluids in response to dry mouth can contribute to weight gain. Medications with anticholinergic effects can also precipitate acute angle-closure glaucoma (Lachkar and Bouassida 2007), although patients with treated glaucoma seem to be able to tolerate these medications with careful monitoring (Bower et al. 2018). Other peripheral side effects of anticholinergic medications can include blurred vision, constipation, tachycardia, urinary retention, and effects on thermoregulation (e.g., hyperthermia in hot weather) (Nasrallah and Tandon 2017; Ozbilen and Adams 2009), and central anticholinergic effects can include impaired learning and memory and slowed cognition (Ang et al. 2017; Vinogradov et al. 2009). Older individuals can be particularly sensitive to these anticholinergic effects and can develop problems such as urinary retention, confusion, fecal impaction, and anticholinergic toxicity (with delirium, somnolence, and hallucinations) (Nasrallah and Tandon 2017). In addition, it is important to consider the anticholinergic side effects associated with other medications that a patient is taking, such as antipsychotic medications, some antidepressant medications, urological medications (e.g., oxybutynin), and nonselective antihistamines (e.g., hydroxyzine, diphenhydramine).

Balancing of Potential Benefits and Harms in Rating the Strength of the Guideline Statement

Benefits

In individuals who have acute dystonia associated with antipsychotic therapy, the use of medications with anticholinergic properties (including diphenhydramine, benztropine, and trihexyphenidyl) can be associated with rapid symptom relief. In addition, continuing treatment with an anticholinergic medication can prevent the return of dystonia until other adjustments to the treatment regimen can be made to minimize the risk of recurrence.

Harms

The harms of using a medication with anticholinergic properties to treat acute dystonia include side effects such as dry mouth, blurred vision, precipitation of acute angle-closure glaucoma, constipation (and in some cases fecal impaction), tachycardia, urinary retention, effects on thermoregulation (e.g., hyperthermia in hot weather), impaired learning and memory, slowed cognition, and anticholinergic toxicity (with delirium, somnolence, and hallucinations). These harms are likely to be greater in older individuals and may be augmented in individuals taking other medications with anticholinergic properties.

Patient Preferences

Clinical experience suggests that acute dystonia associated with antipsychotic therapy is very uncomfortable for patients, and most of them are frightened by it. As a result, patients are typically cooperative with and accepting of acute treatment with an anticholinergic agent. They may also be willing to take one of these medications to prevent the return of dystonia. However, some patients may be troubled by side effects such as blurred vision, dry mouth, and constipation and may wish to avoid more significant side effects associated with anticholinergic medications.

Balancing of Benefits and Harms

The potential benefits of this guideline statement were viewed as far outweighing the potential harms. For the majority of patients who are experiencing acute dystonia associated with antipsychotic therapy, the rapid relief of symptoms with anticholinergic treatment outweighs the side effects associated with these medications, at least on a short-term basis. In patients who experience acute laryngeal dystonia, rapid administration of a medication with anticholinergic properties, such as diphenhydramine, can be lifesaving. Nevertheless, the long-term benefits and harms of anticholinergic medications are less clear, and, in this context, harms may outweigh benefits. For additional discussion of the research evidence, see Appendix C, Statement 11.

Differences of Opinion Among Writing Group Members

Eight writing group members voted to recommend this statement. One writing group member disagreed with this statement out of concern that a reduction in antipsychotic medication dose or a change in medication may be preferable to immediate use of an anticholinergic medication in some situations. In addition, one writing group member expressed concern that the use of the phrase "anticholinergic medication" in the statement may be misleading because diphenhydramine is typically viewed as an antihistamine but may be preferable to other anticholinergic medications to treat acute dystonia.

Review of Available Guidelines From Other Organizations

The guidelines of the WFSBP are in agreement with this recommendation, noting that acute dystonia responds dramatically to administration of anticholinergic or antihistaminic medication (Hasan et al. 2013). The guideline of the BAP notes that use for acute dystonia "should be determined on an individual basis, taking account of factors such as the patient's history of extrapyramidal side effects and the risk of anticholinergic side effects" (Barnes et al. 2011, p. 7).

Quality Measurement Considerations

This guideline statement is not appropriate for use as a quality measure or as part of electronic clinical decision support. Even with short-term treatment, some patients could have the potential to develop significant anticholinergic side effects, which would need to be incorporated into exclusion and exemption criteria. With reductions in the use of high doses of high-potency FGAs, the frequency of acute dystonia is significantly reduced. Any measure would apply only to a small number of individuals, which would complicate testing for feasibility, usability, reliability, and validity.

STATEMENT 12: Treatments for Parkinsonism

APA *suggests* (2C) the following options for patients who have parkinsonism associated with antipsychotic therapy: lowering the dosage of the antipsychotic medication, switching to another antipsychotic medication, or treating with an anticholinergic medication.

Implementation

Medication-induced parkinsonism, which is termed neuroleptic-induced parkinsonism and other medication-induced parkinsonism in DSM-5, is defined as

> [p]arkinsonian tremor, muscular rigidity, akinesia (i.e., loss of movement or difficulty initiating movement), or bradykinesia (i.e., slowing movement) developing within a few weeks of starting or raising the dosage of a medication (e.g., a neuroleptic) or after reducing the dosage of a medication used to treat extrapyramidal symptoms. (American Psychiatric Association 2013a, p. 709)

These symptoms of medication-induced parkinsonism are dose-dependent and generally resolve with discontinuation of antipsychotic medication. It is important to appreciate that medication-induced parkinsonism can affect emotional and cognitive function, at times in the absence of detectable motor symptoms. As a result, it can be difficult to distinguish the negative symptoms of schizophrenia or concomitant depression from medication-induced parkinsonism. In addition, emotional and cognitive features of medication-induced parkinsonism can be subjectively unpleasant and can contribute to poor medication adherence (Acosta et al. 2012; Ascher-Svanum et al. 2006).

A number of approaches can be taken when a patient is experiencing medication-induced parkinsonism. A reduction in the dose of the antipsychotic medication, if feasible, is often helpful in reducing parkinsonism. In some individuals, it may be appropriate to change the antipsychotic medication to one with a lower likelihood of parkinsonism (see Statement 4, Table 6). For individuals who are highly sensitive to medication-induced parkinsonism, clozapine may be considered. However, before reducing the dose of medication or changing to another antipsychotic medication, the benefits of reduced parkinsonism should be weighed against the potential for an increase in psychotic symptoms. Careful monitoring for symptom recurrence is always important when making changes or reducing doses of antipsychotic medications, and use of quantitative measures can be helpful in this regard, as described in Statement 2.

The use of an anticholinergic medication is another option, either on a short-term basis, until a change in dose or a change in medication can occur, or on a longer-term basis, if a change in dose or change in medication is not feasible. In most circumstances, an anticholinergic medication will be started only after parkinsonian symptoms are apparent. However, some individuals may be at increased risk of developing parkinsonism (e.g., those with significant parkinsonism with prior treatment), and prophylactic use of an anticholinergic medication may occasionally be warranted.

Typically, a medication such as benztropine or trihexyphenidyl is used to treat medication-induced parkinsonism because diphenhydramine has a shorter half-life and greater likelihood of sedation.

However, oral or intramuscular diphenhydramine can also be used on an acute basis. Additional details on these medications are provided in Table 10. It should also be noted that different symptoms of parkinsonism (e.g., rigidity, tremors, akinesia) may have a differential response to anticholinergic medications, and different treatment approaches may be needed to address each of these symptoms. Parkinsonism should also be distinguished from tardive dyskinesia, which can be worsened by use of anticholinergic medications (Bergman and Soares-Weiser 2018; Cogentin 2013).

If an anticholinergic medication is used, it is important to adjust the medication to the lowest dose that is able to treat the parkinsonian symptoms. In addition, it is also important to use the medication for the shortest time necessary. After several weeks to months, anticholinergic medications can sometimes be reduced or withdrawn without recurrence of parkinsonism or worsening of other antipsychotic-induced neurological symptoms (Desmarais et al. 2012). Medications with anticholinergic effects can result in multiple difficulties for patients, including impaired quality of life, impaired cognition, and significant health complications (Salahudeen et al. 2015). Dry mouth due to anticholinergic effects is associated with an increased risk for multiple dental complications (Singh and Papas 2014), and drinking high-calorie fluids in response to dry mouth can contribute to weight gain. Medications with anticholinergic effects can also precipitate acute angle-closure glaucoma (Lachkar and Bouassida 2007), although patients with treated glaucoma seem to be able to tolerate these medications with careful monitoring (Bower et al. 2018).

Other peripheral side effects of anticholinergic medications can include blurred vision, constipation, tachycardia, urinary retention, and effects on thermoregulation (e.g., hyperthermia in hot weather) (Nasrallah and Tandon 2017; Ozbilen and Adams 2009), and central anticholinergic effects can include impaired learning and memory and slowed cognition (Ang et al. 2017; Vinogradov et al. 2009). Older individuals can be particularly sensitive to these anticholinergic effects and can develop problems such as urinary retention, confusion, fecal impaction, and anticholinergic toxicity (with delirium, somnolence, and hallucinations) (Nasrallah and Tandon 2017). In addition, it is important to consider the anticholinergic side effects associated with other medications that a patient is taking, such as antipsychotic medications, some antidepressant medications, urological medications (e.g., oxybutynin), and nonselective antihistamines (e.g., hydroxyzine, diphenhydramine).

Amantadine is an alternative to using an anticholinergic medication to treat medication-induced parkinsonism. Studies of amantadine have had small samples, but the available evidence and clinical experience suggest that amantadine may have comparable or somewhat less benefit than anticholinergic agents in treating medication-induced parkinsonism (Ananth et al. 1975; Borison 1983; DiMascio et al. 1976; Fann and Lake 1976; Greenblatt et al. 1977; Kelly et al. 1974; König et al. 1996; McEvoy 1987; McEvoy et al. 1987; Mindham et al. 1972; Silver et al. 1995). With the absence of anticholinergic properties, side effects, including cognitive impairment, are less prominent with amantadine than with anticholinergic agents. Common adverse effects with amantadine include nausea, dizziness, insomnia, nervousness, impaired concentration, fatigue, and livedo reticularis. Hallucinations and suicidal thoughts have also been reported, as has an increased seizure frequency in individuals with preexisting seizure disorder (Micromedex 2019).

Balancing of Potential Benefits and Harms in Rating the Strength of the Guideline Statement

Benefits

In individuals who have medication-induced parkinsonism, a reduction in signs and symptoms such as rigidity, tremor, and bradykinesia can be of significant benefit, whether such a reduction is achieved by reducing the dose of antipsychotic medication, changing to another antipsychotic medication that has less propensity to cause parkinsonism, or using medications with anticholinergic properties to treat the parkinsonism.

TABLE 10. **Medications for treatment of medication-induced parkinsonism[a]**

	Amantadine	Benztropine mesylate	Diphenhydramine	Trihexyphenidyl hydrochloride
Trade name[b]	Symmetrel	Cogentin	Benadryl	Artane
Typical use	Parkinsonism	Acute dystonia, parkinsonism	Acute dystonia, parkinsonism	Acute dystonia, parkinsonism
Mechanism of action	Uncompetitive NMDA receptor antagonist (weak)	Muscarinic antagonist	Histamine H_1 antagonist	Muscarinic antagonist
Available formulations (mg, unless otherwise noted)	Tablet: 100 Tablet, extended release: 129, 193, 258 Capsule: 100 Capsule, liquid filled: 100 Capsule, extended release: 68.5, 137 Oral syrup: 50/5 mL	Tablet: 0.5, 1, 2 Solution, injection: 1/mL (2 mL)	Capsule: 25, 50 Oral elixir: 12.5/5 mL Oral solution: 12.5/5 mL, 6.25/1 mL Tablet: 25, 50 Solution, injection: 50/1 mL Other brand-name formulations are available for allergy relief	Oral elixir: 0.4/mL (473 mL) Tablet: 2, 5
Typical dose range (mg/day)	Immediate-release tablet or capsule: 100–300 Extended-release tablet: 129–322	Tablet: 0.5–6.0 Solution, injection: 1–2	Oral: 75–200 Solution, injection: 10–50	Oral: 5–15
Bioavailability	86%–94%	29%	40%–70%	100%
Time to peak level (hours)	Immediate release: 2–4 Extended release: 7.5–12	Oral: 7 IM: minutes	1–4	1.3
Protein binding	67%	95%	76%–85%	Not known
Metabolism	Primarily renal	Hepatic	Hepatic	Not known
Metabolic enzymes/ transporters	Substrate of organic cation transporter 2	Substrate of CYP2D6 (minor)	Extensively hepatic N-demethylation via CYP2D6; minor demethylation via CYP1A2, CYP2C9, and CYP2C19; inhibits CYP2D6 (weak)	None known
Metabolites	Multiple; unknown activity	Not known	Inactive	Not known
Elimination half-life (hours)	16–17	7	4–8	4
Excretion	Urine 85% unchanged; 0.6% fecal	Urine	Urine (as metabolites and unchanged drug)	Urine and bile
Hepatic impairment	No dose adjustments noted in labeling	No dose adjustments noted in labeling	No dose adjustments noted in labeling	No dose adjustments noted in labeling

	Amantadine	Benztropine mesylate	Diphenhydramine	Trihexyphenidyl hydrochloride
Renal impairment	Elimination half-life increases with renal impairment	No dose adjustments noted in labeling	No dose adjustments noted in labeling; however, dosing interval may need to be increased or dosage reduced in older individuals and those with renal impairments	No dose adjustments noted in labeling
Comments	Negligible removal by dialysis; do not crush or divide extended-release products	Onset of action with IV dose is comparable to IM	Total daily dose typically divided into 3–4 doses per day Maximum daily dose 300 mg for oral and 400 mg for IM/IV, with 100 mg maximum dose for IV/IM IV dose at a rate of 25 mg/minute; IM dose by deep IM injection because subcutaneous or intradermal injection can cause local necrosis	

[a]This table includes information compiled from multiple sources. Detailed information on such issues as dose regimen, dose adjustments, medication administration procedures, handling precautions, and storage can be found in product labeling. It is recommended that readers consult product labeling information for authoritative information on these medications.

[b]The most common U.S. trade names are included for reference only. At the time of publication, some of these products may be manufactured only as generic products. Other medications or other formulations of the listed medications may be available in Canada.

Abbreviations. CYP=cytochrome P450; NMDA=N-methyl-D-aspartate.

Source. Amantadine hydrochloride capsules 2015; Amantadine hydrochloride oral solution 2015; Amantadine hydrochloride tablets 2019; Benadryl 2018; Benztropine injection 2017; Benztropine tablets 2017; Cogentin 2013; Diphenhydramine hydrochloride injection 2019; Lexicomp 2019; Micromedex 2019; Pendopharm 2015; Procyshyn et al. 2019; Trihexyphenidyl hydrochloride oral solution 2010; Trihexyphenidyl hydrochloride tablets 2015.

Harms

Reducing the dose of an antipsychotic medication or changing to a different antipsychotic medication can be associated with an increase in psychotic symptoms. The harms of using a medication with anticholinergic properties to treat medication-induced parkinsonism include side effects such as dry mouth, blurred vision, precipitation of acute angle-closure glaucoma, constipation (and in some cases fecal impaction), tachycardia, urinary retention, effects on thermoregulation (e.g., hyperthermia in hot weather), impaired learning and memory, slowed cognition, and anticholinergic toxicity (with delirium, somnolence, and hallucinations). These harms are likely to be greater in older individuals and may be augmented in individuals taking other medications with anticholinergic properties.

Patient Preferences

Clinical experience suggests that most patients are bothered by medication-induced parkinsonism and would like to minimize or eliminate this side effect of antipsychotic medication. However, most patients will also want to minimize the chance that psychotic symptoms will increase. Many patients are also troubled by side effects such as blurred vision, dry mouth, and constipation and may wish to avoid more significant side effects associated with anticholinergic medications. Consequently, the balance of these possible risks and benefits of different approaches to addressing medication-induced parkinsonism is likely to vary for each individual and his or her risk factors and personal preferences.

Balancing of Benefits and Harms

The potential benefits of this guideline statement were viewed as likely to outweigh the potential harms because medication-induced parkinsonism can affect the patient's quality of life, and patients would prefer to address it, if feasible. However, each of the available options for decreasing or eliminating medication-induced parkinsonism has associated risks and characteristics, and preferences of each patient need to be taken into consideration. In addition, the long-term benefits and harms of anticholinergic medications are less clear, and harms of long-term use may outweigh benefits. For additional discussion of the research evidence, see Appendix C, Statement 12.

Differences of Opinion Among Writing Group Members

Eight writing group members voted to suggest this statement. One writing group member disagreed with this statement, believing that a reduction in antipsychotic medication dose or a change in medication would be preferable to use of an anticholinergic medication.

Review of Available Guidelines From Other Organizations

Statements from other guidelines vary in their approach to medication-induced parkinsonism. The WFSBP guideline notes that use of SGAs or reductions in medication doses should be the primary treatment for medication-induced parkinsonism (Hasan et al. 2013). The BAP guideline notes that decisions about the use of anticholinergic medications for medication-induced parkinsonism should be made on an individual basis, but these medications should not be given prophylactically (Barnes et al. 2011). The PORT guideline notes that prophylactic use of antiparkinsonian agents is not warranted in patients treated with SGAs but may be indicated on an individual basis in patients treated with FGAs (Buchanan et al. 2010).

Quality Measurement Considerations

As a suggestion, this statement is not appropriate for use as a quality measure. It is also not appropriate for incorporation into electronic decision support.

STATEMENT 13: Treatments for Akathisia

APA *suggests* **(2C)** the following options for patients who have akathisia associated with antipsychotic therapy: lowering the dosage of the antipsychotic medication, switching to another antipsychotic medication, adding a benzodiazepine medication, or adding a beta-adrenergic blocking agent.

Implementation

Medication-induced acute akathisia is defined in DSM-5 as

> [s]ubjective complaints of restlessness, often accompanied by observed excessive movements (e.g., fidgety movements of the legs, rocking from foot to foot, pacing, inability to sit or stand still), developing within a few weeks of starting or raising the dosage of a medication (such as a neuroleptic) or after reducing the dosage of a medication used to treat extrapyramidal symptoms. (American Psychiatric Association 2013a, p. 711)

Akathisia is sometimes difficult to distinguish from psychomotor agitation associated with psychosis, leading to a cycle of increasing doses of antipsychotic medication that lead to further increases in akathisia. Even in mild forms in which the patient is able to control most movements, akathisia is often extremely distressing to patients and is a frequent cause of nonadherence with antipsychotic treatment. If allowed to persist, akathisia can contribute to feelings of dysphoria and, in some instances, suicidal behaviors. The reported rates of akathisia vary from 10%–15% to as many as one-third of patients treated with antipsychotic medication, even when SGAs are used (Juncal-Ruiz et al. 2017; Martino et al. 2018; Mentzel et al. 2017; Miller et al. 2008).

A number of approaches can be taken when a patient is experiencing antipsychotic-induced akathisia. A reduction in the dose of the antipsychotic medication, if feasible, is often helpful in reducing akathisia. In some individuals, it may be appropriate to change the antipsychotic medication to one with a lower likelihood of akathisia (see Statement 4, Table 6). However, before reducing the dose of medication or changing to another antipsychotic medication, the benefits of reduced akathisia should be weighed against the potential for an increase in psychotic symptoms. Careful monitoring for symptom recurrence is always important when making changes or reducing doses of antipsychotic medications, and use of quantitative measures can be helpful in this regard, as described in Statement 2.

Benzodiazepine medications, including lorazepam and clonazepam, can also be helpful in the treatment of akathisia. Among other side effects, somnolence and cognitive difficulties can be associated with benzodiazepine use (Lexicomp 2019; Micromedex 2019). In addition, problems with coordination as a result of benzodiazepines can contribute to falls, particularly in older individuals (Donnelly et al. 2017). Although benzodiazepines are much safer than older sedative agents, respiratory depression can be seen with high doses of a benzodiazepine, particularly in combination with alcohol, other sedating medications, or opioids (Hirschtritt et al. 2017). Caution may also be indicated in prescribing benzodiazepines to individuals with sleep apnea, although few studies are available (Mason et al. 2015). Individuals who are treated with a benzodiazepine may also take them in higher amounts or more frequently than intended. In some patients, a sedative, hypnotic, or anxiolytic use disorder may develop, particularly in individuals with a past or current diagnosis of alcohol use disorder or another substance use disorder.

Another option for treatment of akathisia is the β-adrenergic blocking agent propranolol (Pringsheim et al. 2018), which is typically administered in divided doses, with a total daily dose of 30–120 mg. When using propranolol, it is important to monitor blood pressure with increases in dose and recognize that taking propranolol with protein-rich foods can increase bioavailability by 50%. In addition, propranolol is metabolized by CYP1A2, CYP2D6, CYP2C19, and CYP3A4, which can contribute to drug-drug interactions. Some literature also suggests that mirtazapine may reduce akathisia in some patients (Perry et al. 2018; Poyurovsky and Weizman 2018; Praharaj et al. 2015). In contrast, akathisia tends not to respond to anticholinergic agents (Pringsheim et al. 2018; Rathbone and Soares-Weiser 2006).

Balancing of Potential Benefits and Harms in Rating the Strength of the Guideline Statement

Benefits

In individuals who have akathisia associated with antipsychotic medication, a reduction in symptoms can be of significant benefit, whether such a reduction is achieved by reducing the dose of antipsychotic medication, changing to another antipsychotic medication that has less propensity to cause akathisia, or using a benzodiazepine or a β-adrenergic blocking agent to treat akathisia.

Harms

Reducing the dose of an antipsychotic medication or changing to a different antipsychotic medication can be associated with an increase in psychotic symptoms. The harms of using a benzodiazepine can include somnolence, cognitive difficulties, problems with coordination, and risk of misuse or develop-ment of a sedative use disorder. In high doses and particularly in combination with alcohol, other se-dating medications, or opioids, respiratory depression may occur. With use of a β-adrenergic blocking agent, such as propranolol, the primary harm relates to lowering of blood pressure.

Patient Preferences

Clinical experience suggests that most patients are bothered by akathisia and, in some instances, very distressed by it. Thus, almost all patients would like to minimize or eliminate this side effect of antipsychotic medication. However, most patients will also want to minimize the chance that psychotic symptoms will increase. They may also be concerned about the possible side effects of medications such as benzodiazepines and β-adrenergic blocking agents. Consequently, the balance of these possible risks and benefits of different approaches to addressing akathisia are likely to vary for each individual and his or her risk factors and personal preferences.

Balancing of Benefits and Harms

The potential benefits of this guideline statement were viewed as likely to outweigh the potential harms because akathisia can affect the patient's quality of life, and patients would prefer to address it, if feasible. However, each of the available options for decreasing or eliminating akathisia has as-sociated risks and characteristics, and the preferences of each patient need to be taken into consid-eration. For additional discussion of the research evidence, see Appendix C, Statement 13.

Differences of Opinion Among Writing Group Members

There were no differences of opinion. The writing group voted unanimously in favor of this suggestion.

Review of Available Guidelines From Other Organizations

The WFSBP guideline notes that there is some evidence that benzodiazepines are effective in the treatment of akathisia and that there is very limited evidence to support the use of centrally active β-adrenergic blocking agents in the treatment of akathisia (Hasan et al. 2013).

Quality Measurement Considerations

As a suggestion, this statement is not appropriate for use as a quality measure. It is also not appro-priate for incorporation into electronic decision support.

STATEMENT 14: VMAT2 Medications for Tardive Dyskinesia

APA *recommends* **(1B)** that patients who have moderate to severe or disabling tardive dyskinesia as-sociated with antipsychotic therapy be treated with a reversible inhibitor of the vesicular mono-amine transporter 2 (VMAT2).

Implementation

Tardive syndromes are persistent abnormal involuntary movement disorders caused by sustained exposure to antipsychotic medication, the most common of which are tardive dyskinesia, tardive dystonia, and tardive akathisia (Frei et al. 2018). They begin later in treatment than acute dystonia, akathisia, or medication-induced parkinsonism, and they persist and may even increase, despite re-duction in dose or discontinuation of the antipsychotic medication. Typically, tardive dyskinesia presents as "[i]nvoluntary athetoid or choreiform movements (lasting at least a few weeks) gener-ally of the tongue, lower face and jaw, and extremities (but sometimes involving the pharyngeal, diaphragmatic, or trunk muscles)" (American Psychiatric Association 2013a, p. 712), whereas tardive dystonia and tardive akathisia resemble their acute counterparts in phenomenology.

Tardive dyskinesia has been reported after exposure to any of the available antipsychotic medications (Carbon et al. 2017, 2018). It occurs at a rate of approximately 4%–8% per year in adult patients treated with FGAs (Carbon et al. 2018; Woods et al. 2010), a risk that appears to be at least three times that observed with SGAs (Carbon et al. 2018; O'Brien 2016; Woods et al. 2010). Various factors are associated with greater vulnerability to tardive dyskinesia, including age greater than 55 years; female sex; white or African race/ethnicity; presence of a mood disorder, intellectual disability, or central nervous system injury; and past or current akathisia, clinically significant parkinsonism, or acute dystonic reactions (Patterson-Lomba et al. 2019; Solmi et al. 2018a).

Evaluation for the presence of tardive syndromes is important in order to identify them, minimize worsening, and institute clinically indicated treatment. However, evaluation of the risk of tardive dyskinesia is complicated by the fact that dyskinetic movements may be observed with a reduction in antipsychotic medication dose, which is termed a withdrawal-emergent dyskinesia (American Psychiatric Association 2013a). Fluctuations in symptoms are also common and may be influenced by such factors as psychosocial stressors. Furthermore, spontaneous dyskinesias, which are clinically indistinguishable from tardive dyskinesia, have been described in elderly patients before the advent of antipsychotic medications and in up to 20% of never-medicated patients with chronic schizophrenia (Blanchet et al. 2004; Crow et al. 1982; Fenton et al. 1997; Saltz et al. 1991).

Regular assessment of patients for tardive syndromes through clinical examination or through the use of a structured evaluative tool can aid in identifying tardive syndromes, clarifying their likely etiology, monitoring their longitudinal course, and determining the effects of medication changes or treatments for tardive dyskinesia (see Statement 1, Table 2). The AIMS and the DISCUS are examples of such tools (Guy 1976; Kalachnik and Sprague 1993; Munetz and Benjamin 1988). When using scales such as the AIMS or the DISCUS, it should be noted that there is no specific score threshold that suggests a need for intervention, although ranges of scores are noted to correspond with mild, moderate, and severe symptoms. In addition, the same total score can be associated with significantly different clinical manifestations and varying impacts on the patient. Patients, family members, and other persons of support may be able to provide information about the onset of movements; their longitudinal course in relation to treatment or other precipitants; and their impact on functioning, health status (including dentition), and quality of life.

Although the majority of patients who develop tardive dyskinesia have mild symptoms, a small proportion will develop symptoms of moderate or severe degree. In such circumstances, assessment for other contributors to a movement disorder is also warranted (Jinnah and Factor 2015; Mehta et al. 2015; Poewe and Djamshidian-Tehrani 2015; Preskorn et al. 2015; Waln and Jankovic 2015). In addition to a neurological examination and complete history of motor symptoms and past and current medications, history and laboratory testing may include liver function tests, thyroid function tests, serum calcium, complete blood count, and antiphospholipid antibodies. Depending on the results of the history and evaluation, additional studies may be indicated (e.g., ceruloplasmin for Wilson's disease; brain MRI for basal ganglia changes with Huntington's disease, stroke, or other lesions; lumbar puncture for anti-NMDA receptor encephalitis). If dyskinetic movements have begun or have increased in the context of antipsychotic dose reduction, it is important to assess the longitudinal course of symptoms for up to several months because spontaneous reductions or resolution of the dyskinesia may occur.

If no contributing etiology is identified and moderate to severe or disabling tardive dyskinesia persists, treatment is recommended with a reversible inhibitor of the VMAT2. Treatment with a VMAT2 inhibitor can also be considered for patients with mild tardive dyskinesia on the basis of such factors as patient preference, associated impairment, or effect on psychosocial functioning. Table 11 shows the characteristics of VMAT2 inhibitors that are currently available in the United States.

TABLE 11. Reversible inhibitors of human vesicular monoamine transporter type 2[a]

	Deutetrabenazine	Tetrabenazine	Valbenazine
Trade name[b]	Austedo	Xenazine	Ingrezza
Available formulations (mg)	Tablet: 6, 9, 12	Tablet: 12.5, 25	Capsule: 40, 80
Typical dose range (mg/day)	12–48	25–75	40–80
Bioavailability	80%	75%	49%
Time to peak level (hours)	3–4	1–2	0.5–1
Protein binding	60%–68% (α-HTBZ) 59%–63% (β-HTBZ)	82%–85% 60%–68% (α-HTBZ) 59%–63% (β-HTBZ)	>99% 64% α-HTBZ
Metabolism	Hepatic	Hepatic	Hepatic
Metabolic enzymes/ transporters	Major substrate of CYP2D6, minor substrate of CYP1A2 and CYP3A4	Major substrate of CYP2D6	Major substrate of CYP3A4, minor substrate of CYP2D6
Metabolites	Deuterated α-HTBZ and β-HTBZ: active	α-HTBZ, β-HTBZ, and O-dealkylated HTBZ: active	α-HTBZ: active
Elimination half-life (hours)	Deuterated α-HTBZ and β-HTBZ: 9–10	α-HTBZ: 4–8 β-HTBZ: 2–4	15–22
Excretion	Urine: ~75%–85% changed Feces: ~8%–11%	Urine: ~75% changed Feces: ~7%–16%	Urine: 60% Feces: 30%
Hepatic impairment	Contraindicated	Contraindicated	Maximum dose of 40 mg daily with moderate to severe impairment (Child-Pugh score 7–15)
Renal impairment	No information available	No information available	Use not recommended in severe renal impairment (CrCl<30 mL/minute)
Common adverse effects	Sedation	Sedation, depression, extrapyramidal effects, insomnia, akathisia, anxiety, nausea, falls	Sedation
Effect of food on bioavailability	Food affects maximal concentration. Administer with food. Swallow tablets whole and do not chew, crush, or break.	Unaffected by food	Can be taken with or without food. High-fat meals decrease the C_{max} and AUC for valbenazine, but values for the active metabolite (α-HTBZ) are unchanged.

	Deutetrabenazine	Tetrabenazine	Valbenazine
Comments[c]	Give in divided doses; increase from initial dose of 12 mg/day by 6 mg/week to maximum dose of 48 mg/day. Retitrate dose for treatment interruptions of more than 1 week. Follow product labeling if switching from tetrabenazine to deutetrabenazine. Do not exceed total daily dosage of 36 mg/day (18 mg/dose) in poor CYP2D6 metabolizers or patients taking a strong CYP2D6 inhibitor. Assess ECG before and after increasing the daily dose above 24 mg in patients at risk for QTc prolongation. Avoid use in patients with congenital long QT syndrome, with arrhythmias associated with a prolonged QT interval, or with other risks for QTc prolongation (e.g., drugs known to prolong QTc intervals, reduced metabolism via CYP2D6).	Give in divided doses; increase from initial dose of 25–50 mg/day by 12.5 mg/week to maximum of 150–200 mg/day. Retitrate dose for treatment interruptions of more than 5 days. Test for CYP2D6 metabolizer status before giving doses >50 mg/day. Do not exceed 50 mg/day in poor metabolizers or in patients treated with a strong inhibitor of CYP2D6. Avoid use in patients with congenital long QT syndrome, with arrhythmias associated with a prolonged QT interval, or with other risks for QTc prolongation (e.g., drugs known to prolong QTc intervals, reduced metabolism via CYP2D6).	Initiate at 40 mg/day and increase to 80 mg/day after 1 week. Continuation of 40 mg/day may be considered for some patients. Use is not recommended with strong CYP3A4 inducer. A reduced dose is recommended with concomitant use of strong CYP3A4 or CYP2D6 inhibitors or in poor CYP2D6 metabolizers. Avoid use in patients with congenital long QT syndrome, with arrhythmias associated with a prolonged QT interval, or with other risks for QTc prolongation (e.g., drugs known to prolong QTc intervals, reduced metabolism via CYP2D6 or CYP3A4).

ᵃThis table includes information compiled from multiple sources. Detailed information on such issues as dose regimen, dose adjustments, medication administration procedures, handling precautions, and storage can be found in product labeling. It is recommended that readers consult product labeling information for authoritative information on these medications.

ᵇThe most common U.S. trade names are included for reference only. At the time of publication, some of these products may be manufactured only as generic products.

ᶜAll VMAT2 inhibitors are contraindicated within 2 weeks of a monoamine oxidase inhibitor, within 20 days of reserpine, or in patients with active suicidal ideas or untreated depression. Tetrabenazine and deutetrabenazine carry a boxed warning related to depression and suicidal ideation in patients with Huntington's disease.

Abbreviations. AUC=area under the curve; C_{max}=maximum plasma concentration; CrCl=creatinine clearance; CYP=cytochrome P450; ECG=electrocardiogram; HTBZ=dihydrotetrabenazine.

Source. Austedo 2019; Ingrezza 2019; Lexicomp 2019; Micromedex 2019; Xenazine 2018.

In general, deutetrabenazine or valbenazine is preferred over tetrabenazine because of the greater evidence base supporting their use. In addition, tetrabenazine has a shorter half-life and greater rates of associated depression when used in the treatment of patients with Huntington's disease. Other factors that may influence choice of a VMAT2 inhibitor relate to hepatic or renal function; tetrabenazine and deutetrabenazine are contraindicated in individuals with hepatic impairment, whereas valbenazine is not recommended for use in individuals with severe renal impairment. The metabolism of these medications is also somewhat different. Although all of these medications are substrates for CYP2D6 and CYP3A4, tetrabenazine and deutetrabenazine are major substrates for CYP2D6, whereas valbenazine is a major substrate for CYP3A4. Consequently, the patient's CYP2D6 metabolizer status or use of concomitant medications that influence these metabolic enzymes may affect the choice of a VMAT2 inhibitor. In terms of side effects, these medications are generally well tolerated, with sedation being most common. In initial studies of tetrabenazine in patients with Huntington's disease, significant rates of depression were noted as well as concerns about suicidal ideas and behaviors (Shen et al. 2013). However, in studies of deutetrabenazine and valbenazine in patients with tardive dyskinesia, there were no apparent increases in depression or suicidal ideas either in the randomized portions of the clinical trials or in longer open-label extension periods (Solmi et al. 2018b). Nevertheless, depression or suicidal ideas could occur during treatment for tardive dyskinesia, and clinicians will want to be alert to this possibility.

Small clinical trials and case series have examined other treatments for tardive dyskinesia. A lower dose of antipsychotic medication can be considered, although evidence for this approach is minimal (Bergman et al. 2017), and the potential for benefit needs to be weighed against the possibility of recurrent symptoms or relapse. Some benefits have been noted with benzodiazepines (Bergman et al. 2018a), although the potential for benefits must be weighed against the potential side effects of these medications, including somnolence, cognitive difficulties, problems with coordination, and risk of misuse or development of a sedative use disorder. In high doses and particularly in combination with alcohol, other sedating medications, or opioids, respiratory depression may occur. A change in antipsychotic therapy to a lower-potency medication (particularly clozapine) may also be associated with a reduction in tardive dyskinesia, particularly for individuals with moderate to severe symptoms (Mentzel et al. 2018). Again, however, the potential benefits of changing medication should be considered in light of the possibility of symptom recurrence.

In general, giving a higher dose of an antipsychotic may suppress movements of tardive dyskinesia in the short term but would be expected to escalate further development of tardive dyskinesia in the long term. Nevertheless, there may be life-threatening circumstances (e.g., patients with constant movement, gagging, or choking) in which rapid suppression of dyskinesia is needed, and judicious use of an antipsychotic may be appropriate. Anticholinergic medications do not improve and may even worsen tardive dyskinesia (Bergman and Soares-Weiser 2018; Cogentin 2013) in addition to producing significant side effects.

For individuals with other tardive syndromes, other approaches may be helpful on an individual basis. For example, depending on the muscle group that is affected, injections of botulinum toxin have been used to treat tardive dystonia (Brashear et al. 1998; Jinnah and Factor 2015; Kiriakakis et al. 1998). In addition, tardive dystonia may respond to β-adrenergic blocking agents (Hatcher-Martin et al. 2016), and in rare cases of severe intractable tardive dystonia, deep brain stimulation might be considered (Paschen and Deuschl 2018). High doses of anticholinergic agents have also been used to treat severe tardive dystonia (Burke et al. 1982; Kang et al. 1986; Wojcik et al. 1991), although these medications are not useful in treating tardive dyskinesia (Bergman and Soares-Weiser 2018; Cogentin 2013). Reserpine, which also depletes monoamines, should not be used to treat tardive syndromes because it has high rates of associated depression and suicidal ideas and lowers blood pressure (Micromedex 2019). Other treatments, such as vitamin B_6 or vitamin E, are less likely to be associated with harms but do not appear to be associated with benefits in treating tardive dyskinesia (Adelufosi et al. 2015; Soares-Weiser et al. 2018a).

Balancing of Potential Benefits and Harms in Rating the Strength of the Guideline Statement

Benefits

In individuals with moderate to severe or disabling tardive dyskinesia associated with antipsychotic therapy, VMAT2 inhibitors can be associated with significant reductions in motor signs and symptoms of tardive dyskinesia. These medications may also be effective in other tardive syndromes.

Harms

The harms of treatment with VMAT2 inhibitors include sedation and, with tetrabenazine, extrapyramidal effects, akathisia, insomnia, anxiety, nausea, and falls. Depression and suicidal ideas have been reported in individuals who were administered VMAT2 inhibitors for treatment of Huntington's disease. Such effects are possible in individuals treated for tardive dyskinesia, although they were not reported in clinical trials.

Patient Preferences

Clinical experience suggests that most patients with moderate to severe or disabling tardive dyskinesia wish to have a diminution of their motor signs and symptoms. Most patients would be willing to take medication to achieve a reduction in motor signs and symptoms, particularly if it is well tolerated.

Balancing of Benefits and Harms

The potential benefits of this guideline statement were viewed as far outweighing the potential harms. The majority of individuals with moderate to severe or disabling tardive dyskinesia would have a greater likelihood of experiencing benefits of a VMAT2 inhibitor than experiencing harms. Patient preferences to reduce motor signs and symptoms are also likely to favor treatment. For additional discussion of the research evidence, see Appendix C, Statement 14.

Differences of Opinion Among Writing Group Members

There were no differences of opinion. The writing group voted unanimously in favor of this recommendation.

Review of Available Guidelines From Other Organizations

The WFSBP guideline notes that tetrabenazine might have positive effects on tardive dyskinesia (Hasan et al. 2013). It also notes that the risk of tardive dyskinesia is less with SGAs than with FGAs and that there is limited evidence of benefit with clozapine for tardive dyskinesia. Information on a range of other treatments is noted to be even less conclusive. The practice guideline of the American Academy of Neurology, which was published before the availability of deutetrabenazine and valbenazine, notes that tetrabenazine might be considered as a treatment for tardive syndromes (Bhidayasiri et al. 2013).

Quality Measurement Considerations

If a quality measure on VMAT2 inhibitor treatment of tardive syndromes is considered at the provider, facility, health plan, integrated delivery system, or population level, testing of feasibility, usability, reliability, and validity would be essential prior to use for purposes of accountability. However, it may be possible and preferable to incorporate this recommendation into internal facility or health plan initiatives focused on enhanced identification and treatment of tardive syndromes.

Electronic decision support using passive alerts may be able to prompt clinicians to consider a VMAT2 inhibitor, although such prompts would depend on accurate and consistent entry of structured information about the presence of a tardive syndrome, its severity, and its associated degree of disability. Nevertheless, in combination with rating scale data (e.g., AIMS), electronic decision support could help identify individuals with a tardive syndrome who may benefit from a trial of a VMAT2 inhibitor. Information from laboratory data, diagnoses, or problem lists would also be helpful to incorporate in terms of potential contraindications to VMAT2 inhibitor treatment (e.g., tetrabenazine and deutetrabenazine are contraindicated in the presence of hepatic impairment; valbenazine is not recommended for use in individuals with severe renal impairment).

Psychosocial Interventions

STATEMENT 15: Coordinated Specialty Care Programs

APA *recommends* **(1B)** that patients with schizophrenia who are experiencing a first episode of psychosis be treated in a coordinated specialty care program.*

Implementation

For individuals with a first episode of psychosis, coordinated specialty care (CSC) programs have been developed that integrate a number of evidence-based interventions into a comprehensive treatment package. For example, the NAVIGATE program, which was developed for the Recovery After an Initial Schizophrenia Episode (RAISE) Early Treatment research initiative, uses a collaborative, shared decision-making approach that incorporates family involvement and education, individual resiliency training, supported employment and education, and individualized medication treatment (Mueser et al. 2015; National Institute of Mental Health 2019a). Similar CSC programs, which are sometimes referred to as team-based, multicomponent interventions, have also been used in other countries for treatment of early psychosis (Anderson et al. 2018; Craig et al. 2004; Secher et al. 2015). These treatment programs often include individuals with diagnoses other than schizophrenia but have been associated with a number of benefits, including lower mortality (Anderson et al. 2018), lower rates of relapse, better quality of life, better global function, and greater likelihood of working or being in school after receiving up to 2 years of treatment (McDonagh et al. 2017). Patients in such programs may also experience a greater sense of empowerment and support for their autonomy (Browne et al. 2017). Programs are also available that are aimed at early identification and treatment of attenuated psychosis syndrome or related syndromes of high psychosis risk (J. Addington et al. 2017; Cotton et al. 2016); however, these programs are not within the scope of this guideline recommendation because they include individuals who do not have a psychiatric diagnosis or who have diagnoses other than schizophrenia at later follow-up times (Fusar-Poli et al. 2016; Iorfino et al. 2019).

The main barriers to implementing this recommendation in practice relate to the limited availability of first-episode, multicomponent treatment programs. For state health agencies, health systems, or organizations that are implementing these programs, barriers include such issues as funding, training, and implementation support. However, consultation and implementation materials are available to help guide the establishment of new programs with evidence-based approaches (National Institute of Mental Health 2019b; NAVIGATE 2019; OnTrackNY 2019). Tools are also available to assess fidelity of CSC programs to intended implementation principles (Addington et al. 2016, 2018; Durbin et al. 2019; Essock and Addington 2018).

Balancing of Potential Benefits and Harms in Rating the Strength of the Guideline Statement

Benefits

Use of a CSC program for individuals with a first episode of psychosis can be associated with lower mortality, lower rates of relapse, better quality of life, better global function, and greater likelihood of working or being in school after receiving up to 2 years of treatment (low to moderate strength of research evidence).

---

*This guideline statement should be implemented in the context of a person-centered treatment plan that includes evidence-based nonpharmacological and pharmacological treatments for schizophrenia.

Harms

The harms of a CSC program for individuals with a first episode of psychosis are not well delineated but are likely to be small.

Patient Preferences

Clinical experience suggests that many patients with a first episode of psychosis are cooperative with and accepting of a CSC program; however, other patients may not wish to take part in such a program out of a belief that they do not have a condition that requires treatment or because of logistical barriers that influence their ability to access the more intensive treatment provided by such a program.

Balancing of Benefits and Harms

The potential benefits of this guideline statement were viewed as far outweighing the potential harms. CSC treatment programs are generally viewed positively by patients, and they improve a number of patient-oriented outcomes with minimal risk of harms. For additional discussion of the research evidence, see Appendix C, Statement 15.

Differences of Opinion Among Writing Group Members

There were no differences of opinion. The writing group voted unanimously in favor of this recommendation.

Review of Available Guidelines From Other Organizations

Other guidelines did not specifically address the use of CSC programs, but they do endorse many of the individual elements of such programs (e.g., family engagement, psychoeducation, supported employment, medication treatment).

Quality Measurement Considerations

More patients may benefit from CSC programs in the United States than currently receive it. Consequently, state mental health agencies, health plans, and health organizations may wish to implement initiatives to increase the use of a CSC program among individuals with a first episode of psychosis.

This guideline statement would not be appropriate for a performance-based quality measure unless it were tested for feasibility, usability, reliability, and validity. Factors such as geographic variations in treatment availability would need to be considered in testing any quality measures related to CSC program use. It may also be difficult to determine whether a patient is receiving appropriate CSC services.

Electronic decision support using passive alerts may be able to prompt clinicians to consider referral to a CSC program if the presence of a first episode of schizophrenia and the patient's history of prior treatment were accurately and consistently entered into the electronic record as structured data. The electronic record could also incorporate reference information on the location and referral processes for CSC treatment programs in the local area.

STATEMENT 16: Cognitive-Behavioral Therapy

APA *recommends* **(1B)** that patients with schizophrenia be treated with cognitive-behavioral therapy for psychosis (CBTp).*

---

*This guideline statement should be implemented in the context of a person-centered treatment plan that includes evidence-based nonpharmacological and pharmacological treatments for schizophrenia.

Implementation

The use of cognitive-behavioral therapy (CBT) for individuals with schizophrenia has a number of potential benefits, including improvements in quality of life and global, social, and occupational function and reductions in core symptoms of illness, such as positive symptoms. However, it is important to appreciate that these benefits have been found in studies of CBT that is adapted to use for individuals with psychosis (CBTp), which has some differences from CBT that is focused on other indications. More specifically, CBTp focuses on guiding patients to develop their own alternative explanations for maladaptive cognitive assumptions that are healthier and realistic and do not perpetuate the patient's convictions regarding the veracity of delusional beliefs or hallucinatory experiences. Thus, the overall approach with CBTp includes developing a collaborative and nonjudgmental therapeutic relationship in which patients can learn to monitor relationships between thoughts, feelings, behaviors, and symptoms and to evaluate the perceptions, beliefs, and thought processes that contribute to symptoms (Beck and Rector 2005; Beck et al. 2009; Beck Institute 2019; Hardy 2019; Kingdon and Turkington 2019; Landa 2019; Lecomte et al. 2016; Morrison 2017; Turkington et al. 2006; Wright et al. 2009). (Videos that demonstrate some of the approaches to CBTp are available at I Can Feel Better, www.icanfeelbetter.org/cbtpskills.) Through this dual focus on monitoring and evaluation, patients can develop beneficial coping strategies and improve functioning, with behavioral self-monitoring serving as a basis for graded task assignments or activity scheduling. In addition, symptoms can be discussed as being within a range of normal experiences (e.g., hearing a loved one's voice in the context of grief), and alternative explanations for symptoms can be developed that help reduce associated stress (Turkington et al. 2006).

CBTp can be started in any treatment setting, including inpatient settings, and during any phase of illness (Turkington et al. 2006), although some initial reduction in symptoms may be needed for optimal participation (Burns et al. 2014; Valmaggia et al. 2008). It can also be conducted in group as well as in individual formats, either in person or via Web-based delivery platforms. CBTp can also be made available to family members or other persons of support (Turkington and Spencer 2019). Although patient preferences and treatment availability may influence choice of a delivery method, there do not appear to be clear-cut differences in the treatment benefits of group as compared with individual CBTp (McDonagh et al. 2017; Wykes et al. 2008).

The duration of treatment with CBTp has varied in research and clinical practice, with a range from 8 weeks to 5 years of treatment reported in the literature (McDonagh et al. 2017). However, guidelines from other countries recommend a minimum treatment duration of 16 sessions of CBTp (National Institute for Health and Care Excellence 2014; Norman et al. 2017; Scottish Intercollegiate Guidelines Network 2013). Although the available research suggests that treatment benefits are no longer significant when assessed more than 6 months after the end of a CBTp course (McDonagh et al. 2017), it is unclear whether longer durations of treatment with CBTp will result in greater benefits or will help in maintaining treatment-related improvements.

Issues with implementation of CBTp have also been examined. Although the methodological rigor of most studies has been low (Ince et al. 2016), common barriers to CBTp have been identified. For example, some individuals with schizophrenia may be too symptomatic or are experiencing too many side effects (e.g., sedation) to allow effective participation, particularly in inpatient settings. From a patient-centered perspective, CBTp was sometimes viewed as more emotionally challenging and requiring more effort (e.g., homework) than other psychological therapies (Wood et al. 2015). However, engagement strategies, such as motivational interviewing, can be useful in helping patients explore whether CBTp might have potential benefits for them that would offset such concerns.

Attitudinal barriers of staff and organizational management were also found to be common and included a lack of understanding of CBTp and negative expectancies about its value. In addition to inadequate availability of trained staff, staff reported difficulty in identifying patients who were most likely to benefit from CBTp as well as a lack of dedicated time to provide CBTp. Insufficient initial training and insufficient reinforcement of training were also common. Thus, for CBTp to be effective, individuals who are providing CBTp should have appropriate training using established approaches, supervision in CBTp techniques, and experience in treating individuals with schizophrenia. In addition, concerted efforts may be needed to foster positive attitudes and assure adequate time to deliver CBTp. At organizational or health system levels, attention to enhancing the availability of CBTp is also important given the limited availability of CBTp in the United States. Stepped-care approaches, learning collaborative models, and other approaches to best-practice consultations show promise as ways to enhance delivery of CBTp in community settings (Creed et al. 2014; Kopelovich et al. 2019a, 2019b; Stirman et al. 2010).

Balancing of Potential Benefits and Harms in Rating the Strength of the Guideline Statement

Benefits

Use of CBTp in the treatment of schizophrenia can be associated with overall reductions in core illness symptoms, such as positive symptoms (moderate strength of research evidence). CBTp can also be associated with short-term improvements (e.g., for up to 6 months) in quality of life (low strength of research evidence) and global, social, and occupational function (moderate strength of research evidence).

Harms

The harms of CBTp in the treatment of schizophrenia are not well delineated or systematically studied but are likely to be small based on the small number of reported harms in clinical trials.

Patient Preferences

Clinical experience suggests that many patients are cooperative with and accepting of CBTp as part of a treatment plan; however, other patients may not wish to participate in CBTp, may be reluctant to adhere to assignments between sessions, or may experience logistical barriers (e.g., time, access to transportation, childcare, cost) to attending CBTp sessions.

Balancing of Benefits and Harms

The potential benefits of this guideline statement were viewed as far outweighing the potential harms. Specifically, the potential for modest benefits in important patient-centered outcomes during and for periods of up to 6 months after CBTp treatment seemed to outweigh the minimal harms of CBTp treatment. For additional discussion of the research evidence, see Appendix C, Statement 16.

Differences of Opinion Among Writing Group Members

There were no differences of opinion. The writing group voted unanimously in favor of this recommendation.

Review of Available Guidelines From Other Organizations

Statements from other practice guidelines are consistent with this recommendation. The RANZCP and NICE guidelines recommend the use of CBTp for all individuals with schizophrenia (Galletly et al. 2016; National Institute for Health and Care Excellence 2014), whereas the SIGN, CSG, and PORT guidelines recommend CBTp for individuals who have persistent symptoms despite treatment with an antipsychotic medication (Dixon et al. 2010; Norman et al. 2017; Scottish Intercollegiate Guidelines Network 2013). The NICE, SIGN, and CSG guidelines note that CBTp should include at least 16 planned sessions (National Institute for Health and Care Excellence 2014; Norman et al. 2017; Scottish Intercollegiate Guidelines Network 2013).

Quality Measurement Considerations

This guideline statement may not be appropriate for a performance-based quality measure because of the impact of logistical barriers to CBTp, including geographic variations in availability of CBTp, and the difficulty in identifying whether delivered psychotherapy is CBTp. Reminders about CBTp are also not well suited to incorporation into electronic health record clinical decision support. Anecdotal observations suggest that use of CBTp is infrequent in the United States (Kopelovich et al. 2019b). Consequently, health organizations and health plans may wish to implement programs to increase the use of CBTp among individuals with schizophrenia.

STATEMENT 17: Psychoeducation

APA *recommends* (1B) that patients with schizophrenia receive psychoeducation.*

Implementation

Elements of psychoeducation are an integral part of good clinical practice. For example, APA's *Practice Guidelines for the Psychiatric Evaluation of Adults* emphasizes the importance of involving patients in treatment-related decision-making and recommends providing the patient with education about the differential diagnosis, risks of untreated illness, treatment options, and benefits and risks of treatment (American Psychiatric Association 2016a). In addition, these informal approaches to psychoeducation have been expanded into formal, systematically delivered programs of psychoeducation that have been evaluated through clinical trials (Pekkala and Merinder 2002; Xia et al. 2011).

The psychoeducational programs that have been studied have varied in their format, duration, and scope. Some psychoeducational programs are delivered on an individual basis, whereas others are delivered in a group format, often in conjunction with family members or other individuals who are involved in the patient's life. In clinical trials, a 12-session program of psychoeducation is the norm; however, briefer psychoeducation programs of 10 sessions or fewer have also been studied (Pekkala and Merinder 2002; Xia et al. 2011). Typically, psychoeducation is conducted on an outpatient basis, but elements of formal psychoeducation programs can also be incorporated into care in inpatient settings.

Information that is commonly conveyed in a psychoeducation program includes key information about diagnosis, symptoms, psychosocial interventions, medications, and side effects as well as information about stress and coping, crisis plans, early warning signs, and suicide and relapse prevention (Bäuml et al. 2006). Teaching of illness management or self-management strategies (Substance Abuse and Mental Health Services Administration 2010a), as discussed in Statement 21, is often incorporated into psychoeducation. In addition to conveying empathy and respect for the individual, psychoeducation is delivered in a manner that aims to stimulate hope, reassurance, resilience, and empowerment. Typically, psychoeducation incorporates multiple educational modalities, such as workbooks (McCrary et al. 2019), pamphlets, videos, and individual or group discussions in achieving the goals of psychoeducation. Information that may be useful to patients and families as a part of psychoeducation is available through SMI Adviser (https://smiadviser.org). Barriers to providing psychoeducation as a part of the treatment plan relate primarily to program availability. Online delivery of psychoeducation may be one approach to enhancing availability.

---

*This guideline statement should be implemented in the context of a person-centered treatment plan that includes evidence-based nonpharmacological and pharmacological treatments for schizophrenia.

Balancing of Potential Benefits and Harms in Rating the Strength of the Guideline Statement

Benefits

Use of psychoeducation in the treatment of schizophrenia can be associated with a number of potential benefits, including improvements in global function (low strength of research evidence) and reductions in relapse rates (moderate strength of research evidence). Enhancements in treatment adherence and improved satisfaction with mental health services have also been noted in some studies.

Harms

The harms of psychoeducation are likely to be minimal on the basis of results from clinical trials that show no differences in the rate of harms experienced by individuals treated with psychoeducation as compared with usual care (low strength of research evidence).

Patient Preferences

Clinical experience suggests that most patients are interested in receiving information about their diagnosis and potential treatments as part of their care. In addition, most patients are accepting of more formal and systematic approaches to psychoeducation. However, some patients may not wish to participate in psychoeducation or may experience logistical barriers (e.g., time, access to transportation, childcare, costs) in attending psychoeducation sessions.

Balancing of Benefits and Harms

The potential benefits of this guideline statement were viewed as far outweighing the potential harms. Specifically, any minimal harms of psychoeducation seem to be outweighed by the potential for modest benefits in important patient-centered outcomes such as improvements in global function and reductions in relapse rates. For additional discussion of the research evidence, see Appendix C, Statement 17.

Differences of Opinion Among Writing Group Members

There were no differences of opinion. The writing group voted unanimously in favor of this recommendation.

Review of Available Guidelines From Other Organizations

Guidelines from other organizations, including CSG, RANZCP, and SIGN, note the value of psychoeducation for individuals with schizophrenia, including information about diagnosis (Galletly et al. 2016; Norman et al. 2017; Scottish Intercollegiate Guidelines Network 2013).

Quality Measurement Considerations

This guideline statement may not be appropriate for a performance-based quality measure because of the diversity of psychoeducational approaches and services and uncertainty regarding linking specific patient needs for psychoeducation with markers of delivery of psychoeducation. Reminders about psychoeducation are also not well suited to incorporation into electronic health record clinical decision support. However, health organizations and health plans may wish to implement quality improvement efforts to increase the use of formal psychoeducational programs among individuals with schizophrenia.

STATEMENT 18: Supported Employment Services

APA *recommends* **(1B)** that patients with schizophrenia receive supported employment services.*

Implementation

Supported employment differs from other vocational rehabilitation services in providing assistance in searching for and maintaining competitive employment concurrently with job training, embedded job support, and mental health treatment (Becker and Drake 2003; Frederick and VanderWeele 2019; Substance Abuse and Mental Health Services Administration 2010b). In contrast, other vocational rehabilitation approaches focus on training before placement and put greater emphasis on placement in sheltered and transitional employment rather than in a competitive employment setting (Marino and Dixon 2014). For individuals whose goals are related to educational advancement prior to pursuit of employment, supported educational services may also be pursued (Substance Abuse and Mental Health Services Administration 2012b).

Of approaches to supported employment, the bulk of studies involve individual placement and support (IPS; Becker and Drake 2003; Frederick and VanderWeele 2019; McDonagh et al. 2017; Substance Abuse and Mental Health Services Administration 2010b). In addition to a focus on rapid attainment of competitive employment, IPS emphasizes patient preferences in the types of jobs sought, the nature of the services that are delivered, and the outreach that occurs with potential employers (Marino and Dixon 2014). Patient preferences also guide whether to disclose the presence of a psychiatric illness to the employer, with more than half of individuals choosing to disclose this information (DeTore et al. 2019). Services are offered to anyone who is interested, with no exclusion criteria for participation. Additional principles of IPS include individualized long-term job support and integration of employment specialists with the clinical team. Employment specialists also develop relationships with community employers and provide personalized benefits counseling to participants.

Evidence consistently shows that supported employment is associated with greater rates of competitive employment than transitional employment or prevocational training, although prevocational training is superior to no vocational intervention at all (Marshall et al. 2014; McDonagh et al. 2017; Metcalfe et al. 2018; Modini et al. 2016; Richter and Hoffmann 2019; Suijkerbuijk et al. 2017). Augmenting supported employment with symptom-related skills training, training in workplace fundamentals, or cognitive training may assist in gaining and maintaining competitive employment (Dewa et al. 2018; Suijkerbuijk et al. 2017). Other benefits of supported employment include greater number of hours worked per week, a longer duration of each job, a longer duration of total employment, and an increase in earnings (McDonagh et al. 2017). Individuals receiving supported employment are also more likely to obtain job-related accommodations than individuals with mental illness who are not receiving supported employment (McDowell and Fossey 2015). Such accommodations typically relate to assistance from the supported employment coach but may also include flexible scheduling, reduced hours, modified job duties, and modified training and supervision. In addition to job-related benefits of supported employment, there is some evidence of modest reductions in symptoms and a reduced risk of hospitalization associated with obtaining a job (Bouwmans et al. 2015; Burns et al. 2007; Charzyńska et al. 2015; Hoffmann et al. 2014; Luciano et al. 2014).

Among individuals who receive supported employment, factors that may be associated with a greater likelihood of success include lower levels of symptoms, higher levels of cognitive function-

---

*This guideline statement should be implemented in the context of a person-centered treatment plan that includes evidence-based nonpharmacological and pharmacological treatments for schizophrenia.

ing (e.g., attention, memory, executive functioning, psychomotor speed), greater work success in the past, higher levels of educational attainment, and greater interest in obtaining employment (Kirsh 2016). Peer support and support from families and others in the patient's social network may also be associated with better outcomes, although these factors have been less well studied (Kirsh 2016). Even when individuals do not experience initial success with supported employment, addition of cognitive remediation may improve vocational outcomes (McGurk et al. 2015, 2016).

There are a number of barriers to supported employment, including economic and regulatory factors (Kirsh 2016; Metcalfe et al. 2018; Modini et al. 2016) and the limited number of available programs (Marshall et al. 2014; Sherman et al. 2017). Although data are limited, employers may be reluctant to participate in supported employment out of concern about the impact of providing work-related accommodations and because of discrimination and bias toward individuals with serious mental illness (Kirsh 2016). Treating clinicians may also serve as a barrier by having inappropriately limited expectations (Kirsh 2016) and being unaware that some individuals with schizophrenia are able to function at high levels of occupational achievement (Cohen et al. 2017). In addition, concerns about losing disability benefits or health insurance may lead some individuals to forgo supported employment opportunities (Kirsh 2016). Such concerns are not entirely unrealistic because many of the competitive jobs that individuals do obtain are entry-level and/or part-time positions without health insurance benefits (Kirsh 2016). Within supported employment programs, organizational barriers to success have included poor fidelity to supported employment principles (Marshall et al. 2014); insufficient time devoted to leading and management of the programs; and insufficient training, skills, and business and public relations knowledge of program staff (Kirsh 2016; Swanson et al. 2013). Each of these barriers is important to address at individual, systems, and policy levels so that more patients can benefit from supported employment interventions.

For clinicians and organizations wishing to learn more about supported employment or develop supported employment programs, additional information is available through SMI Adviser (https://smiadviser.org), NAVIGATE (https://navigateconsultants.org/manuals), and the Boston University Center for Psychiatric Rehabilitation (https://cpr.bu.edu).

Balancing of Potential Benefits and Harms in Rating the Strength of the Guideline Statement

Benefits

Use of supported employment as part of the treatment of schizophrenia can be associated with significantly better employment outcomes, including a significantly greater likelihood of obtaining competitive employment, a significantly greater likelihood of working more than 20 hours per week, more weeks of employment, and greater earnings relative to vocational training or no vocational interventions (moderate strength of research evidence).

Harms

The harms of supported employment in the treatment of schizophrenia are not well delineated or systematically reported but are likely to be small.

Patient Preferences

Clinical experience suggests that few patients are currently receiving supported employment, but a significant number of individuals may be interested in supported employment if it were readily available and offered to them. However, some individuals may be in school, have responsibilities at home, or already be employed. Others would rather not seek employment or may have concerns about losses of benefits or health insurance if they did pursue competitive employment. Logistical barriers (e.g., access to transportation, childcare) may also affect patient preferences related to supported employment.

Balancing of Benefits and Harms

The potential benefits of this guideline statement were viewed as far outweighing the potential harms. Specifically, the potential for benefits in important patient-centered outcomes related to employment seemed to outweigh the minimal harms of supported employment programs. For additional discussion of the research evidence, see Appendix C, Statement 18.

Differences of Opinion Among Writing Group Members

There were no differences of opinion. The writing group voted unanimously in favor of this recommendation.

Review of Available Guidelines From Other Organizations

Guidelines from other organizations are generally consistent with this recommendation. NICE and PORT recommend that supported employment be offered to individuals with schizophrenia who wish to find or return to work (Dixon et al. 2010; National Institute for Health and Care Excellence 2014), and RANZCP recommends IPS services for individuals with first-episode psychosis (Galletly et al. 2016). RANZCP, NICE, and CSG also emphasize the appropriateness of other occupational or educational activities for individuals with schizophrenia (Galletly et al. 2016; National Institute for Health and Care Excellence 2014; Norman et al. 2017).

Quality Measurement Considerations

This guideline statement may not be appropriate for a performance-based quality measure because of the barriers to supported employment, including variations in availability, and difficulty identifying when patients desire competitive employment. Reminders about supported employment are also not well suited to incorporation into electronic health record clinical decision support. However, given the infrequent availability of supported employment in the United States, health organizations and health plans may wish to implement programs to increase the use of supported employment among individuals with schizophrenia.

STATEMENT 19: Assertive Community Treatment

APA *recommends* **(1B)** that patients with schizophrenia receive assertive community treatment if there is a history of poor engagement with services leading to frequent relapse or social disruption (e.g., homelessness; legal difficulties, including imprisonment).*

Implementation

ACT, sometimes referred to as programs of assertive community treatment, is a multidisciplinary, team-based approach in which patients receive individualized care outside a formal clinical setting. Thus, individuals may be engaged in their homes, workplaces, or other community locations. Continuity of care is enhanced because individuals work with an assigned team, which has 24/7 availability, rather than being assigned to a designated clinician for care. Team members typically include a psychiatrist, nurse, and social worker or case manager. Peer specialists, vocational specialists, and clinicians with expertise in substance use treatment are often part of the team as well.

Other features of ACT include its provision of personalized and flexible care that addresses the patient's needs and preferences without time limits or other constraints on services. Particularly in rural

---

*This guideline statement should be implemented in the context of a person-centered treatment plan that includes evidence-based nonpharmacological and pharmacological treatments for schizophrenia.

areas, some ACT teams are augmenting face-to-face visits with telepsychiatry visits, although research will be needed to determine whether such an approach alters the benefits of ACT (Swanson and Trestman 2018). ACT teams also work with a smaller number of individuals than traditional outpatient clinicians or case managers do, which contributes to the ability to provide frequent visits and a more personalized and comprehensive approach to care. For these reasons, ACT is often used in individuals who have a history of poor engagement with services that leads to frequent relapse or social disruption (e.g., homelessness; legal difficulties, including imprisonment), although it can also be used for individuals who are better engaged but still have high rates of service utilization. Many individuals who are referred for ACT are also at risk for poor adherence and may benefit from consideration of an LAI antipsychotic medication (see Statement 10).

Studies of ACT suggest that it is associated with symptom improvement comparable to other treatment delivery approaches and that individuals who receive ACT are more likely to be domiciled, living independently, and working and less likely to be hospitalized as compared with individuals who receive treatment as usual (McDonagh et al. 2017). Although ACT has multiple strengths that would make it an attractive approach in individuals with co-occurring disorders and schizophrenia, the impact of ACT on physical health has not been well studied (Vanderlip et al. 2017). Also, in individuals with a concomitant substance use disorder, research to date has not shown associated improvements in functioning, mortality, or substance use as compared with usual care (McDonagh et al. 2017).

In terms of implementation barriers, there is often limited availability of ACT programs. Funding these programs can be challenging because the comprehensive and multidisciplinary nature of ACT services is not well aligned with payment models in the U.S. health care delivery system (Monroe-DeVita et al. 2012). Effective delivery of ACT services is also dependent on having a high level of fidelity to ACT program standards (Monroe-DeVita et al. 2012; Thorning et al. 2016), and this requires considerable training as well as ongoing mentoring, collaboration, and consultation with individuals who are skilled in ACT implementation. Attention to outcomes and organizational culture is also important in providing a team-based approach that is warm, flexible, pragmatic, collaborative, and supportive of patients' recovery (Monroe-DeVita et al. 2012). For organizations or state mental health systems that are implementing ACT programs, a number of resources are available (Center for Evidence-Based Practices 2019; Substance Abuse and Mental Health Services Administration 2008; Thorning et al. 2016).

Balancing of Potential Benefits and Harms in Rating the Strength of the Guideline Statement

Benefits

Use of ACT in the treatment of schizophrenia can be associated with a number of benefits as compared with treatment as usual, including a greater likelihood of being domiciled, living independently, or working and a lower likelihood of being hospitalized (low to moderate strength of research evidence).

Harms

The harms of ACT in the treatment of schizophrenia are not well delineated but are likely to be small.

Patient Preferences

Clinical experience suggests that most patients are cooperative with and accepting of ACT, particularly once they have engaged with treatment. In some circumstances, patients may be reluctant to accept ACT services because of impaired awareness of a need for treatment. In this context, ACT may be used as one component of court-mandated care (e.g., assisted outpatient treatment, community treatment order, outpatient commitment). However, in the few studies that have examined patient perceptions, ACT is generally viewed as supporting patients and building relationships in a recovery-oriented fashion (Appelbaum and Le Melle 2008; Morse et al. 2016).

Balancing of Benefits and Harms

The potential benefits of this guideline statement were viewed as far outweighing the potential harms. ACT is generally viewed positively by patients, and it improves a number of patient-oriented outcomes with minimal risk of harms. For additional discussion of the research evidence, see Appendix C, Statement 19.

Differences of Opinion Among Writing Group Members

There were no differences of opinion. The writing group voted unanimously in favor of this recommendation.

Review of Available Guidelines From Other Organizations

This guideline recommendation is consistent with the SIGN recommendation to offer assertive outreach to individuals with schizophrenia who "make high use of inpatient services, who show residual psychotic symptoms and who have a history of poor engagement with services leading to frequent relapse and/or social breakdown (for example homelessness)" (Scottish Intercollegiate Guidelines Network 2013, p. 8). The PORT guideline also notes that ACT should be included in systems of care that serve individuals with schizophrenia and that it "should be provided to individuals who are at risk for repeated hospitalizations or have recent homelessness" (Dixon et al. 2010, p. 49). In addition, RANZCP recommends the use of ACT "after initial contact, during crises and after discharge from hospital" in individuals with schizophrenia (Galletly et al. 2016, p. 29).

Quality Measurement Considerations

This guideline statement may not be appropriate for a performance-based quality measure because of the impact of logistical barriers to ACT, including geographic variations in availability. Reminders about ACT are also not well suited to incorporation into electronic health record clinical decision support because of the multiple patient-specific factors that may contribute to a decision to recommend ACT. However, anecdotal observations suggest that more patients may benefit from ACT in the United States than currently receive it. Consequently, state mental health agencies, health plans, and health organizations may wish to implement programs to increase the use of ACT among individuals with schizophrenia who have had a history of poor engagement with services, leading to frequent relapse or social disruption (e.g., homelessness; legal difficulties, including imprisonment).

STATEMENT 20: Family Interventions

APA *suggests* **(2B)** that patients with schizophrenia who have ongoing contact with family receive family interventions.*

Implementation

An important aspect of good psychiatric treatment is involvement of family members, person(s) of support, and other individuals who play a key role in the patient's life. In addition to spouses, par-

---

*This guideline statement should be implemented in the context of a person-centered treatment plan that includes evidence-based nonpharmacological and pharmacological treatments for schizophrenia.

ents, children, or other biological or nonbiological relatives, such individuals may include people who reside with the patient, intimate partners, and close friends who are an integral part of the patient's support network. Such individuals benefit from discussion of such topics as diagnosis and management of schizophrenia, types of support that are available, and ways to plan for and access help in a crisis. Other goals include helping individuals repair or strengthen their connections with family members and other members of their support system.

Family interventions are systematically delivered, extend beyond conveying of information, and focus on the future rather than on past events (Mueser et al. 2013). The family interventions that are suggested in this guideline statement go beyond the basics of family involvement and illness education that are important for good clinical care. They may include structured approaches to problem-solving, training in how to cope with illness symptoms, assistance with improving family communication, provision of emotional support, and strategies for reducing stress and enhancing social support networks (McDonagh et al. 2017; McFarlane 2016; Mueser et al. 2013). Family interventions can be particularly important early in the course of schizophrenia (McFarlane 2016) but can also be helpful during any phase of treatment.

Most patients want family to be involved in their treatment (Cohen et al. 2013). Nevertheless, even when a patient does not wish for a specific person to be involved in his or her care, the clinician may listen to information provided by that individual, as long as confidential information is not provided to the informant (American Psychiatric Association 2016a). Although some health professionals may be unsure about legal or regulatory aspects of sharing information, general information that is not specific to the patient can be provided (e.g., common approaches to treatment, general information about medications and their side effects, available support and emergency assistance). Also, to prevent or lessen a serious and imminent threat to the health or safety of the patient or others, the "Principles of Medical Ethics" (American Psychiatric Association 2013f) and HIPAA (Office for Civil Rights 2017a, 2017b) permit clinicians to disclose necessary information about a patient to family members, caregivers, law enforcement, or other persons involved with the patient. HIPAA also permits health care providers to disclose necessary information to the patient's family, friends, or other persons involved in the patient's care or payment for care when such disclosure is judged to be in the best interests of the patient and the patient is not present or is unable to agree or object to a disclosure because of incapacity or emergency circumstances (Office for Civil Rights 2017b).

The family interventions that have been studied include a variety of formats and approaches (McDonagh et al. 2017; McFarlane 2016). Interventions may or may not include the patient and can be conducted with a single family or a multifamily group. In many early studies, family interventions included the patient and were led by a member of the patient's clinical care team. This approach allowed a liaison to develop among the care team, the patient, members of the family, and other person(s) of support. Other studies have been conducted independent of the patient's care team. In terms of approach, some family interventions focus on psychoeducation, whereas other interventions incorporate other treatment elements (e.g., motivational interviewing, goal setting, cognitive-behavioral intervention, behavioral family therapy, support groups, social network development, communication training, role-playing, stress management, relaxation training). Given the diversity of options for family interventions, the selection of a specific approach should consider the preferences of the patient and family in collaboration with the clinician.

Benefits of family interventions include reductions in core symptoms of illness and reductions in relapses, including rehospitalization (McDonagh et al. 2017). Some studies have also shown benefits for family members such as reductions in levels of burden and distress or improvements in relationships among family members (McFarlane 2016; Sin et al. 2017a). Evidence suggests that benefits of family interventions are greatest when more than 10 treatment sessions are delivered over a period of at least 7 months (McDonagh et al. 2017). However, the Family-to-Family intervention available through the National Alliance on Mental Illness has shown significant benefits using a 12-week program consisting of weekly sessions of 2–3 hours each (Dixon et al. 2011; Lucksted et al. 2013; Marcus et al. 2013; Toohey et al. 2016).

A common barrier to implementing family interventions relates to program availability. However, guidance is available on developing family intervention programs focused on psychoeducation (Glynn et al. 2014; Substance Abuse and Mental Health Services Administration 2009). In addition, the National Alliance on Mental Illness has reduced this barrier through its Family-to-Family program, which has led to a significant expansion in the availability of family interventions (National Alliance on Mental Illness 2019b). Additional barriers include constraints of family members (e.g., work schedules, access to transportation, childcare, health issues) that may limit their ability to be involved in frequent family sessions. Similar logistical barriers can exist for patients when family interventions incorporate patient participation. Other implementation barriers include organizational and clinician-focused barriers such as time and cost constraints and insufficient understanding of the potential benefits of family intervention (Ince et al. 2016).

Balancing of Potential Benefits and Harms in Rating the Strength of the Guideline Statement

Benefits

Use of family interventions in the treatment of schizophrenia can reduce the likelihood of relapse (low to moderate strength of research evidence) and reduce core illness symptoms (low strength of research evidence).

Harms

The harms of family interventions in the treatment of schizophrenia are not well documented but appear to be minimal.

Patient Preferences

Clinical experience suggests that many patients are cooperative with and accepting of family interventions as part of a treatment plan; however, other patients may have had difficulties in relationships with family members in the past and may not want family members to be involved in their treatment.

Balancing of Benefits and Harms

The potential benefits of this guideline statement were viewed as likely to outweigh the potential harms. For patients who have ongoing contact with their families, including relatives and significant others, there are distinct benefits to family interventions. However, some patients may not be in favor of family involvement even when they do have some ongoing contact with family members, and, for this reason, the statement was suggested rather than being recommended for all individuals. For additional discussion of the research evidence, see Appendix C, Statement 20.

Differences of Opinion Among Writing Group Members

Eight writing group members voted in favor of this suggestion. One writing group member disagreed with this statement as worded and felt that it would be preferable for the guideline statement to make specific mention of other persons of support who may be involved with the patient and are commonly included in such interventions in addition to family members.

Review of Available Guidelines From Other Organizations

This guideline statement is consistent with guidelines from other organizations. CSG, NICE, RANZCP, SIGN, and PORT guidelines all recommend offering family interventions when an individual with schizophrenia reside with or are in close contact with family (Dixon et al. 2010; Galletly et al. 2016; National Institute for Health and Care Excellence 2014; Norman et al. 2017; Scottish Intercollegiate Guidelines Network 2013). These guidelines also emphasize the importance of providing information to family and others involved in the patient's care on such topics as diagnosis and management of schizophrenia, types of support that are available, and ways to access help in a crisis.

Quality Measurement Considerations

As a suggestion, this guideline statement is not appropriate for use as a performance-based quality measure or for incorporation into electronic decision support. Nevertheless, given the potential benefits of this approach, health care organizations and health plans may wish to track the availability and utilization of family interventions.

STATEMENT 21: Self-Management Skills and Recovery-Focused Interventions

APA *suggests* **(2C)** that patients with schizophrenia receive interventions aimed at developing self-management skills and enhancing person-oriented recovery.*

Implementation

Illness self-management training programs have been applied to help address many chronic conditions and are designed to improve knowledge about one's illness and management of symptoms (Grady and Gough 2014). Goals include reducing the risk of relapse, recognizing signs of relapse, developing a relapse prevention plan, and enhancing coping skills to address persistent symptoms, with the aim of improving quality of life and social and occupational functioning. In the studies included in the AHRQ review (McDonagh et al. 2017), self-management training was generally delivered in a group setting with sessions of 45–90 minutes each, and the number of intervention sessions ranged from 7 to 48 sessions. However, the evidence suggested better outcomes in patients who participated in at least 10 self-management intervention sessions. Self-management sessions were typically facilitated by clinicians, although peer-facilitated sessions have also been used. In addition, some studies have used individually targeted interventions, either face-to-face or via computer-based formats (Lean et al. 2019). Self-management approaches have also been used to address co-occurring medical conditions in individuals with serious mental illness, including schizophrenia, with benefits that included increased patient activation and improved health-related quality of life (Druss et al. 2010; Goldberg et al. 2013; Muralidharan et al. 2019).

Recovery-focused interventions have also been developed that focus on fostering self-determination in relation to a patient's personal goals, needs, and strengths. Such approaches may include elements of self-management skill development, psychoeducation, and peer-based interventions but also include components and activities that allow participants to share experiences and receive support, learn and practice strategies for success, and identify and take steps toward reaching personal goals. Studies of peer-based interventions are limited (Castelein et al. 2015; Chien et al. 2019), and studies of recovery-focused interventions have also been small in number. Nevertheless, the available information suggests that these interventions may promote increased recovery, hope, and empowerment among individuals with serious mental illnesses (Le Boutillier et al. 2011; Mueser et al. 2013; Thomas et al. 2018).

The most common barrier to implementing this guideline statement is the availability of programs for developing self-management skills and enhancing person-oriented recovery. However, a toolkit for developing illness management and recovery-based programs in mental health is available through the

---

*This guideline statement should be implemented in the context of a person-centered treatment plan that includes evidence-based nonpharmacological and pharmacological treatments for schizophrenia.

Substance Abuse and Mental Health Services Administration (https://store.samhsa.gov/product/Illness-Management-and-Recovery-Evidence-Based-Practices-EBP-KIT/sma09-4463). Other resources are available through the Boston University Center for Psychiatric Rehabilitation (https://cpr.bu.edu), the Center on Integrated Health Care and Self-Directed Recovery (www.center4healthandsdc.org), Digital Opportunities for Outcomes in Recovery Services (https://skills.digitalpsych.org), Mental Health America (www.mhanational.org/self-help-tools), the National Alliance on Mental Illness (www.nami.org), NAVIGATE (https://navigateconsultants.org/manuals), SMI Adviser (https://smiadviser.org/individuals-families), and the Temple University Collaborative on Community Inclusion (www.tucollaborative.org).

Balancing of Potential Benefits and Harms in Rating the Strength of the Guideline Statement

Benefits

Use of interventions aimed at developing self-management skills and enhancing person-oriented recovery in individuals with schizophrenia can be associated with reductions in symptom severity and risk of relapse and an increased sense of hope and empowerment (low to moderate strength of research evidence). Self-management approaches that are aimed at addressing co-occurring medical conditions in individuals with serious mental illness also have benefits that include increased patient activation and improved health-related quality of life.

Harms

The harms of interventions aimed at developing self-management skills and enhancing person-oriented recovery in the treatment of schizophrenia are not well studied but are likely to be minimal.

Patient Preferences

Clinical experience suggests that most patients are cooperative with and accepting of interventions aimed at developing self-management skills and enhancing person-oriented recovery. However, some patients may not wish to take part in such interventions because of personal preferences or logistical barriers to attending group sessions (e.g., access to transportation, childcare).

Balancing of Benefits and Harms

The potential benefits of this guideline statement in terms of patient engagement, empowerment, and beneficial outcomes were viewed as likely to outweigh the potential harms, which were viewed as minimal. For additional discussion of the research evidence, see Appendix C, Statement 21.

Differences of Opinion Among Writing Group Members

There were no differences of opinion. The writing group voted unanimously in favor of this suggestion.

Review of Available Guidelines From Other Organizations

This guideline statement is consistent with recommendations of other guidelines (RANZCP, NICE) that support the use of self-management and peer-support programs in the treatment of individuals with schizophrenia (Galletly et al. 2016; National Institute for Health and Care Excellence 2014).

Quality Measurement Considerations

As a suggestion, this guideline statement is not appropriate for use as a performance-based quality measure or for incorporation into electronic decision support. Nevertheless, given the potential benefits of such interventions, health care organizations and health plans may wish to track the availability and utilization of programs to develop self-management skills and enhance person-oriented recovery.

STATEMENT 22: Cognitive Remediation

APA *suggests* **(2C)** that patients with schizophrenia receive cognitive remediation.*

Implementation

Cognitive remediation approaches are intended to address cognitive difficulties that can accompany schizophrenia, with the aim of enhancing function and quality of life. A number of different cognitive remediation approaches have been used, typically in group or computer-based formats, in an effort to enhance cognitive processes such as attention, memory, executive function, social cognition, or meta-cognition (Delahunty and Morice 1996; Medalia et al. 2018; Reeder et al. 2016; Wykes et al. 2011). Some programs have focused on improving cognitive flexibility (e.g., shifting cognitive sets), working memory (e.g., sequencing, multitasking, delayed recall), and planning (e.g., sequencing and chunking, active coding), whereas meta-cognitive approaches have attempted to teach patients how and when particular strategies that bypass specific cognitive limitations can be used. Some programs add aspects of social and communication skills to neurocognitive elements of remediation (Pentaraki et al. 2017).

Although this variability in program format and content confounds interpretation of the evidence, cognitive remediation does seem to result in improvements in cognition, symptoms, and function in individuals with schizophrenia, at least on a short-term basis (Harvey et al. 2018; McDonagh et al. 2017; Revell et al. 2015). Although long-term follow-up studies of cognitive remediation are not available in individuals with schizophrenia, data from healthy older individuals show long-term improvements as a result of cognitive training (Rebok et al. 2014). Beneficial effects on psychosocial outcomes seem particularly robust when cognitive remediation is used as a component of or adjunct to other forms of psychiatric rehabilitation rather than being delivered as a stand-alone intervention (McGurk et al. 2007; Revell et al. 2015; van Duin et al. 2019; Wykes et al. 2011). However, some apparent improvements in cognitive performance may result from practicing specific tasks and may not produce generalizable changes in other contexts. Furthermore, the specific elements of a particular cognitive remediation program may influence the benefits that are observed (Cella and Wykes 2019).

The primary barriers to use of cognitive remediation are related to program availability. Online delivery of cognitive remediation may be one way to overcome these barriers. Information and training on developing cognitive remediation programs are available (Medalia 2019; Medalia et al. 2018). In addition, Web-based programs have been used in clinical trials and may provide options for patients without access to in-person cognitive remediation programs (Jahshan et al. 2019; Kukla et al. 2018).

Balancing of Potential Benefits and Harms in Rating the Strength of the Guideline Statement

Benefits

Use of cognitive remediation is associated with moderate improvements in specific aspects of cognition (Harvey et al. 2018; Wykes et al. 2011) as well as small positive effects on social, occupational,

---

*This guideline statement should be implemented in the context of a person-centered treatment plan that includes evidence-based nonpharmacological and pharmacological treatments for schizophrenia.

and global function (low strength of research evidence); core illness symptoms (low strength of research evidence); and negative symptoms (moderate strength of research evidence) compared with usual care over approximately 16 weeks of treatment (McDonagh et al. 2017).

Harms

The harms of cognitive remediation in the treatment of schizophrenia are not well studied but are likely to be small.

Patient Preferences

Evidence from research trials suggests that patients are likely to be cooperative with and accepting of cognitive remediation as part of a treatment plan (Reeder et al. 2016); however, other patients may not wish to participate because of logistical barriers (e.g., time, cost, access to transportation, childcare).

Balancing of Benefits and Harms

The potential benefits of this guideline statement were viewed as likely to outweigh the potential harms, which were viewed as minimal. Differences in patient preferences, variability in the appropriateness of cognitive remediation for individuals with schizophrenia, and the unclear durability of benefits led to suggesting cognitive remediation rather than recommending it. For additional discussion of the research evidence, see Appendix C, Statement 22.

Differences of Opinion Among Writing Group Members

There were no differences of opinion. The writing group voted unanimously in favor of this suggestion.

Review of Available Guidelines From Other Organizations

The RANZCP guideline recommends that cognitive remediation be available to individuals with schizophrenia if cognitive impairment is present and should be specifically "offered when cognitive deficits are affecting recovery and function" (Galletly et al. 2016, p. 20). The SIGN and CSG guidelines note that cognitive remediation "may be considered for individuals diagnosed with schizophrenia who have persisting problems associated with cognitive difficulties" (Norman et al. 2017, p. 621; Scottish Intercollegiate Guidelines Network 2013, p. 28).

Quality Measurement Considerations

As a suggestion, this guideline statement is not appropriate for use as a performance-based quality measure or for incorporation into electronic decision support.

STATEMENT 23: Social Skills Training

APA *suggests* **(2C)** that patients with schizophrenia who have a therapeutic goal of enhanced social functioning receive social skills training.*

Implementation

Social skills training in the treatment of schizophrenia can improve social function, core illness symptoms, and negative symptoms more than usual care can (McDonagh et al. 2017). Reductions in relapse rates, including rehospitalization rates, have also been noted in some studies (McDonagh et al. 2017).

---

*This guideline statement should be implemented in the context of a person-centered treatment plan that includes evidence-based nonpharmacological and pharmacological treatments for schizophrenia.

Social skills training has an overarching goal of improving interpersonal and social skills but can be delivered using a number of approaches (Almerie et al. 2015; Kopelowicz et al. 2006; Turner et al. 2018). These include cognitive-behavioral, social-cognitive, interpersonal, and functional adaptive skills training. Social skills training is delivered in a group format and includes homework assignments to facilitate skill acquisition. Other specific elements of the intervention will vary with the theoretical emphasis of the training. However, examples of techniques that can be used in social skills training include role-playing, modeling, and feedback approaches to enhance interpersonal interactions; behaviorally oriented exercises in assertiveness, appropriate contextual responses, and verbal and nonverbal communication; and instruction and practice with social and emotional perceptions (Almerie et al. 2015; Kopelowicz et al. 2006; Turner et al. 2018). These techniques are aimed at generating improvements in typical social behaviors such as making eye contact, smiling at appropriate times, actively listening to others, and sustaining conversations. In some social skills training programs, group sessions are augmented with video or technologically based interventions, in vivo community trips to practice social skills (Glynn et al. 2002; Mueser et al. 2010), and involvement of support people who are accessible, pleasant, and knowledgeable about the local environments' resources and limitations (Mueser et al. 2010; Tauber et al. 2000).

As with other psychosocial interventions, availability of social skills training is a common barrier to its incorporation into treatment. However, information about social skills training is available for organizations that wish to develop such programs (Bellack and Goldberg 2019; Bellack et al. 2004; Granholm et al. 2016).

Balancing of Potential Benefits and Harms in Rating the Strength of the Guideline Statement

Benefits

Social skills training in the treatment of schizophrenia can improve social function, core illness symptoms, and negative symptoms more than usual care can (low strength of research evidence).

Harms

The harms of social skills training in the treatment of schizophrenia have not been well documented but appear to be minimal.

Patient Preferences

Clinical experience suggests that many patients are cooperative with and accepting of social skills training as part of a treatment plan; however, other patients may not wish to take part in social skills training because of logistical barriers (e.g., time, cost, access to transportation, childcare) or having goals for treatment that are unrelated to social skills.

Balancing of Benefits and Harms

The potential benefits of this guideline statement were viewed as likely to outweigh the potential harms. Although the harms appear to be minimal, there is a low strength of research evidence for benefits, and patient preferences may differ in terms of desiring to focus on social skills as a part of treatment. Consequently, this guideline statement was rated as a suggestion. For additional discussion of the research evidence, see Appendix C, Statement 23.

Differences of Opinion Among Writing Group Members

There were no differences of opinion. The writing group voted unanimously in favor of this suggestion.

Review of Available Guidelines From Other Organizations

Other guidelines are generally consistent with this guideline statement. The PORT, RANZCP, CSG, and SIGN guidelines suggest offering social skills training to individuals with schizophrenia who have deficits in social skills (Buchanan et al. 2010; Galletly et al. 2016; Norman et al. 2017; Scottish Intercollegiate Guidelines Network 2013). However, the NICE guideline notes that social skills training should not be routinely offered to individuals with schizophrenia (National Institute for Health and Care Excellence 2014).

Quality Measurement Considerations

As a suggestion, this guideline statement is not appropriate for use as a performance-based quality measure or for incorporation into electronic decision support. Nevertheless, given the potential benefits of such an approach for some patients, health care organizations and health plans may wish to track the availability and utilization of social skills training for individuals with schizophrenia.

STATEMENT 24: Supportive Psychotherapy

APA *suggests* (2C) that patients with schizophrenia be treated with supportive psychotherapy.*

Implementation

Supportive psychotherapy is commonly a part of the treatment plan in individuals with schizophrenia who are not receiving other modes of psychotherapy (e.g., CBTp). Because the evidence related to its benefits is limited, supportive psychotherapy should not take precedence over other evidence-based psychosocial treatments (e.g., CSC, CBTp, psychoeducation). When compared with treatment as usual, no advantage was seen for supportive psychotherapy in terms of global or social function (L. A. Buckley et al. 2015; McDonagh et al. 2017); however, these findings are difficult to interpret given the frequent use of supportive psychotherapy techniques as part of usual care. When compared with insight-oriented psychotherapies, a small number of early studies suggested that supportive psychotherapy might be associated with better outcomes in coping skills, adherence, and relapse (Fenton 2000; Hogarty et al. 1997; Stanton et al. 1984).

The focus of supportive psychotherapy is reality based and present centered (Kates and Rockland 1994; Novalis et al. 1993; Winston 2014; Winston et al. 2012). It commonly aims to help patients cope with symptoms, improve adaptive skills, and enhance self-esteem, although descriptions of the goals of supportive psychotherapy have varied. Examples of techniques used to foster these goals include reassurance; praise; encouragement; explanation; clarification; reframing; guidance; suggestion; and use of a conversational, nonconfrontational style of communication. Many of the common elements that have been identified in effective psychotherapies, including a positive therapeutic alliance, are also integral to supportive psychotherapy (Frank and Frank 1991; Wampold 2015). Typically, supportive psychotherapy is conducted in conjunction with medication management at a frequency that can vary from weekly to every few months depending on the needs of the individual patient. Other psychosocial treatments can also be used as part of the treatment plan in conjunction with these modalities.

---

*This guideline statement should be implemented in the context of a person-centered treatment plan that includes evidence-based nonpharmacological and pharmacological treatments for schizophrenia.

Balancing of Potential Benefits and Harms in Rating the Strength of the Guideline Statement

Benefits

Use of supportive psychotherapy in the treatment of schizophrenia was not associated with relative benefits in global or social function as compared with treatment as usual (low strength of research evidence). However, treatment as usual already incorporates supportive psychotherapy under most circumstances. In addition, clinical experience suggests that supportive psychotherapy may be associated with such benefits as strengthening the therapeutic alliance, reducing demoralization, and developing practical coping strategies in the treatment of individuals with schizophrenia.

Harms

The harms of using supportive psychotherapy in the treatment of schizophrenia appear to be small, although evidence is limited. However, if supportive psychotherapy is used preferentially instead of a treatment that is associated with more robust evidence of benefit, there may be indirect negative effects.

Patient Preferences

Clinical experience suggests that most patients are cooperative with and accepting of supportive psychotherapy as part of a treatment plan, even when they are reluctant to engage in other psychosocial interventions. However, some patients may not wish to engage in psychotherapy or may have logistical barriers (e.g., time, access to transportation, financial considerations) that make it difficult to attend psychotherapy sessions.

Balancing of Benefits and Harms

The potential benefits of this guideline statement were viewed as likely to outweigh the potential harms. In clinical practice, the use of supportive psychotherapy is commonplace as part of the treatment of schizophrenia, which makes it challenging to interpret the research comparisons of supportive psychotherapy versus treatment as usual. Given the limited evidence of any harms of supportive psychotherapy, the potential benefits of supportive psychotherapy appear to be greater than the harms. For additional discussion of the research evidence, see Appendix C, Statement 24.

Differences of Opinion Among Writing Group Members

There were no differences of opinion. The writing group voted unanimously in favor of this suggestion.

Review of Available Guidelines From Other Organizations

The NICE guideline notes that supportive psychotherapy should not be offered routinely to individuals with schizophrenia if other psychosocial treatments that have greater efficacy are available (National Institute for Health and Care Excellence 2014). However, the NICE guideline also notes that patient preferences should be taken into account, particularly if other psychosocial interventions are not available locally.

Quality Measurement Considerations

As a suggestion, this guideline statement is not appropriate for use as a performance-based quality measure or for incorporation into electronic decision support.

Areas for Further Research in Individuals With Schizophrenia

Overall

- Improve the generalizability of study populations
- Enhance study recruitment approaches and use a priori specification of subgroup analyses to obtain data on treatment effects in inpatients, minority groups, women, older individuals, individuals with multiple psychiatric or physical health conditions, and individuals with severe and/or treatment-resistant illness
- Assure that sample sizes are adequate to achieve statistical power
- Assure that studies report data in a consistent fashion and prespecify outcomes of interest
- Assure that studies identify the magnitude of change in scale scores that constitutes a clinically meaningful difference
- Increase collection of data on patient-centered outcomes (e.g., quality of life, social functioning, physical health, recovery)
- Improve systematic collection of information on harms, including in studies of psychosocial interventions
- Identify approaches (e.g., pharmacogenomics, biomarkers, symptom clusters, and other predictive variables) for optimizing treatment selection
- Determine efficient, valid, and reliable approaches to quantitative measurement of positive symptoms, negative symptoms, functioning, quality of life, and treatment-related side effects
- Determine ways in which demographic or sociocultural factors influence treatment outcomes
- Determine the durability of treatment effects and potential for long-term harms through long-term studies (e.g., at least 1 year of treatment with follow-up assessments at 3–5 years)
- Determine the benefits, harms, and appropriate use of treatments in individuals with co-occurring disorders (e.g., stimulants in co-occurring ADHD; benzodiazepines with co-occurring anxiety; smoking cessation interventions, including medication and nonmedication approaches with co-occurring nicotine dependence)
- Identify methods that will allow information from mobile technologies, wearable technology, and large-scale data analytics to inform assessment, treatment, and future research
- Determine optimal monitoring frequencies and approaches to detect treatment-related benefits and side effects
- Identify optimal approaches to improving physical health in individuals with schizophrenia
- Identify optimal approaches to treatment of co-occurring substance use disorders in individuals with schizophrenia
- Identify approaches to redesigning workflows and models of care delivery to improve the use of best practices in the treatment of schizophrenia
- Identify approaches to determining the optimal setting of care (e.g., inpatient, partial hospital, intensive outpatient, psychosocial rehabilitation, Clubhouse models)
- Identify optimal approaches to integrate recovery-based and peer-based programs into other models of care delivery
- Identify optimal approaches to care coordination and case management, including intensive case management

Medications and Other Somatic Interventions

- Determine the comparative effectiveness of newer SGAs (including LAI formulations) versus comparable doses of other SGAs and some FGAs
- Determine the comparative harms of antipsychotic medications, including long-term harms and rare but serious harms
- Determine optimal antipsychotic treatment approaches for individuals with suicidal or aggressive behaviors, including additional studies of clozapine for aggressive behavior
- Identify risks and benefits of using other medications (e.g., lithium, anticonvulsants, antidepressants, stimulants, benzodiazepines, other sedative-hypnotics) in combination with antipsychotic medications to address specific target symptoms or treatment nonresponse
- Identify risks and benefits of concomitant use of more than one antipsychotic medication
- Identify risks and benefits of strategies to minimize or treat side effects of antipsychotic medications, including use of concomitant medications, reductions in antipsychotic dose, or changing to a different antipsychotic medication
- Determine optimal approaches to making medication changes (i.e., switching from one antipsychotic to another) to minimize risk of relapse and reduce potential for treatment-related side effects
- Identify optimal clinical approaches for determining when a treatment trial is adequate and when treatment resistance is present
- Determine relationships between blood levels of antipsychotic medications (including active metabolites) and therapeutic response that can be used to guide dose titration and determination of treatment adequacy
- Identify whether there are subgroups of patients for whom medication discontinuation may be possible
- Determine whether intermittent treatment or early relapse is associated with increased long-term harms (e.g., greater treatment resistance, neurobiological changes)
- Determine optimal approaches to prevention and treatment of specific side effects of antipsychotic medications, including neurological side effects, weight gain, diabetes, metabolic syndrome, and cardiovascular disease
- Determine the optimal duration of treatments for neurological side effects (e.g., VMAT2 inhibitors for tardive dyskinesia, anticholinergic agents for parkinsonism)
- Determine the efficacy and comparative effectiveness of neurostimulation approaches (e.g., ECT, TMS) in conjunction with other treatments for schizophrenia

Psychosocial Interventions

- Assure that psychosocial interventions are clearly defined and described and that measurements of fidelity to the intervention model are incorporated into the study design
- Conduct research on optimizing long-term outcomes with psychosocial interventions (e.g., use of booster treatment sessions or continued treatment at a lower frequency for maintenance of therapeutic benefits in those with a good initial response)
- Develop approaches to reduce the heterogeneity in usual care groups, which makes it difficult to interpret and compare studies of psychosocial interventions that use usual care as a control comparison
- Assure that studies of psychosocial interventions determine the intensity, frequency, and duration of treatment that is needed to optimize outcomes

- Develop methods to study psychosocial interventions to identify key contributors to benefit (e.g., clinician experience, treatment fidelity, use of shared decision-making, clinician-patient alliance, family engagement, setting of care)
- Investigate the benefits and harms of other psychosocial interventions (e.g., mindfulness, acceptance and commitment therapy, metacognitive reflection and insight therapy, Open Dialogue, exercise, music and dance therapies)
- Determine benefits, harms, and optimal approaches for implementation of peer-based services, recovery-oriented programs, and self-management strategies
- Determine the components of multicomponent interventions (e.g., CSC) that are crucial to positive outcomes
- Determine the effectiveness and sustainability of CSC with longer-term program participation
- Determine the elements of supported employment programs that are most likely to foster long-term competitive employment

Guideline Development Process

This guideline was developed using a process intended to meet standards of the Institute of Medicine (2011) (now known as the National Academy of Medicine). The process is fully described in a document available on the American Psychiatric Association (APA) website at www.psychiatry.org/psychiatrists/practice/clinical-practice-guidelines/guideline-development-process.

Management of Potential Conflicts of Interest

Members of the Guideline Writing Group (GWG) are required to disclose all potential conflicts of interest before appointment, before and during guideline development, and on publication. If any potential conflicts are found or disclosed during the guideline development process, the member must recuse himself or herself from any related discussion and voting on a related recommendation. The members of both the GWG and the Systematic Review Group (SRG) reported no conflicts of interest. The "Disclosures" section includes more detailed disclosure information for each GWG and SRG member involved in the guideline's development.

Guideline Writing Group Composition

The GWG was initially composed of eight psychiatrists with general research and clinical expertise and a psychiatric resident (A.D.). This non-topic-specific group was intended to provide diverse and balanced views on the guideline topic in order to minimize potential bias. One psychiatrist (P.B.) and one psychologist (M.F.L.) were added to provide subject matter expertise in schizophrenia. An additional member (A.S.Y.) provided input on quality measure considerations. The vice-chair of the GWG (L.J.F.) provided methodological expertise on such topics as appraising the strength of research evidence. The GWG was also diverse and balanced with respect to other characteristics, such as geographic location and demographic background. The National Alliance on Mental Illness, Mental Health America, and the Schizophrenia and Related Disorders Alliance of America reviewed the draft and provided perspective from patients, families, and other care partners.

Systematic Review Methodology

The Agency for Healthcare Research and Quality's (AHRQ) systematic review, *Treatments for Schizophrenia in Adults* (McDonagh et al. 2017), served as the predominant source of information for this guideline. APA also conducted a search of additional systematic reviews and meta-analyses to include consideration of placebo-controlled trials that were not part of the AHRQ review. An additional search was conducted in MEDLINE (PubMed) and PsycINFO on treatments for neurological side effects of antipsychotic medications, including acute dystonia, parkinsonism, akathisia, and tardive syndromes. The search terms, limits used, and dates of these searches are available in Appendix B. Results were limited to English-language, adult (18 and older), and human-only studies. These titles and abstracts were reviewed for relevance by one individual (L.J.F.). Available guidelines from other organizations were also reviewed (Addington et al. 2017a, 2017b; Barnes et al. 2011; Buchanan et al. 2010; Crockford and Addington 2017; Galletly et al. 2016; Hasan et al. 2012; National Institute for Health and Care Excellence 2014; Pringsheim et al. 2017; Scottish Intercollegiate Guidelines Network 2013).

Rating the Strength of Supporting Research Evidence

Strength of supporting research evidence describes the level of confidence that findings from scientific observation and testing of an effect of an intervention reflect the true effect. Confidence is enhanced by such factors as rigorous study design and minimal potential for study bias.

Ratings were determined, in accordance with the AHRQ's "Methods Guide for Effectiveness and Comparative Effectiveness Reviews" (Agency for Healthcare Research and Quality 2014), by the methodologist (L.J.F.) and reviewed by members of the SRG and GWG. Available clinical trials were assessed across four primary domains: risk of bias, consistency of findings across studies, directness of the effect on a specific health outcome, and precision of the estimate of effect.

The ratings are defined as follows:

- High (denoted by the letter A)=high confidence that the evidence reflects the true effect. Further research is very unlikely to change our confidence in the estimate of effect.
- Moderate (denoted by the letter B)=moderate confidence that the evidence reflects the true effect. Further research may change our confidence in the estimate of effect and may change the estimate.
- Low (denoted by the letter C)=low confidence that the evidence reflects the true effect. Further research is likely to change our confidence in the estimate of effect and is likely to change the estimate.

The AHRQ has an additional category of *insufficient* for evidence that is unavailable or does not permit estimation of an effect. APA uses the *low* rating when evidence is insufficient because there is low confidence in the conclusion and further research, if conducted, would likely change the estimated effect or confidence in the estimated effect.

Rating the Strength of Guideline Statements

Each guideline statement is separately rated to indicate strength of recommendation and strength of supporting research evidence. *Strength of recommendation* describes the level of confidence that potential benefits of an intervention outweigh potential harms. This level of confidence is a consensus judgment of the authors of the guideline and is informed by available evidence, which includes evidence from clinical trials as well as expert opinion and patient values and preferences.

There are two possible ratings: recommendation or suggestion. A *recommendation* (denoted by the numeral 1 after the guideline statement) indicates confidence that the benefits of the intervention clearly outweigh harms. A *suggestion* (denoted by the numeral 2 after the guideline statement) indicates greater uncertainty. Although the benefits of the statement are still viewed as outweighing the harms, the balance of benefits and harms is more difficult to judge, or the benefits or the harms may be less clear. With a suggestion, patient values and preferences may be more variable, and this can influence the clinical decision that is ultimately made. These strengths of recommendation correspond to ratings of *strong* or *weak* (also termed *conditional*) as defined under the Grading of Recommendations Assessment, Development and Evaluation (GRADE) method for rating recommendations in clinical practice guidelines (described in publications such as Guyatt et al. 2008 and others available on the website of the GRADE working group at www.gradeworkinggroup.org).

When a negative statement is made, ratings of strength of recommendation should be understood as meaning the inverse of the above (e.g., *recommendation* indicates confidence that harms clearly outweigh benefits).

The GWG determined ratings of strength of recommendation by a modified Delphi method using blind, iterative voting and discussion. In order for the GWG members to be able to ask for clarifications about the evidence, the wording of statements, or the process, the vice-chair of the GWG served as a resource and did not vote on statements. All other formally appointed GWG members, including the chair, voted.

In weighing potential benefits and harms, GWG members considered the strength of supporting research evidence, their own clinical experiences and opinions, and patient preferences. For recommendations, at least 10 out of 11 members must have voted to recommend the intervention or assessment after three rounds of voting, and at most 1 member was allowed to vote other than "recommend" the intervention or assessment. On the basis of the discussion among the GWG members, adjustments to the wording of recommendations could be made between the voting rounds. If this level of consensus was not achieved, the GWG could have agreed to make a suggestion rather than a recommendation. No suggestion or statement could have been made if 3 or more members voted "no statement." Differences of opinion within the GWG about ratings of strength of recommendation, if any, are described in the subsection "Balancing of Potential Benefits and Harms in Rating the Strength of the Guideline Statement" for each statement.

Use of Guidelines to Enhance Quality of Care

Clinical practice guidelines can help enhance quality by synthesizing available research evidence and delineating recommendations for care on the basis of the available evidence. In some circumstances, practice guideline recommendations will be appropriate to use in developing quality measures. Guideline statements can also be used in other ways, such as educational activities or electronic clinical decision support, to enhance the quality of care that patients receive. Furthermore, when availability of services is a major barrier to implementing guideline recommendations, improved tracking of service availability and program development initiatives may need to be implemented by health organizations, health insurance plans, federal or state agencies, or other regulatory programs.

Typically, guideline recommendations that are chosen for development into quality measures will advance one or more aims of the Institute of Medicine's report on *Crossing the Quality Chasm* (Institute of Medicine Committee on Quality of Health Care in America 2001) and the ongoing work guided by the multistakeholder-integrated, AHRQ-led National Quality Strategy by facilitating care that is safe, effective, patient centered, timely, efficient, and equitable. To achieve these aims, a broad range of quality measures (Watkins et al. 2015) is needed that spans the entire continuum of care (e.g., prevention, screening, assessment, treatment, continuing care), addresses the different levels of the health system hierarchy (e.g., system-wide, organization, program/department, individual clinicians), and includes measures of different types (e.g., process, outcome, patient-centered experience). Emphasis is also needed on factors that influence the dissemination and adoption of evidence-based practices (Drake et al. 2008; Greenhalgh et al. 2004; Horvitz-Lennon et al. 2009).

Measure development is complex and requires detailed development of specification and pilot testing (Center for Health Policy/Center for Primary Care and Outcomes Research and Battelle Memorial Institute 2011; Fernandes-Taylor and Harris 2012; Iyer et al. 2016; Pincus et al. 2016; Watkins et al. 2011). Generally, however, measure development should be guided by the available evidence and focused on measures that are broadly relevant and meaningful to patients, clinicians, and policy makers. Measure feasibility is another crucial aspect of measure development but is often decided on the basis of current data availability, which limits opportunities for development of novel measurement concepts. Furthermore, innovation in workflow and data collection systems can benefit from looking beyond practical limitations in the early development stages in order to foster development of meaningful measures.

Often, quality measures will focus on gaps in care or on care processes and outcomes that have significant variability across specialties, health care settings, geographic areas, or patients' demographic characteristics. Administrative databases, registries, and data from electronic health records can help to identify gaps in care and key domains that would benefit from performance improvements (Acevedo et al. 2015; Patel et al. 2015; Watkins et al. 2016). Nevertheless, for some guideline statements, evidence of practice gaps or variability will be based on anecdotal observations if the typical practices of psychiatrists and other health professionals are unknown. Variability in the use of guideline-recommended approaches may reflect appropriate differences that are tailored to the patient's preferences, treatment of co-occurring illnesses, or other clinical circumstances that may not have been studied in the available research. On the other hand, variability may indicate a need to strengthen clinician knowledge or address other barriers to adoption of best practices (Drake et al. 2008; Greenhalgh et al. 2004; Horvitz-Lennon et al. 2009). When performance is compared among organizations, variability may reflect a need for quality improvement initiatives to improve overall outcomes but could also reflect case-mix differences such as socioeconomic factors or the prevalence of co-occurring illnesses.

When a guideline recommendation is considered for development into a quality measure, it must be possible to define the applicable patient group (i.e., the denominator) and the clinical action or outcome of interest that is measured (i.e., the numerator) in validated, clear, and quantifiable terms. Furthermore, the health system's or clinician's performance on the measure must be readily ascertained from chart review, patient-reported outcome measures, registries, or administrative data. Documentation of quality measures can be challenging and, depending on the practice setting, can pose practical barriers to meaningful interpretation of quality measures based on guideline recommendations. For example, when recommendations relate to patient assessment or treatment selection, clinical judgment may need to be used to determine whether the clinician has addressed the factors that merit emphasis for an individual patient. In other circumstances, standardized instruments can facilitate quality measurement reporting, but it is difficult to assess the appropriateness of clinical judgment in a validated, standardized manner. Furthermore, utilization of standardized assessments remains low (Fortney et al. 2017), and clinical findings are not routinely documented in a standardized format. Many clinicians appropriately use free text prose to describe symptoms, response to treatment, discussions with family, plans of treatment, and other aspects of care and clinical decision-making. Reviewing these free text records for measurement purposes would be impractical, and it would be difficult to hold clinicians accountable to such measures without significant increases in electronic medical record use and advances in natural language processing technology.

Conceptually, quality measures can be developed for purposes of accountability, for internal or health system–based quality improvement, or both. Accountability measures require clinicians to report their rate of performance of a specified process, intermediate outcome, or outcome in a specified group of patients. Because these data are used to determine financial incentives or penalties based on performance, accountability measures must be scientifically validated, have a strong evidence base, and fill gaps in care. In contrast, internal or health system–based quality improvement measures are typically designed by and for individual providers, health systems, or payers. They typically focus on measurements that can suggest ways for clinicians or administrators to improve efficiency and delivery of services within a particular setting. Internal or health system–based quality improvement programs may or may not link performance with payment, and, in general, these measures are not subject to strict testing and validation requirements.

Quality improvement activities, including performance measures derived from these guidelines, should yield improvements in quality of care to justify any clinician burden (e.g., documentation burden) or related administrative costs (e.g., for manual extraction of data from charts, for modifications of electronic medical record systems to capture required data elements). Possible unintended consequences of any derived measures also need to be addressed in testing of a fully specified measure in a variety of practice settings. For example, highly specified measures may lead to overuse of standardized language that does not accurately reflect what has occurred in practice. If multiple discrete fields are used to capture information on a paper or electronic record form, data will be easily retrievable and reportable, but oversimplification is a possible unintended consequence of measurement. Just as guideline developers must balance the benefits and harms of a particular guideline recommendation, developers of performance measures must weigh the potential benefits, burdens, and unintended consequences in optimizing quality measure design and testing.

External Review

This guideline was made available for review in May–June 2019 by stakeholders, including the APA membership, scientific and clinical experts, allied organizations, and the public. In addition, a number of patient advocacy organizations were invited for input. A total of 98 individuals and 20 organizations submitted comments on the guideline (for a list of the names, see the section "Individuals and Organizations That Submitted Comments"). The chair and co-chair of the GWG reviewed and addressed all comments received; substantive issues were reviewed by the GWG.

Funding and Approval

This guideline development project was funded and supported by the APA without any involvement of industry or external funding. The guideline was submitted to the APA Assembly and APA Board of Trustees and approved on November 17, 2019 and December 15, 2019, respectively.

Glossary of Terms

Adequate dose   The dose of a medication at which therapeutic effects occurred when tested in clinical trials in a comparable population of subjects. This dose will differ for each medication and may need to be adjusted in an individual patient to address factors that would influence drug absorption, metabolism, elimination, or other pharmacokinetic properties.

Adequate response   A reduction in symptoms as a result of treatment that is associated with clinically significant benefit in functioning and/or quality of life. A reduction in symptoms of 50% or more is sometimes used as a threshold for adequacy of response.

Antipsychotic medication   One of a group of medications used in the treatment of psychosis. Some of the antipsychotic medications are also approved for use in other conditions such as mood disorders or Tourette's syndrome. The first-generation antipsychotic (FGA) medications, sometimes referred to as *typical* antipsychotic medications, were the initial medications to be discovered. The FGAs include, but are not limited to, chlorpromazine, droperidol, fluphenazine, haloperidol, loxapine, molindone, perphenazine, pimozide, thioridazine, thiothixene, and trifluoperazine. The second-generation antipsychotic (SGA) medications, sometimes referred to as *atypical* antipsychotic medications, include, but are not limited, to aripiprazole, asenapine, brexpiprazole, cariprazine, clozapine, iloperidone, lurasidone, olanzapine, paliperidone, quetiapine, risperidone, and ziprasidone. In terms of the Neuroscience-based Nomenclature (www.nbn2.org), antipsychotic medications are categorized as follows:

- Dopamine D_2 receptor antagonists: fluphenazine, haloperidol, perphenazine, pimozide
- D_2 and serotonin type 2 (5-HT_2) receptor antagonists: chlorpromazine, iloperidone, loxapine, lurasidone, olanzapine, thioridazine, trifluoperazine, ziprasidone
- D_2 and 5-HT_{1A} receptor partial agonist and 5-HT_{2A} receptor antagonist: aripiprazole, brexpiprazole
- 5-HT_2, D_2, and norepinephrine (NE) α_2 receptor antagonist: asenapine
- D_2, 5-HT_2, and NE α_2 receptor antagonists: clozapine, paliperidone, risperidone
- D_2 and 5-HT_2 receptor antagonist and NE transporter reuptake inhibitor: quetiapine

Within each group of antipsychotic medications, there is significant variability in the pharmacological properties and side-effect profiles of specific drugs.

Assessment   The process of obtaining information about a patient through any of a variety of methods, including face-to-face interview, review of medical records, physical examination (by the psychiatrist, another physician, or a medically trained clinician), diagnostic testing, or history taking from collateral sources (American Psychiatric Association 2016a).

Capacity for decision making   The ability of an individual, when faced with a specific clinical or treatment-related decision, "to communicate a choice, to understand the relevant information, to appreciate the medical consequences of the situation, and to reason about treatment choices" (Appelbaum 2007, p. 1835).

Comprehensive and person-centered treatment plan   A plan of treatment that is developed as an outgrowth of the psychiatric evaluation and is modified as clinically indicated. A comprehensive treatment plan can include nonpharmacological treatments, pharmacological treatments, or both. It is individualized to the patient's clinical presentation, safety-related needs, concomitant medical conditions, personal background, relationships, life circumstances, and strengths and vulnerabilities. There is no prescribed format that a comprehensive treatment plan must follow. The breadth and depth of the initial treatment plan will depend on the amount of time and extent of information that are available, as well as the needs of the patients and the care setting. Additions and modifications to the treatment plan are made as additional information accrues (e.g., from family, staff, medical records, and other collateral sources) and the patient's responses to clinical interventions are observed.

Contraindication   A situation in which a drug or procedure should not be used because it may be harmful to the patient.

Delusion   A false belief based on incorrect inference about external reality that is firmly held despite what almost everyone else believes and despite what constitutes incontrovertible and obvious proof or evidence to the contrary. The belief is not ordinarily accepted by other members of the person's culture or subculture (i.e., it is not an article of religious faith) (American Psychiatric Association 2013e). The content of a delusion may include a variety of themes (e.g., persecutory, referential, somatic, religious, grandiose) (American Psychiatric Association 2013a).

Disorganized thinking   Disorganized thinking (also referred to as formal thought disorder) is typically inferred from the individual's speech and must be severe enough to substantially impair effective communication. The individual may switch from one topic to another (derailment or loose associations), provide answers to questions in an obliquely related or completely unrelated fashion (tangentiality), or exhibit severely disorganized and nearly incomprehensible speech that resembles receptive aphasia in its linguistic disorganization (incoherence or "word salad") (adapted from American Psychiatric Association 2013a).

Grossly disorganized or abnormal motor behavior   Grossly disorganized or abnormal motor behavior may manifest itself in a variety of ways, ranging from childlike "silliness" to unpredictable agitation. Problems may be noted in any form of goal-directed behavior, leading to difficulties in performing activities of daily living. Catatonic behavior is another manifestation of abnormal motor behavior and can range from resistance to instructions (negativism); to maintaining a rigid, inappropriate, or bizarre posture; to a complete lack of verbal and motor responses (mutism and stupor). It can also include purposeless and excessive motor activity without obvious cause (catatonic excitement). Other features are repeated stereotyped movements, staring, grimacing, mutism, and the echoing of speech (adapted from American Psychiatric Association 2013a).

Hallucination   Perception-like experiences that occur without an external stimulus. Hallucinations are vivid and clear, with the full force and impact of normal perceptions, and not under voluntary control. They may occur in any sensory modality (American Psychiatric Association 2013a).

Hepatic failure   Deterioration of liver function that results in coagulation abnormality (usually an international normalized ratio greater than or equal to 1.5) and any degree of mental alteration (encephalopathy). Although there is no identifiable cause in approximately 15% of cases of acute hepatic failure, typical etiologies include drug-induced liver injury, viral hepatitis, autoimmune liver disease, and shock or hypoperfusion (Lee et al. 2011).

Hepatic impairment   Inability of the liver to function normally; typically defined in severity according to laboratory values and clinical characteristics as reflected by the Child-Pugh score or the Model for End-Stage Liver Disease (MELD) score (Ghany and Hoofnagle 2018; U.S. Food and Drug Administration 2003).

Hopelessness   Feeling of despair about the future out of the belief that there is no possibility of a solution to current problems or a positive outcome.

I^2 A statistical estimate of the proportion of the variance that is due to heterogeneity.

Impulsivity   Acting on the spur of the moment in response to immediate stimuli, acting on a momentary basis without a plan or consideration of outcomes, difficulty establishing and following plans, or having a sense of urgency and exhibiting self-harming behavior under emotional distress (American Psychiatric Association 2013f).

Initial psychiatric evaluation   A comprehensive assessment of a patient that has the following aims: identify the reason that the patient is presenting for evaluation; establish rapport with the patient; understand the patient's background, relationships, current life circumstances, and strengths and vulnerabilities; establish whether the patient has a psychiatric condition; collect information needed to develop a differential diagnosis and clinical formulation; identify immediate concerns for patient safety; and develop an initial treatment plan or revise an existing plan in collaboration with the patient. Relevant information may be obtained by interviewing the patient; reviewing prior records; or obtaining collateral information from treating clinicians, family members, or others involved in the patient's life. Physical examination, laboratory studies, imaging, psychological or neuropsychological testing, or other assessments may also be included. The psychiatric evaluation may occur in a variety of settings, including inpatient or outpatient psychiatric settings and other medical settings. The evaluation is usually time intensive. The amount of time spent depends on the complexity of the problem, the clinical setting, and the patient's ability and willingness to cooperate with the assessment. Several meetings with the patient (and family or others) over time may be necessary. Psychiatrists may conduct other types of evaluations that have other goals (e.g., forensic evaluations) or that may be more focused and circumscribed than a psychiatric evaluation as defined here. Guidelines are not intended to address such evaluations (American Psychiatric Association 2016a).

Negative symptoms   Negative symptoms can be prominent in schizophrenia and can include diminution of emotional expression (eye contact; intonation of speech; and movements of the hand, head, and face), decrease in motivated self-initiated purposeful activities (avolition), diminution of speech output (alogia), decrease in the ability to experience pleasure from positive stimuli (anhedonia), or apparent lack of interest in social interactions (asociality) (adapted from American Psychiatric Association 2013a).

Over-the-counter medications or supplements   Drugs or supplements that can be bought without a prescription.

Person-centered care   Care that is respectful of and responsive to individual preferences, needs, and values and ensures that an individual's values guide all clinical decisions; sometimes referred to as patient-centered care (Institute of Medicine Committee on Quality of Health Care in America 2001). In person-centered care, patients, families, and other persons of support are provided with information that allows them to make informed decisions (Institute of Medicine 2006). Evidence-based interventions should be adapted to meet individual needs and preferences where possible (van Dulmen et al. 2015), and shared decision-making and self-management approaches are encouraged (Institute of Medicine 2006). Person-centered care is achieved through a dynamic and collaborative relationship among individuals, families, other persons of support, and treating clinicians that supports the individual's realistic health and life goals and informs decision-making to the extent that the individual desires (American Geriatrics Society Expert Panel on Person-Centered Care 2016).

Renal impairment   Inability of the kidney(s) to function normally, typically described in terms of reductions in creatinine clearance or estimated glomerular filtration rate (eGFR). An eGFR of 60–89 mL/min/1.73 m^2 indicates mildly reduced kidney function; an eGFR of 30–59 mL/min/1.73 m^2 indicates moderately reduced kidney function; an eGFR of 15–29 mL/min/1.73 m^2 indicates severely reduced kidney function; and an eGFR of less than 15 mL/min/1.73 m^2 indicates a very severe reduction in kidney function or end-stage renal disease (Kidney Disease: Improving Global Outcomes [KDIGO] CKD Work Group 2013).

Suicidal ideas   Thoughts of serving as the agent of one's own death.

Suicide   Death caused by self-directed injurious behavior with any intent to die as a result of the behavior (Crosby et al. 2011).

Suicide attempt   A nonfatal, self-directed, potentially injurious behavior with any intent to die as a result of the behavior. A suicide attempt may or may not result in injury (Crosby et al. 2011). It may be aborted by the individual or interrupted by another individual.

Suicide intent   Subjective expectation and desire for a self-injurious act to end in death.

Suicide means   The instrument or object used to engage in self-inflicted injurious behavior with any intent to die as a result of the behavior.

Suicide method   The mechanism used to engage in self-inflicted injurious behavior with any intent to die as a result of the behavior.

Suicide plan   Delineation of the method, means, time, place, or other details for engaging in self-inflicted injurious behavior with any intent to die as a result of the behavior.

Therapeutic alliance   A characteristic of the relationship between the patient and clinician that describes the sense of collaboration in pursuing therapeutic goals as well as the patient's sense of attachment to the clinician and perception of whether the clinician is helpful (Gabbard 2009).

Trauma history   A history of events in the patient's life with the potential to have been emotionally traumatic, including but not limited to exposure to actual or threatened death, serious injury, illness, or sexual violence. Exposure may occur through direct experience or by observing an event in person or through technology (e.g., television, audio or video recording) or by learning of an event that occurred to a close family member or close friend. Trauma could also include early adversity, neglect, maltreatment, emotional abuse, physical abuse, or sexual abuse occurring in childhood; exposure to natural or man-made disasters; exposure to combat situations; being a victim of a violent crime; involvement in a serious motor vehicle accident; or having serious or painful or prolonged medical experiences (e.g., intensive care unit stay).

Treatment as usual   Treatment that is consistent with care received for a specific condition in a real-world nonresearch context. Treatment as usual, sometimes referred to as usual care or standard care, is often used as an active comparison condition for studies of new interventions. Elements of treatment as usual are heterogeneous and differ with each study but can include medication treatment, medication management, case management, rehabilitation services, and psychotherapy (McDonagh et al. 2017).

References

Abilify (aripiprazole) [product monograph]. Saint-Laurent, QC, Canada, Otsuka Canada Pharmaceutical, November 2017

Abilify (aripiprazole) [prescribing information]. Rockville, MD, Otsuka America Pharmaceutical, August 2019

Abilify Maintena (aripiprazole) [prescribing information]. Rockville, MD, Otsuka America Pharmaceutical, March 2018. Available at: www.otsuka-us.com/media/static/Abilify-M-PI.pdf. Accessed January 20, 2019.

Abilify Mycite (aripiprazole) [prescribing information]. Rockville, MD, Otsuka America Pharmaceutical, November 2017

Acevedo A, Garnick DW, Dunigan R, et al: Performance measures and racial/ethnic disparities in the treatment of substance use disorders. J Stud Alcohol Drugs 76(1):57–67, 2015 25486394

Achtyes E, Simmons A, Skabeev A, et al: Patient preferences concerning the efficacy and side-effect profile of schizophrenia medications: a survey of patients living with schizophrenia. BMC Psychiatry 18(1):292, 2018 30223804

ACOG Committee on Practice Bulletins—Obstetrics: ACOG Practice Bulletin: Clinical management guidelines for obstetrician-gynecologists number 92. Use of psychiatric medications during pregnancy and lactation. Obstet Gynecol 111(4):1001–1020, 2008 18378767

Acosta FJ, Hernández JL, Pereira J, et al: Medication adherence in schizophrenia. World J Psychiatry 2(5):74–82, 2012 24175171

Addington D, McKenzie E, Smith H, et al: Conformance to evidence-based treatment recommendations in schizophrenia treatment services. Can J Psychiatry 57(5):317–323, 2012 22546064

Addington DE, Norman R, Bond GR, et al: Development and testing of the First-Episode Psychosis Services Fidelity Scale. Psychiatr Serv 67(9):1023–1025, 2016 27032665

Addington D, Abidi S, Garcia-Ortega I, et al: Canadian guidelines for the assessment and diagnosis of patients with schizophrenia spectrum and other psychotic disorders. Can J Psychiatry 62(9):594–603, 2017a 28730847

Addington D, Anderson E, Kelly M, et al: Canadian practice guidelines for comprehensive community treatment for schizophrenia and schizophrenia spectrum disorders. Can J Psychiatry 62(9):662–672, 2017b 28886669

Addington D, Birchwood M, Jones P, et al: Fidelity scales and performance measures to support implementation and quality assurance for first episode psychosis services. Early Interv Psychiatry 12(6):1235–1242, 2018 29882236

Addington J, Addington D, Abidi S, et al: Canadian treatment guidelines for individuals at clinical high risk of psychosis. Can J Psychiatry 62(9):656–661, 2017 28730848

Adelufosi AO, Abayomi O, Ojo TM: Pyridoxal 5 phosphate for neuroleptic-induced tardive dyskinesia. Cochrane Database Syst Rev April 13(4):CD010501, 2015 25866243

Agency for Healthcare Research and Quality: Methods guide for effectiveness and comparative effectiveness reviews (AHRQ Publ No 10(14)-EHC063-EF). Rockville, MD, Agency for Healthcare Research and Quality, January 2014. Available at: www.effectivehealthcare.ahrq.gov/search-for-guides-reviews-and-reports/?pageaction=displayproduct&productid=318. Accessed February 15, 2017.

Agerwala SM, McCance-Katz EF: Integrating screening, brief intervention, and referral to treatment (SBIRT) into clinical practice settings: a brief review. J Psychoactive Drugs 44(4):307–317, 2012 23210379

Aggarwal NK, Lewis-Fernández R: An introduction to the Cultural Formulation Interview. Focus 13(4):426–431, 2015

Ahalt C, Williams B: Reforming solitary-confinement policy: heeding a presidential call to action. N Engl J Med 374(18):1704–1706, 2016 27144846

Ahalt C, Haney C, Rios S, et al: Reducing the use and impact of solitary confinement in corrections. Int J Prison Health 13(1):41–48, 2017 28299967

Ahmed S, Khan AM, Mekala HM, et al: Combined use of electroconvulsive therapy and antipsychotics (both clozapine and non-clozapine) in treatment resistant schizophrenia: a comparative meta-analysis. Heliyon 3(11):e00429, 2017 29264404

Ajmal A, Joffe H, Nachtigall LB: Psychotropic-induced hyperprolactinemia: a clinical review. Psychosomatics 55(1):29–36, 2014 24140188

Alabed S, Latifeh Y, Mohammad HA, Bergman H: Gamma-aminobutyric acid agonists for neuroleptic-induced tardive dyskinesia. Cochrane Database Syst Rev Apr 17 4(4):CD000203, 2018 29663328

Alastal Y, Hasan S, Chowdhury MA, et al: Hypertriglyceridemia-induced pancreatitis in psychiatric patients: a case report and review of literature. Am J Ther 23(3):e947–949, 2016 24987947

Alban RF, Nuño M, Ko A, et al: Weaker gun state laws are associated with higher rates of suicide secondary to firearms. J Surg Res 221:135–142, 2018 29229119

Alberti KG, Eckel RH, Grundy SM, et al: Harmonizing the metabolic syndrome: a joint interim statement of the International Diabetes Federation Task Force on Epidemiology and Prevention; National Heart, Lung, and Blood Institute; American Heart Association; World Heart Federation; International Atherosclerosis Society; and International Association for the Study of Obesity. Circulation 120(16):1640–1645, 2009 19805654

Aleman A, Enriquez-Geppert S, Knegtering H, Dlabac-de Lange JJ: Moderate effects of noninvasive brain stimulation of the frontal cortex for improving negative symptoms in schizophrenia: meta-analysis of controlled trials. Neurosci Biobehav Rev 89:111–118, 2018 29471017

Ali SA, Mathur N, Malhotra AK, Braga RJ: Electroconvulsive therapy and schizophrenia: a systematic review. Mol Neuropsychiatry 5(2):75–83, 2019 31192220

Alldredge BK: Seizure risk associated with psychotropic drugs: clinical and pharmacokinetic considerations. Neurology 53(5 suppl 2):S68–S75, 1999 10496236

Allen JG, Frueh BC, Ellis TE, et al: Integrating outcomes assessment and research into clinical care in inpatient adult psychiatric treatment. Bull Menninger Clin 73(4):259–295, 2009 20025425

Almerie MQ, Al Marhi MO, Jawoosh M, et al: Social skills programmes for schizophrenia. Cochrane Database Syst Rev Jun 9(6):CD009006, 2015 26059249

Al-Rousan T, Rubenstein L, Sieleni B, et al: Inside the nation's largest mental health institution: a prevalence study in a state prison system. BMC Public Health 17(1):342, 2017 28427371

Alvarez-Jimenez M, Gonzalez-Blanch C, Crespo-Facorro B, et al: Antipsychotic-induced weight gain in chronic and first-episode psychotic disorders: a systematic critical reappraisal. CNS Drugs 22(7):547–562, 2008 18547125

Alvir JM, Lieberman JA, Safferman AZ, et al: Clozapine-induced agranulocytosis: incidence and risk factors in the United States. N Engl J Med 329(3):162–167, 1993 8515788

Amantadine hydrochloride capsules [prescribing information]. High Point, NC, Banner Life Sciences, December 2015

Amantadine hydrochloride oral solution [prescribing information]. Farmville, NC, CMP Pharma, January 2015

Amantadine hydrochloride tablets [prescribing information]. Yardley, PA, Vensun Pharmaceuticals, January 2019

American Academy of Pediatrics and the American College of Obstetricians and Gynecologists: Guidelines for Perinatal Care, 8th Edition. Elk Grove Village, IL, American Academy of Pediatrics; Washington, DC, American College of Obstetricians and Gynecologists, 2017

American College of Correctional Physicians: Restricted housing of mentally ill inmates. Marion, MA, American College of Correctional Physicians, 2013. Available at: http://accpmed.org/restricted_housing_of_mentally.php. Accessed September 22, 2019.

American College of Obstetricians and Gynecologists: ACOG Committee Opinion No. 736: Optimizing postpartum care. Obstet Gynecol 131(5):e140–e150, 2018 29683911

American College of Obstetricians and Gynecologists' Committee on Obstetric Practice; Breastfeeding Expert Work Group: Committee Opinion No. 658: Optimizing support for breastfeeding as part of obstetric practice. Obstet Gynecol 127(2):e86–92, 2016 26942393

American Diabetes Association: 2. Classification and diagnosis of diabetes: standards of medical care in diabetes—2018. Diabetes Care 41 (suppl 1):S13–S27, 2018 29222373

American Geriatrics Society Expert Panel on Person-Centered Care: Person-centered care: a definition and essential elements. J Am Geriatr Soc 64(1):15–18, 2016 26626262

American Psychiatric Association: Diagnostic and Statistical Manual of Mental Disorders, 4th Edition, Text Revision. Washington, DC, American Psychiatric Association, 2000

American Psychiatric Association: Practice Guideline for the Treatment of Patients With Schizophrenia, 2nd Edition. Arlington, VA, American Psychiatric Publishing, 2004

American Psychiatric Association: Position statement on treatment of substance use disorders in the criminal justice system. Arlington, VA, American Psychiatric Association, 2007. Available at: www.psychiatry.org/File%20Library/About-APA/Organization-Documents-Policies/Policies/Position-2007-Substance-Abuse-Criminal-Justice.pdf. Accessed September 22, 2019.

American Psychiatric Association: Guideline Watch: Practice Guideline for the Treatment of Patients With Schizophrenia. Arlington, VA, American Psychiatric Publishing, 2009a

American Psychiatric Association: Position statement on atypical antipsychotic medications. Arlington, VA, American Psychiatric Association, 2009b. Available at: www.psychiatry.org/File%20Library/About-APA/Organization-Documents-Policies/Policies/Position-2009-Atypical-Antipsychotics.pdf. Accessed September 22, 2019.

American Psychiatric Association: Outpatient services for the mentally ill involved in the criminal justice system. Arlington, VA, American Psychiatric Association, 2009c. Available at: www.psychiatry.org/File%20 Library/Psychiatrists/Directories/Library-and-Archive/task-force-reports/tfr2009_outpatient.pdf. Accessed September 27, 2019.

American Psychiatric Association: Diagnostic and Statistical Manual of Mental Disorders, 5th Edition. Arlington, VA, American Psychiatric Association, 2013a

American Psychiatric Association: Clinician-rated dimensions of psychosis symptom severity, in Diagnostic and Statistical Manual of Mental Disorders, 5th Edition. Arlington, VA, American Psychiatric Association, 2013b, pp 743–744. Available at: www.psychiatry.org/File%20Library/Psychiatrists/Practice/DSM/APA_DSM5_Clinician-Rated-Dimensions-of-Psychosis-Symptom-Severity.pdf. Accessed November 10, 2019.

American Psychiatric Association: DSM-5 self-rated level 1 cross-cutting symptom measure—adult, in Diagnostic and Statistical Manual of Mental Disorders, 5th Edition. Arlington, VA, American Psychiatric Association, 2013c, pp 738–739. Available at: www.psychiatry.org/File%20Library/Psychiatrists/Practice/DSM/APA_DSM5_Level-1-Measure-Adult.pdf. Accessed November 10, 2019.

American Psychiatric Association: WHODAS 2.0 (World Health Organization Disability Assessment Schedule 2.0): 36-item version, self-administered, in Diagnostic and Statistical Manual of Mental Disorders, 5th Edition. Arlington, VA, American Psychiatric Association, 2013d, pp 747–748. Available at: www.psychiatry.org/psychiatrists/practice/dsm/educational-resources/assessment-measures. Accessed November 10, 2019.

American Psychiatric Association: Glossary of technical terms, in Diagnostic and Statistical Manual of Mental Disorders, 5th Edition. Arlington, VA, American Psychiatric Association, 2013e, pp 817–831

American Psychiatric Association: The Principles of Medical Ethics With Annotations Especially Applicable to Psychiatry, 2013 Edition. Arlington, VA, American Psychiatric Association, 2013f. Available at: www.psychiatry.org/File%20Library/Psychiatrists/Practice/Ethics/principles-medical-ethics.pdf. Accessed November 18, 2018.

American Psychiatric Association: Resource document on involuntary outpatient commitment and related programs of assisted outpatient treatment. Arlington, VA, American Psychiatric Association, 2015. Available at: www.psychiatry.org/psychiatrists/search-directories-databases/library-and-archive/resource-documents. Accessed October 2, 2019.

American Psychiatric Association: Practice Guidelines for the Psychiatric Evaluation of Adults, 3rd Edition. Arlington, VA, American Psychiatric Association Publishing, 2016a

American Psychiatric Association: Psychiatric Services in Correctional Facilities, 3rd Edition. Arlington, VA, American Psychiatric Association Publishing, 2016b

American Psychiatric Association: Position statement on segregation of prisoners with mental illness. Arlington, VA, American Psychiatric Association, 2017. Available at: www.psychiatry.org/File%20Library/About-APA/Organization-Documents-Policies/Policies/Position-2012-Prisoners-Segregation.pdf. Accessed September 22, 2019.

American Psychiatric Association: Position statement on solitary confinement (restricted housing) of juveniles. Washington, DC, American Psychiatric Association, 2018. Available at: www.psychiatry.org/File%20Library/About-APA/Organization-Documents-Policies/Policies/Position-2018-Solitary-Confinement-Restricted-Housing-of-Juveniles.pdf. Accessed October 3, 2019.

American Public Health Association: Solitary confinement as a public health issue. Washington, DC, American Public Health Association, 2013. Available at: www.apha.org/policies-and-advocacy/public-health-policy-statements/policy-database/2014/07/14/13/30/solitary-confinement-as-a-public-health-issue. Accessed on September 22, 2019.

Ananth J, Sangani H, Noonan JP: Amantadine in drug-induced extrapyramidal signs: a comparative study. Int J Clin Pharmacol Biopharm 11(4):323–326, 1975 239908

Anderson GD, Chan LN: Pharmacokinetic drug interactions with tobacco, cannabinoids and smoking cessation products. Clin Pharmacokinet 55(11):1353–1368, 2016 27106177

Anderson KE, Stamler D, Davis MD, et al: Deutetrabenazine for treatment of involuntary movements in patients with tardive dyskinesia (AIM-TD): a double-blind, randomised, placebo-controlled, phase 3 trial. Lancet Psychiatry 4(8):595–604, 2017 28668671

Anderson KK, Norman R, MacDougall A, et al: Effectiveness of early psychosis intervention: comparison of service users and nonusers in population-based health administrative data. Am J Psychiatry 175(5):443–452, 2018 29495897

Andorn A, Graham J, Csernansky J, et al: Monthly extended-release risperidone (RBP-7000) in the treatment of schizophrenia: results from the phase 3 program. J Clin Psychopharmacol 39(5):428–433, 2019 31343440

Andreasen NC: Scale for the Assessment of Negative Symptoms. Iowa City, University of Iowa, 1984a

Andreasen NC: Scale for the Assessment of Positive Symptoms. Iowa City, University of Iowa, 1984b

Andrews JC, Schünemann HJ, Oxman AD, et al: GRADE guidelines: 15. Going from evidence to recommendation—determinants of a recommendation's direction and strength. J Clin Epidemiol 66(7):726–735, 2013 23570745

Anestis MD, Houtsma C: The association between gun ownership and statewide overall suicide rates. Suicide Life Threat Behav 48(2):204–217, 2018 28294383

Ang MS, Abdul Rashid NA, Lam M, et al: The impact of medication anticholinergic burden on cognitive performance in people with schizophrenia. J Clin Psychopharmacol 37(6):651–656, 2017 29016375

Angell B, Matthews E, Barrenger S, et al: Engagement processes in model programs for community reentry from prison for people with serious mental illness. Int J Law Psychiatry 37(5):490–500, 2014 24650496

Angus S, Sugars J, Boltezar R, et al: A controlled trial of amantadine hydrochloride and neuroleptics in the treatment of tardive dyskinesia. J Clin Psychopharmacol 17(2):88–91, 1997 10950469

Appelbaum PS: Clinical practice: assessment of patients' competence to consent to treatment. N Engl J Med 357(18):1834–1840, 2007

Appelbaum PS, Le Melle S: Techniques used by assertive community treatment (ACT) teams to encourage adherence: patient and staff perceptions. Community Ment Health J 44(6):459–464, 2008 18516679

Arana GW, Goff DC, Baldessarini RJ, Keepers GA: Efficacy of anticholinergic prophylaxis for neuroleptic-induced acute dystonia. Am J Psychiatry 145(8):993–996, 1988 2899403

Aripiprazole orally disintegrating tablets [prescribing information]. Bridgewater, NJ, Alembic Pharmaceuticals, November 2018

Aripiprazole solution [prescribing information]. Weston, FL, Apotex, November 2016

Aristada (aripiprazole lauroxil) [prescribing information]. Waltham, MA, Alkermes, August 2019

Aristada Initio (aripiprazole lauroxil) [prescribing information]. Waltham, MA, Alkermes, August 2019

Ascher-Svanum H, Zhu B, Faries D, et al: A prospective study of risk factors for nonadherence with antipsychotic medication in the treatment of schizophrenia. J Clin Psychiatry 67(7):1114–1123, 2006 16889456

Aune D, Sen A, Norat T, et al: Body mass index, abdominal fatness, and heart failure incidence and mortality: a systematic review and dose-response meta-analysis of prospective studies. Circulation 133(7):639–649, 2016 26746176

Austedo (deutetrabenazine) tablets [prescribing information]. North Wales, PA, Teva Pharmaceuticals USA, July 2019

Aytemir K, Maarouf N, Gallagher MM, et al: Comparison of formulae for heart rate correction of QT interval in exercise electrocardiograms. Pacing Clin Electrophysiol 22(9):1397–1401, 1999 10527023

Bachmann CJ, Aagaard L, Bernardo M, et al: International trends in clozapine use: a study in 17 countries. Acta Psychiatr Scand 136(1):37–51, 2017 28502099

Bai YM, Ting Chen T, Chen JY, et al: Equivalent switching dose from oral risperidone to risperidone long-acting injection: a 48-week randomized, prospective, single-blind pharmacokinetic study. J Clin Psychiatry 68(8):1218–1225, 2007 17854246

Baillargeon J, Binswanger IA, Penn JV, et al: Psychiatric disorders and repeat incarcerations: the revolving prison door. Am J Psychiatry 166(1):103–109, 2009a 19047321

Baillargeon J, Penn JV, Thomas CR, et al: Psychiatric disorders and suicide in the nation's largest state prison system. J Am Acad Psychiatry Law 37(2):188–193, 2009b 19535556

Baillargeon J, Hoge SK, Penn JV: Addressing the challenge of community reentry among released inmates with serious mental illness. Am J Community Psychol 46(3–4):361–375, 2010 20865315

Bak M, Fransen A, Janssen J, et al: Almost all antipsychotics result in weight gain: a meta-analysis. PLoS One 9(4):e94112, 2014 24763306

Balon R, Berchou R: Hematologic side effects of psychotropic drugs. Psychosomatics 27(2):119–120, 125–127, 1986 2869545

Balshem H, Helfand M, Schünemann HJ, et al: GRADE guidelines: 3. Rating the quality of evidence. J Clin Epidemiol 64(4):401–406, 2011 21208779

Barber S, Olotu U, Corsi M, Cipriani A: Clozapine combined with different antipsychotic drugs for treatment-resistant schizophrenia. Cochrane Database Syst Rev (3):CD006324, 2017 28333365

Barnes TR; Schizophrenia Consensus Group of British Association for Psychopharmacology: Evidence-based guidelines for the pharmacological treatment of schizophrenia: recommendations from the British Association for Psychopharmacology. J Psychopharmacol 25(5):567–620, 2011 21292923

Barnhill JW: The psychiatric interview and mental status examination, in The American Psychiatric Publishing Textbook of Psychiatry, 6th Edition. Edited by Hales RE, Yudofsky SC, Roberts LW. Arlington, VA, American Psychiatric Association, 2014, pp 3–30

Barrowclough C, Tarrier N, Lewis S, et al: Randomised controlled effectiveness trial of a needs-based psychosocial intervention service for carers of people with schizophrenia. Br J Psychiatry 174:505–511, 1999 10616628

Bartels SJ, Pratt SI, Mueser KT, et al: Long-term outcomes of a randomized trial of integrated skills training and preventive healthcare for older adults with serious mental illness. Am J Geriatr Psychiatry 22(11):1251–1261, 2014 23954039

Bartels SJ, Pratt SI, Aschbrenner KA, et al: Pragmatic replication trial of health promotion coaching for obesity in serious mental illness and maintenance of outcomes. Am J Psychiatry 172(4):344–352, 2015 25827032

Bassett AS, Chow EW: 22q11 deletion syndrome: a genetic subtype of schizophrenia. Biol Psychiatry 46(7):882–891, 1999 10509171

Bassett AS, Lowther C, Merico D, et al: International 22q11.2DS Brain and Behavior Consortium: rare genome-wide copy number variation and expression of schizophrenia in 22q11.2 deletion syndrome. Am J Psychiatry 174(11):1054–1063, 2017 28750581

Bäuml J, Froböse T, Kraemer S, et al: Psychoeducation: a basic psychotherapeutic intervention for patients with schizophrenia and their families. Schizophr Bull 32 (suppl 1):S1–S9, 2006 16920788

Bebbington P, Jakobowitz S, McKenzie N, et al: Assessing needs for psychiatric treatment in prisoners, 1: prevalence of disorder. Soc Psychiatry Psychiatr Epidemiol 52(2):221–229, 2017 27878322

Bech P, Austin SF, Timmerby N, et al: A clinimetric analysis of a BPRS-6 scale for schizophrenia severity. Acta Neuropsychiatr 30(4):187–191, 2018 29409548

Beck AT, Rector NA: Cognitive approaches to schizophrenia: theory and therapy. Annu Rev Clin Psychol 1:577–606, 2005 17716100

Beck AT, Rector NA, Stolar N, Grant P: Schizophrenia: Cognitive Theory, Research, and Therapy. New York, Guilford, 2009, p 418

Beck Institute: CBT for schizophrenia. Bala Cynwyd, PA, Beck Institute, 2019. Available at: https://beck institute.org/workshop/cbt-for-schizophrenia. Accessed May 6, 2020.

Becker DR, Drake RE: A Working Life for People With Severe Mental Illness. New York, Oxford University Press, 2003

Bellack AS, Goldberg RW: VA Psychosocial Rehabilitation Training Program: social skills training for serious mental illness. Baltimore, MD, MIRECC VISN 5, 2019. Available at: www.mirecc.va.gov/visn5/training/sst/sst_clinicians_handbook.pdf. Accessed April 11, 2019.

Bellack AS, Mueser KT, Gingerich S, Agresta J: Social Skills Training for Schizophrenia: A Step-by-Step Guide, 2nd Edition. New York, Guilford, 2004

Bellissima BL, Tingle MD, Cicović A, et al: A systematic review of clozapine-induced myocarditis. Int J Cardiol 259:122–129, 2018 29579587

Bellou V, Belbasis L, Tzoulaki I, Evangelou E: Risk factors for type 2 diabetes mellitus: an exposure-wide umbrella review of meta-analyses. PLoS One 13(3):e0194127, 2018 29558518

Benadryl (diphenhydramine) [prescribing information]. Fort Washington, PA, McNeil Consumer Healthcare, June 2018

Benztropine injection [prescribing information]. Lake Forest, IL, Akorn, November 2017

Benztropine tablets [prescribing information]. Livonia, MI, Major Pharmaceuticals, October 2017

Bergamo C, Sigel K, Mhango G, et al: Inequalities in lung cancer care of elderly patients with schizophrenia: an observational cohort study. Psychosom Med 76(3):215–220, 2014 24677164

Bergman H, Soares-Weiser K: Anticholinergic medication for antipsychotic-induced tardive dyskinesia. Cochrane Database Syst Rev Jan 17 1(1):CD000204, 2018 29341071

Bergman H, Walker DM, Nikolakopoulou A, et al: Systematic review of interventions for treating or preventing antipsychotic-induced tardive dyskinesia. Health Technol Assess 21(43):1–218, 2017 28812541

Bergman H, Bhoopathi PS, Soares-Weiser K: Benzodiazepines for antipsychotic-induced tardive dyskinesia. Cochrane Database Syst Rev Jan 20 1(1):CD000205, 2018a 29352477

Bergman H, Rathbone J, Agarwal V, Soares-Weiser K: Antipsychotic reduction and/or cessation and antipsychotics as specific treatments for tardive dyskinesia. Cochrane Database Syst Rev Feb 6 2(2):CD000459, 2018b 29409162

Berman BD: Neuroleptic malignant syndrome: a review for neurohospitalists. Neurohospitalist 1(1):41–47, 2011 23983836

Bertelsen M, Jeppesen P, Petersen L, et al: Suicidal behaviour and mortality in first-episode psychosis: the OPUS trial. Br J Psychiatry Suppl 51:s140–s146, 2007 18055932

Bertilsson L: Metabolism of antidepressant and neuroleptic drugs by cytochrome P450s: clinical and interethnic aspects. Clin Pharmacol Ther 82(5):606–609, 2007 17898711

Bhidayasiri R, Fahn S, Weiner WJ, et al; American Academy of Neurology: Evidence-based guideline: treatment of tardive syndromes: report of the Guideline Development Subcommittee of the American Academy of Neurology. Neurology 81(5):463–469, 2013 23897874

Bird AM, Smith TL, Walton AE: Current treatment strategies for clozapine-induced sialorrhea. Ann Pharmaco-
    ther 45(5):667–675, 2011 21540404

Bishara D, Olofinjana O, Sparshatt A, et al: Olanzapine: a systematic review and meta-regression of the relation-
    ships between dose, plasma concentration, receptor occupancy, and response. J Clin Psychopharmacol
    33(3):329–335, 2013 23609380

Bitter I, Katona L, Zámbori J, et al: Comparative effectiveness of depot and oral second generation antipsy-
    chotic drugs in schizophrenia: a nationwide study in Hungary. Eur Neuropsychopharmacol 23(11):1383–
    1390, 2013 23477752

Blanchet PJ, Abdillahi O, Beauvais C, et al: Prevalence of spontaneous oral dyskinesia in the elderly: a reappraisal.
    Mov Disord 19(8):892–896, 2004 15300653

Bliss SA, Warnock JK: Psychiatric medications: adverse cutaneous drug reactions. Clin Dermatol 31(1):101–109,
    2013 23245981

Bolton JM, Morin SN, Majumdar SR, et al: Association of mental disorders and related medication use with
    risk for major osteoporotic fractures. JAMA Psychiatry 74(6):641–648, 2017 28423154

Bonfioli E, Berti L, Goss C, et al: Health promotion lifestyle interventions for weight management in psychosis: a
    systematic review and meta-analysis of randomised controlled trials. BMC Psychiatry 12:78, 2012 22789023

Bonoldi I, Simeone E, Rocchetti M, et al: Prevalence of self-reported childhood abuse in psychosis: a meta-analysis
    of retrospective studies. Psychiatry Res 210(1):8–15, 2013 23790604

Borison RL: Amantadine in the management of extrapyramidal side effects. Clin Neuropharmacol 6 (suppl 1):
    S57–S63, 1983 6139167

Bouchama A, Dehbi M, Mohamed G, et al: Prognostic factors in heat wave related deaths: a meta-analysis.
    Arch Intern Med 167(20):2170–2176, 2007 17698676

Bousman CA, Dunlop BW: Genotype, phenotype, and medication recommendation agreement among com-
    mercial pharmacogenetic-based decision support tools. Pharmacogenomics J 18(5):613–622, 2018
    29795409

Bouwmans C, de Sonneville C, Mulder CL, Hakkaart-van Roijen L: Employment and the associated impact on
    quality of life in people diagnosed with schizophrenia. Neuropsychiatr Dis Treat 11:2125–2142, 2015
    26316759

Bower T, Samek DA, Mohammed A, et al: Systemic medication usage in glaucoma patients. Can J Ophthalmol
    53(3):242–245, 2018 29784160

Bowie CR, Reichenberg A, Patterson TL, et al: Determinants of real-world functional performance in schizophre-
    nia subjects: correlations with cognition, functional capacity, and symptoms. Am J Psychiatry 163(3):418–
    425, 2006 16513862

Bowtell M, Eaton S, Thien K, et al: Rates and predictors of relapse following discontinuation of antipsychotic
    medication after a first episode of psychosis. Schizophr Res 195:231–236, 2018 29066258

Bradley-Engen MS, Cuddeback GS, Gayman MD, et al: Trends in state prison admission of offenders with serious
    mental illness. Psychiatr Serv 61(12):1263–1265, 2010 21123414

Braham LG, Trower P, Birchwood M: Acting on command hallucinations and dangerous behavior: a critique
    of the major findings in the last decade. Clin Psychol Rev 24(5):513–528, 2004 15325743

Brain C, Kymes S, DiBenedetti DB, et al: Experiences, attitudes, and perceptions of caregivers of individuals
    with treatment-resistant schizophrenia: a qualitative study. BMC Psychiatry 18(1):253, 2018 30103719

Brand RM, McEnery C, Rossell S, et al: Do trauma-focussed psychological interventions have an effect on psy-
    chotic symptoms? A systematic review and meta-analysis. Schizophr Res 195:13–22, 2018 28844432

Brashear A, Ambrosius WT, Eckert GJ, Siemers ER: Comparison of treatment of tardive dystonia and idiopathic
    cervical dystonia with botulinum toxin type A. Mov Disord 13(1):158-161, 1998 9452343

Briggs GG, Freeman RK, Towers CV, Forinash AB: Drugs in Pregnancy and Lactation: A Reference Guide to
    Fetal and Neonatal Risk, 11th Edition. Philadelphia, PA, Wolters Kluwer, 2017

Brito JP, Domecq JP, Murad MH, et al: The Endocrine Society guidelines: when the confidence cart goes before
    the evidence horse. J Clin Endocrinol Metab 98(8):3246–3252, 2013 23783104

Bromet EJ, Kotov R, Fochtmann LJ, et al: Diagnostic shifts during the decade following first admission for psy-
    chosis. Am J Psychiatry 168(11):1186–1194, 2011 21676994

Bromet EJ, Nock MK, Saha S, et al; World Health Organization World Mental Health Survey Collaborators: As-
    sociation between psychotic experiences and subsequent suicidal thoughts and behaviors: a cross-national
    analysis from the World Health Organization World Mental Health Surveys. JAMA Psychiatry 74(11):1136–
    1144, 2017 28854302

Brown JD, Barrett A, Caffery E, et al: State and demographic variation in use of depot antipsychotics by Med-
    icaid beneficiaries with schizophrenia. Psychiatr Serv 65(1):121–124, 2014 24382765

Brown S, Inskip H, Barraclough B: Causes of the excess mortality of schizophrenia. Br J Psychiatry 177:212–
    217, 2000 11040880

Browne J, Penn DL, Bauer DJ, et al: Perceived autonomy support in the NIMH RAISE Early Treatment Program. Psychiatr Serv 68(9):916–922, 2017 28566027

Brunette MF, Mueser KT, Babbin S, et al: Demographic and clinical correlates of substance use disorders in first episode psychosis. Schizophr Res 194:4–12, 2018 28697856

Bruno V, Valiente-Gómez A, Alcoverro O: Clozapine and fever: a case of continued therapy with clozapine. Clin Neuropharmacol 38(4):151–153, 2015 26166236

Buchanan A, Sint K, Swanson J, Rosenheck R: Correlates of future violence in people being treated for schizophrenia. Am J Psychiatry 176(9):694–701, 2019 31014102 Epub ahead of print

Buchanan RW, Kreyenbuhl J, Kelly DL, et al; Schizophrenia Patient Outcomes Research Team (PORT): The 2009 schizophrenia PORT psychopharmacological treatment recommendations and summary statements. Schizophr Bull 36(1):71–93, 2010 19955390

Buckley LA, Maayan N, Soares-Weiser K, Adams CE: Supportive therapy for schizophrenia. Cochrane Database Syst Rev (4):CD004716, 2015 2587146

Buckley PF, Schooler NR, Goff DC, et al: Comparison of SGA oral medications and a long-acting injectable SGA: the PROACTIVE study. Schizophr Bull 41(2):449–459, 2015 24870446

Buckley PF, Schooler NR, Goff DC, et al: Comparison of injectable and oral antipsychotics in relapse rates in a pragmatic 30-month schizophrenia relapse prevention study. Psychiatr Serv 67(12):1370–1372, 2016 27476806

Buhagiar K, Jabbar F: Association of first- vs. second-generation antipsychotics with lipid abnormalities in individuals with severe mental illness: a systematic review and meta-analysis. Clin Drug Investig 39(3):253–273, 2019 30675684

Burke RE, Fahn S, Jankovic J, et al: Tardive dystonia: late-onset and persistent dystonia caused by antipsychotic drugs. Neurology 32(12):1335–1346, 1982 6128697

Burnett AL, Bivalacqua TJ: Priapism: new concepts in medical and surgical management. Urol Clin North Am 38(2):185–194, 2011 21621085

Burns AM, Erickson DH, Brenner CA: Cognitive-behavioral therapy for medication-resistant psychosis: a meta-analytic review. Psychiatr Serv 65(7):874–880, 2014 24686725

Burns T, Catty J, Becker T, et al; EQOLISE Group: The effectiveness of supported employment for people with severe mental illness: a randomised controlled trial. Lancet 370(9593):1146–1152, 2007 17905167

Burns T, Rugkåsa J, Molodynski A, et al: Community treatment orders for patients with psychosis (OCTET): a randomised controlled trial. Lancet 381(9878):1627–1633, 2013 23537605

Bush G, Fink M, Petrides G, et al: Catatonia I: rating scale and standardized examination. Acta Psychiatr Scand 93(2):129–136, 1996a 8686483

Bush G, Fink M, Petrides G, et al: Catatonia II: treatment with lorazepam and electroconvulsive therapy. Acta Psychiatr Scand 93(2):137–143, 1996b 8686484

Bushe C, Paton C: The potential impact of antipsychotics on lipids in schizophrenia: is there enough evidence to confirm a link? J Psychopharmacol 19(6 suppl):76–83, 2005 16280340

Caemmerer J, Correll CU, Maayan L: Acute and maintenance effects of non-pharmacologic interventions for antipsychotic associated weight gain and metabolic abnormalities: a meta-analytic comparison of randomized controlled trials. Schizophr Res 140(1–3):159–168, 2012 22763424

Carbon M, Hsieh CH, Kane JM, Correll CU: Tardive dyskinesia prevalence in the period of second-generation antipsychotic use: a meta-analysis. J Clin Psychiatry 78(3):e264–e278, 2017 28146614

Carbon M, Kane JM, Leucht S, Correll CU: Tardive dyskinesia risk with first-and second-generation antipsychotics in comparative randomized controlled trials: a meta-analysis. World Psychiatry 17(3):330–340, 2018 30192088

Carney R, Cotter J, Firth J, et al: Cannabis use and symptom severity in individuals at ultra high risk for psychosis: a meta-analysis. Acta Psychiatr Scand 136(1):5–15, 2017 28168698

Caroff SN, Mann SC: Neuroleptic malignant syndrome. Psychopharmacol Bull 24(1):25–29, 1988 3290944

Caroff SN, Mann SC, Keck PE Jr, Francis A: Residual catatonic state following neuroleptic malignant syndrome. J Clin Psychopharmacol 20(2):257–259, 2000 10770467

Caroli F, Raymondet P, Izard I, et al: Opinions of French patients with schizophrenia regarding injectable medication. Patient Prefer Adherence 5:165–171, 2011 21573047

Carrillo JA, Herraiz AG, Ramos SI, Benítez J: Effects of caffeine withdrawal from the diet on the metabolism of clozapine in schizophrenic patients. J Clin Psychopharmacol 18(4):311–316, 1998 9690697

Carruthers J, Radigan M, Erlich MD, et al: An initiative to improve clozapine prescribing in New York State. Psychiatr Serv 67(4):369–371, 2016 26725299

Cassidy RM, Yang F, Kapczinski F, Passos IC: Risk factors for suicidality in patients with schizophrenia: a systematic review, meta-analysis, and meta-regression of 96 studies. Schizophr Bull 44(4):787–797, 2018 29036388

Castelein S, Bruggeman R, Davidson L, van der Gaag M: Creating a supportive environment: peer support groups for psychotic disorders. Schizophr Bull 41(6):1211–1213, 2015 26297694.

Catley D, Goggin K, Harris KJ, et al: A randomized trial of motivational interviewing: cessation induction among smokers with low desire to quit. Am J Prev Med 50(5):573–583, 2016 26711164

Cella M, Preti A, Edwards C, et al: Cognitive remediation for negative symptoms of schizophrenia: a network meta-analysis. Clin Psychol Rev 52:43–51, 2017 27930934

Cella M, Wykes T: The nuts and bolts of cognitive remediation: exploring how different training components relate to cognitive and functional gains. Schizophr Res 203:12–16, 2019 28919130

Center for Evidence-Based Practices: Assertive community treatment. Cleveland, OH, Case Western Reserve University, 2019. Available at: www.centerforebp.case.edu/practices/act. Accessed March 31, 2019.

Center for Health Policy/Center for Primary Care and Outcomes Research and Battelle Memorial Institute: Quality Indicator Measure Development, Implementation, Maintenance, and Retirement. Contract No 290-04-0020. Rockville, MD, Agency for Healthcare Research and Quality, May 2011. Available at: www.qualityindicators.ahrq.gov/Downloads/Resources/Publications/2011/QI_Measure_Development_Implementation_Maintenance_Retirement_Full_5-3-11.pdf. Accessed April 2, 2017.

Center for Substance Abuse Treatment: Trauma-Informed Care in Behavioral Health Services. Treatment Improvement Protocol (TIP) Series No 57. Rockville, MD, Substance Abuse and Mental Health Services Administration, 2014. Available at: www.ncbi.nlm.nih.gov/books/NBK207201. Accessed May 10, 2019.

Centers for Disease Control and Prevention: Infection Control Basics: Standard Precautions for All Patient Care. Atlanta, GA, Centers for Disease Control and Prevention, January 26, 2016. Available at: www.cdc.gov/infectioncontrol/basics/standard-precautions.html. Accessed October 4, 2019.

Centers for Disease Control and Prevention: FAQs Regarding Safe Practices for Medical Injections. Atlanta, GA, Centers for Disease Control and Prevention, June 20, 2019a. Available at: www.cdc.gov/injection safety/providers/provider_faqs.html. Accessed July 22, 2020.

Centers for Disease Control and Prevention: Vaccine Recommendations and Guidelines of the ACIP: Vaccine Administration. Atlanta, GA, Centers for Disease Control and Prevention, June 21, 2019b. Available at: www.cdc.gov/vaccines/hcp/acip-recs/general-recs/administration.html. Accessed October 4, 2019.

Centers for Disease Control and Prevention: Tobacco Use and Quitting Among Individuals With Behavioral Health Conditions. Atlanta, GA, Centers for Disease Control and Prevention, 2020. Available at: www.cdc.gov/tobacco/disparities/mental-illness-substance-use/index.htm. Accessed July 8, 2020.

Cerovecki A, Musil R, Klimke A, et al: Withdrawal symptoms and rebound syndromes associated with switching and discontinuing atypical antipsychotics: theoretical background and practical recommendations. CNS Drugs 27(7):545–572, 2013 23821039

Challis S, Nielssen O, Harris A, Large M: Systematic meta-analysis of the risk factors for deliberate self-harm before and after treatment for first-episode psychosis. Acta Psychiatr Scand 127(6):442–454, 2013 23298325

Chapel JM, Ritchey MD, Zhang D, Wang G: Prevalence and medical costs of chronic diseases among adult Medicaid beneficiaries. Am J Prev Med 53(6S2):S143–S154, 2017 29153115

Charzyńska K, Kucharska K, Mortimer A: Does employment promote the process of recovery from schizophrenia? A review of the existing evidence. Int J Occup Med Environ Health 28(3):407–418, 2015 26190722

Chasser Y, Kim AY, Freudenreich O: Hepatitis C treatment: clinical issues for psychiatrists in the post-interferon era. Psychosomatics 58(1):1–10, 2017 27871760

Chatziralli IP, Sergentanis TN: Risk factors for intraoperative floppy iris syndrome: a meta-analysis. Ophthalmology 118(4):730–735, 2011 21168223

Chen SY, Ravindran G, Zhang Q, et al: Treatment strategies for clozapine-induced sialorrhea: a systematic review and meta-analysis. CNS Drugs 33(3):225–238, 2019 30758782

Chien WT, Clifton AV, Zhao S, Lui S: Peer support for people with schizophrenia or other serious mental illness. Cochrane Database Syst Rev April 4 4(4):CD010880, 2019 30946482

Chisolm MS, Payne JL: Management of psychotropic drugs during pregnancy. BMJ 532:h5918, 2016 26791406

Chlorpromazine hydrochloride injection [prescribing information]. Deerfield, IL, Baxter, September 2010

Chlorpromazine hydrochloride injection [prescribing information]. Eatontown, NJ, West-Ward Pharmaceuticals, November 2016

Chlorpromazine hydrochloride tablets [prescribing information]. Bridgewater, NJ, Amneal Pharmaceuticals, January 2018

Cho J, Hayes RD, Jewell A, et al: Clozapine and all-cause mortality in treatment-resistant schizophrenia: a historical cohort study. Acta Psychiatr Scand 139(3):237–247, 2019 30478891

Chouinard G, Jones B, Remington G, et al: A Canadian multicenter placebo-controlled study of fixed doses of risperidone and haloperidol in the treatment of chronic schizophrenic patients. J Clin Psychopharmacol 13(1):25–40, 1993 7683702

Cimo A, Stergiopoulos E, Cheng C, et al: Effective lifestyle interventions to improve type II diabetes self-management for those with schizophrenia or schizoaffective disorder: a systematic review. BMC Psychiatry 12:24, 2012 22443212

Citrome L: Activating and sedating adverse effects of second-generation antipsychotics in the treatment of schizophrenia and major depressive disorder: absolute risk increase and number needed to harm. J Clin Psychopharmacol 37(2):138–147, 2017a 28141623

Citrome L: Valbenazine for tardive dyskinesia: a systematic review of the efficacy and safety profile for this newly approved novel medication—What is the number needed to treat, number needed to harm and likelihood to be helped or harmed? Int J Clin Pract 71(7), 2017b 28497864

Citrome L, Volavka J, Czobor P, et al: Effects of clozapine, olanzapine, risperidone, and haloperidol on hostility among patients with schizophrenia. Psychiatr Serv 52(11):1510–1514, 2001 11684748

Claghorn J, Honigfeld G, Abuzzahab FS Sr, et al: The risks and benefits of clozapine versus chlorpromazine. J Clin Psychopharmacol 7(6):377–384, 1987 3323261

Clarke DE, Wilcox HC, Miller L, et al: Feasibility and acceptability of the DSM-5 Field Trial procedures in the Johns Hopkins Community Psychiatry Programs. Int J Methods Psychiatr Res 23(2):267–278, 2014 24615761

Clausen W, Watanabe-Galloway S, Baerentzen MB, Britigan DH: Health literacy among people with serious mental illness. Community Ment Health J 52(4):399–405, 2016 26443671

Clayton AH, McGarvey EL, Clavet GJ: The Changes in Sexual Functioning Questionnaire (CSFQ): development, reliability, and validity. Psychopharmacol Bull 33(4):731–745, 1997a 9493486

Clayton AH, McGarvey EL, Clavet GJ, Piazza L: Comparison of sexual functioning in clinical and nonclinical populations using the Changes in Sexual Functioning Questionnaire (CSFQ). Psychopharmacol Bull 33(4):747–753, 1997b 9493487

Cloud DH, Drucker E, Browne A, Parsons J: Public health and solitary confinement in the United States. Am J Public Health 105(1):18–26, 2015 25393185

Cloutier M, Aigbogun MS, Guerin A, et al: The economic burden of schizophrenia in the United States in 2013. J Clin Psychiatry 77(6):764–771, 2016 27135986

Clozapine [prescribing information]. Greenville, NC, Mayne Pharma, June 2017

Clozapine REMS Program: Recommended monitoring frequency and clinical decisions by ANC level. Phoenix, AZ, Clozapine REMS Program, December 23, 2014. Available at: www.clozapinerems.com/CpmgClozapineUI/rems/pdf/resources/ANC_Table.pdf. Accessed February 12, 2019.

Clozapine REMS Program: Prescriber certification. Phoenix, AZ, Clozapine REMS Program, 2019a. Available at: www.clozapinerems.com/CpmgClozapineUI/hcpHome.u. Accessed February 12, 2019.

Clozapine REMS Program: Program materials: prescriber. Phoenix, AZ, Clozapine REMS Program, 2019b. Available at: www.clozapinerems.com/CpmgClozapineUI/resources.u#tabr4. Accessed February 12, 2019.

Clozapine REMS Program: Clozapine and the risk of neutropenia: a guide for healthcare providers. Phoenix, AX, Clozpine REMS Program, February 2019c. Available at: www.clozapinerems.com/CpmgClozapineUI/rems/pdf/resources/Clozapine_REMS_A_Guide_for_Healthcare_Providers.pdf. Accessed July 14, 2020.

Clozaril (clozapine) [prescribing information]. East Hanover, NJ, Novartis Pharmaceuticals, January 2017

Clozaril (clozapine) [product monograph]. Etobicoke, ON, Canada, HLS Therapeutics, July 2019

Cogentin (benztropine) injection [prescribing information]. Lake Forest, IL, Akorn, May 2013

Cohen AN, Drapalski AL, Glynn SM, et al: Preferences for family involvement in care among consumers with serious mental illness. Psychiatr Serv 64(3):257–263, 2013 23242515

Cohen AN, Hamilton AB, Saks ER, et al: How occupationally high-achieving individuals with a diagnosis of schizophrenia manage their symptoms. Psychiatr Serv 68(4):324–329, 2017 27842472

Coid JW, Ullrich S, Kallis C, et al: The relationship between delusions and violence: findings from the East London first episode psychosis study. JAMA Psychiatry 70(5):465–471, 2013 23467760

College of Psychiatric and Neurologic Pharmacists: Psychiatric pharmacy essentials: antipsychotic dose equivalents. Lincoln, NE, College of Psychiatric and Neurologic Pharmacists, 2019. Available at: https://cpnp.org/guideline/essentials/antipsychotic-dose-equivalents. Accessed February 25, 2019.

Conley RR, Kelly DL, Richardson CM, et al: The efficacy of high-dose olanzapine versus clozapine in treatment-resistant schizophrenia: a double-blind crossover study. J Clin Psychopharmacol 23(6):668–671, 2003 14624201

Conus P, Cotton S, Schimmelmann BG, et al: Rates and predictors of 18-months remission in an epidemiological cohort of 661 patients with first-episode psychosis. Soc Psychiatry Psychiatr Epidemiol 52(9):1089–1099, 2017 28477070

Cook BL, Wayne GF, Kafali EN, et al: Trends in smoking among adults with mental illness and association between mental health treatment and smoking cessation. JAMA 311(2):172–182, 2014 24399556

Cook JA, Leff HS, Blyler CR, et al: Results of a multisite randomized trial of supported employment interventions for individuals with severe mental illness. Arch Gen Psychiatry 62(5):505–512, 2005 15867103

Cookson J, Hodgson R, Wildgust HJ: Prolactin, hyperprolactinaemia and antipsychotic treatment: a review and lessons for treatment of early psychosis. J Psychopharmacol 26(5 suppl):42–51, 2012 22472310

Copeland ME: Wellness recovery action plan. Occup Ther Ment Health 17:(3–4), 127–150, 2000

Correll CU, Robinson DG, Schooler NR, et al: Cardiometabolic risk in patients with first-episode schizophrenia spectrum disorders: baseline results from the RAISE-ETP study. JAMA Psychiatry 71(12):1350–1363, 2014 25321337

Correll CU, Citrome L, Haddad PM, et al: The use of long-acting injectable antipsychotics in schizophrenia: evaluating the evidence. J Clin Psychiatry 77 (suppl 3):1–24, 2016 27732772

Correll CU, Josiassen RC, Liang GS, et al: Efficacy of valbenazine (NBI-98854) in treating subjects with tardive dyskinesia and mood disorder. Psychopharmacol Bull 47(3):53–60, 2017a 28839340

Correll CU, Rubio JM, Inczedy-Farkas G, et al: Efficacy of 42 pharmacologic cotreatment strategies added to antipsychotic monotherapy in schizophrenia: systematic overview and quality appraisal of the meta-analytic evidence. JAMA Psychiatry 74(7):675–684, 2017b 28514486

Correll CU, Solmi M, Veronese N, et al: Prevalence, incidence and mortality from cardiovascular disease in patients with pooled and specific severe mental illness: a large-scale meta-analysis of 3,211,768 patients and 113,383,368 controls. World Psychiatry 16(2):163–180, 2017c 28498599

Correll CU, Rubio JM, Kane JM: What is the risk-benefit ratio of long-term antipsychotic treatment in people with schizophrenia? World Psychiatry 17(2):149–160, 2018 29856543

Cotton SM, Filia KM, Ratheesh A, et al: Early psychosis research at Orygen, the National Centre of Excellence in Youth Mental Health. Soc Psychiatry Psychiatr Epidemiol 51(1):1–13, 2016 26498752

Couchman L, Morgan PE, Spencer EP, Flanagan RJ: Plasma clozapine, norclozapine, and the clozapine: norclozapine ratio in relation to prescribed dose and other factors: data from a therapeutic drug monitoring service, 1993–2007. Ther Drug Monit 32(4):438–447, 2010 20463634

Coulter C, Baker KK, Margolis RL: Specialized consultation for suspected recent-onset schizophrenia: diagnostic clarity and the distorting impact of anxiety and reported auditory hallucinations. J Psychiatr Pract 25(2):76–81, 2019 30849055

Council of Medical Specialty Societies: Principles for the Development of Specialty Society Clinical Guidelines. Chicago, IL, Council of Medical Specialty Societies, 2012

Craig TK, Garety P, Power P, et al: The Lambeth Early Onset (LEO) Team: randomised controlled trial of the effectiveness of specialised care for early psychosis. BMJ 329(7474):1067, 2004 15485934

Credible Meds: Risk categories for drugs that prolong QT and induce torsades de pointes (TdP). Oro Valley, AZ, Credible Meds, 2019. Available at: https://crediblemeds.org/healthcare-providers/drug-list. Accessed May 6, 2020.

Creed TA, Stirman SW, Evans AC, Beck AT: A model for implementation of cognitive therapy in community mental health: the Beck Initiative. Behav Ther 37(3):56–64, 2014

Crockford D, Addington D: Canadian schizophrenia guidelines: schizophrenia and other psychotic disorders with coexisting substance use disorders. Can J Psychiatry 62(9):624–634, 2017 28886671

Crosby AE, Ortega L, Melanson C: Self-Directed Violence Surveillance: Uniform Definitions and Recommended Data Elements, Version 1.0. Atlanta, GA, National Center for Injury Prevention and Control, Centers for Disease Control and Prevention, February 2011. Available at: www.cdc.gov/violenceprevention/pdf/self-directed-violence-a.pdf. Accessed May 25, 2015.

Crow TJ, Cross AJ, Johnstone EC, et al: Abnormal involuntary movements in schizophrenia: are they related to the disease process or its treatment? Are they associated with changes in dopamine receptors? J Clin Psychopharmacol 2(5):336–340, 1982 7130435

Cunqueiro A, Durango A, Fein DM, et al: Diagnostic yield of head CT in pediatric emergency department patients with acute psychosis or hallucinations. Pediatr Radiol 49(2):240–244, 2019 30291381

Czobor P, Van Dorn RA, Citrome L, et al: Treatment adherence in schizophrenia: a patient-level meta-analysis of combined CATIE and EUFEST studies. Eur Neuropsychopharmacol 25(8):1158–1166, 2015 26004980

D'Amato T, Bation R, Cochet A, et al: A randomized, controlled trial of computer-assisted cognitive remediation for schizophrenia. Schizophr Res 125(2–3):284–290, 2011 21094025

Daod E, Krivoy A, Shoval G, et al: Psychiatrists' attitude towards the use of clozapine in the treatment of refractory schizophrenia: a nationwide survey. Psychiatry Res 275:155–161, 2019 30913436

Das C, Mendez G, Jagasia S, Labbate LA: Second-generation antipsychotic use in schizophrenia and associated weight gain: a critical review and meta-analysis of behavioral and pharmacologic treatments. Ann Clin Psychiatry 24(3):225–239, 2012 22860242

Dauwan M, Begemann MJ, Heringa SM, Sommer IE: Exercise improves clinical symptoms, quality of life, global functioning, and depression in schizophrenia: a systematic review and meta-analysis. Schizophr Bull 42(3):588–599, 2016 26547223

Davidson M: The debate regarding maintenance treatment with antipsychotic drugs in schizophrenia. Dialogues Clin Neurosci 20(3):215–221, 2018 30581291

Davis JM, Chen N: Dose response and dose equivalence of antipsychotics. J Clin Psychopharmacol 24(2):192–208, 2004 15206667

de Boer MK, Castelein S, Wiersma D, et al: A systematic review of instruments to measure sexual functioning in patients using antipsychotics. J Sex Res 51(4):383–389, 2014 24754359

de Boer MK, Castelein S, Wiersma D, et al: The facts about sexual (dys)function in schizophrenia: an overview of clinically relevant findings. Schizophr Bull 41(3):674–686, 2015 25721311

De Hert M, Correll CU, Bobes J, et al: Physical illness in patients with severe mental disorders, I: prevalence, impact of medications and disparities in health care. World Psychiatry 10(1):52–77, 2011 21379357

De Hert M, Peuskens J, Sabbe T, et al: Relationship between prolactin, breast cancer risk, and antipsychotics in patients with schizophrenia: a critical review. Acta Psychiatr Scand 133(1):5–22, 2016 26114737

Delahunty A, Morice R: Rehabilitation of frontal/executive impairments in schizophrenia. Aust N Z J Psychiatry 30(6):760–767, 1996 9034464

de Leon J, Diaz FJ: A meta-analysis of worldwide studies demonstrates an association between schizophrenia and tobacco smoking behaviors. Schizophr Res 76(2–3):135–157, 2005 15949648

Depression and Bipolar Support Alliance: Restoring intimacy. Chicago, IL, Depression and Bipolar Support Alliance, 2019. Available at: www.dbsalliance.org/education/related-concerns/sexual-health-and-mood-disorders/restoring-intimacy. Accessed May 6, 2019.

de Oliveira IR, de Sena EP, Pereira EL, et al: Haloperidol blood levels and clinical outcome: a meta-analysis of studies relevant to testing the therapeutic window hypothesis. J Clin Pharm Ther 21(4):229–236, 1996 8933296

de Silva VA, Suraweera C, Ratnatunga SS, et al: Metformin in prevention and treatment of antipsychotic induced weight gain: a systematic review and meta-analysis. BMC Psychiatry 16(1):341, 2016 27716110

Desmarais JE, Beauclair L, Margolese HC: Anticholinergics in the era of atypical antipsychotics: short-term or long-term treatment? J Psychopharmacol 26(9):1167–1174, 2012 22651987

Deste G, Barlati S, Cacciani P, et al: Persistence of effectiveness of cognitive remediation interventions in schizophrenia: a 1-year follow-up study. Schizophr Res 161(2–3):403–406, 2015 25533593

DeTore NR, Hintz K, Khare C, Mueser KT: Disclosure of mental illness to prospective employers: Clinical, psychosocial, and work correlates in persons receiving supported employment. Psychiatry Res 273:312–317, 2019 30677720

Devinsky O, Pacia SV: Seizures during clozapine therapy. J Clin Psychiatry 55 (suppl B):153–156, 1994 7961562

Devinsky O, Honigfeld G, Patin J: Clozapine-related seizures. Neurology 41(3):369–371, 1991 2006003

de Vries B, van Busschbach JT, van der Stouwe ECD, et al: Prevalence rate and risk factors of victimization in adult patients with a psychotic disorder: a systematic review and meta-analysis. Schizophr Bull 45(1):114–126, 2019 29547958

Dewa CS, Loong D, Trojanowski L, Bonato S: The effectiveness of augmented versus standard individual placement and support programs in terms of employment: a systematic literature review. J Ment Health 27(2):174–183, 2018 28488948

de With SAJ, Pulit SL, Staal WG, et al: More than 25 years of genetic studies of clozapine-induced agranulocytosis. Pharmacogenomics J 17(4):304–311, 2017 28418011

Dickenson R, Momcilovic S, Donnelly L: Anticholinergics vs placebo for neuroleptic-induced parkinsonism. Schizophr Bull 43(1):17, 2017 27585460

Dickerson F, Schroeder J, Katsafanas E, et al: Cigarette smoking by patients with serious mental illness, 1999–2016: an increasing disparity. Psychiatr Serv 69(2):147–153, 2018 28945183

Diener E, Emmons RA, Larsen RJ, Griffin S: The Satisfaction With Life Scale. J Pers Assess 49(1):71–75, 1985 16367493

DiMascio A, Bernardo DL, Greenblatt DJ, Marder JE: A controlled trial of amantadine in drug-induced extrapyramidal disorders. Arch Gen Psychiatry 33(5):599–602, 1976 5066

Diphenhydramine hydrochloride injection [prescribing information]. Lake Forest, IL, Hospira, May 2019

Dixon LB, Dickerson F, Bellack AS, et al; Schizophrenia Patient Outcomes Research Team (PORT): The 2009 schizophrenia PORT psychosocial treatment recommendations and summary statements. Schizophr Bull 36(1):48–70, 2010 19955389

Dixon LB, Lucksted A, Medoff DR, et al: Outcomes of a randomized study of a peer-taught Family-to-Family Education Program for mental illness. Psychiatr Serv 62(6):591–597, 2011 21632725

Dixon LB, Holoshitz Y, Nossel I: Treatment engagement of individuals experiencing mental illness: review and update. World Psychiatry 15(1):13–20, 2016 26833597

Djulbegovic B, Trikalinos TA, Roback J, et al: Impact of quality of evidence on the strength of recommendations: an empirical study. BMC Health Serv Res 9:120, 2009 19622148

Dold M, Li C, Tardy M, et al: Benzodiazepines for schizophrenia. Cochrane Database Syst Rev Nov 14 11(11):CD006391, 2012 23152236

Dold M, Li C, Gillies D, Leucht S: Benzodiazepine augmentation of antipsychotic drugs in schizophrenia: a meta-analysis and Cochrane review of randomized controlled trials. Eur Neuropsychopharmacol 23(9):1023–1033, 2013 23602690

Dold M, Fugger G, Aigner M, et al: Dose escalation of antipsychotic drugs in schizophrenia: a meta-analysis of randomized controlled trials. Schizophr Res 166(1–3):187–193, 2015 26008883

Dollfus S, Lecardeur L, Morello R, Etard O: Placebo response in repetitive transcranial magnetic stimulation trials of treatment of auditory hallucinations in schizophrenia: a meta-analysis. Schizophr Bull 42(2):301–308, 2016 26089351

Dondé C, Vignaud P, Poulet E, et al: Management of depression in patients with schizophrenia spectrum disorders: a critical review of international guidelines. Acta Psychiatr Scand 138(4):289–299, 2018 29974451

Donnelly K, Bracchi R, Hewitt J, et al: Benzodiazepines, Z-drugs and the risk of hip fracture: a systematic review and meta-analysis. PloS One 12(4):e0174730, 2017 28448593

Donoghue K, Doody GA, Murray RM, et al: Cannabis use, gender and age of onset of schizophrenia: data from the ÆSOP study. Psychiatry Res 215(3):528–532, 2014 24461684

Donohoe G, Dillon R, Hargreaves A, et al: Effectiveness of a low support, remotely accessible, cognitive remediation training programme for chronic psychosis: cognitive, functional and cortical outcomes from a single blind randomised controlled trial. Psychol Med 48(5):751–764, 2018 28933314

Dougall N, Maayan N, Soares-Weiser K, et al: Transcranial magnetic stimulation (TMS) for schizophrenia. Cochrane Database Syst Rev Aug 20(8):CD006081, 2015 26289586

Draine J, Blank Wilson A, Metraux S, et al: The impact of mental illness status on the length of jail detention and the legal mechanism of jail release. Psychiatr Serv 61(5):458–462, 2010 20439365

Drake R, Skinner J, Goldman HH: What explains the diffusion of treatments for mental illness? Am J Psychiatry 165(11):1385–1392, 2008 18981070

Drake RE, Gates C, Whitaker A, Cotton PG: Suicide among schizophrenics: a review. Compr Psychiatry 26(1):90–100, 1985 3881217

Drapalski AL, Piscitelli S, Lee RJ, et al: Family involvement in the clinical care of clients with first-episode psychosis in the RAISE Connection Program. Psychiatr Serv 69(3):358–361, 2018 29089013

Druss BG, Bradford DW, Rosenheck RA, et al: Mental disorders and use of cardiovascular procedures after myocardial infarction. JAMA 283(4):506–511, 2000 10659877

Druss BG, Zhao L, von Esenwein SA, et al: The Health and Recovery Peer (HARP) Program: a peer-led intervention to improve medical self-management for persons with serious mental illness. Schizophr Res 118(1–3):264–270, 2010 20185272

Druss BG, Chwastiak L, Kern J, et al: Psychiatry's role in improving the physical health of patients with serious mental illness: a report from the American Psychiatric Association. Psychiatr Serv 69(3):254–256, 2018 29385957

Durbin J, Selick A, Langill G, et al: Using fidelity measurement to assess quality of early psychosis intervention services in Ontario. Psychiatr Serv 70(9):840–844, 2019 31159664

Dyck DG, Short RA, Hendryx MS, et al: Management of negative symptoms among patients with schizophrenia attending multiple-family groups. Psychiatr Serv 51(4):513–519, 2000 10737828

Dzahini O, Singh N, Taylor D, Haddad PM: Antipsychotic drug use and pneumonia: systematic review and meta-analysis. J Psychopharmacol 32(11):1167–1181, 2018 30334664

Easter MM, Swanson JW, Robertson AG, et al: Facilitation of psychiatric advance directives by peers and clinicians on assertive community treatment teams. Psychiatr Serv 68(7):717–723, 2017 28366114

Ekström J, Godoy T, Riva A: Clozapine: agonistic and antagonistic salivary secretory actions. J Dent Res 89(3):276–280, 2010 20093673

Ellison JC, Dufresne RL: A review of the clinical utility of serum clozapine and norclozapine levels. Ment Health Clin 5(2):68–73, 2015

El-Sayeh HG, Rathbone J, Soares-Weiser K, Bergman H: Non-antipsychotic catecholaminergic drugs for antipsychotic-induced tardive dyskinesia. Cochrane Database Syst Rev (1):CD000458, 2018 29342497

Essali A, Rihawi A, Altujjar M, et al: Anticholinergic medication for non-clozapine neuroleptic-induced hypersalivation in people with schizophrenia. Cochrane Database Syst Rev Dec 19(12):CD009546, 2013 24353163

Essock S, Addington D: Coordinated Specialty Care for People With First Episode Psychosis: Assessing Fidelity to the Model. Alexandria, VA, National Association of State Mental Health Program Directors, 2018. Available at: www.nasmhpd.org/sites/default/files/Issue_Brief_Fidelity.pdf. Accessed October 9, 2019.

Essock SM, Covell NH, Davis SM, et al: Effectiveness of switching antipsychotic medications. Am J Psychiatry 163(12):2090–2095, 2006 17151159

Eum S, Lee AM, Bishop JR: Pharmacogenetic tests for antipsychotic medications: clinical implications and considerations. Dialogues Clin Neurosci 18(3):323–337, 2016 27757066

Every-Palmer S, Ellis PM: Clozapine-induced gastrointestinal hypomotility: a 22-year bi-national pharmacovigilance study of serious or fatal 'slow gut' reactions, and comparison with international drug safety advice. CNS Drugs 31(8):699–709, 2017 28623627

Factor SA, Remington G, Comella CL, et al: The effects of valbenazine in participants with tardive dyskinesia: results of the 1-year KINECT 3 extension study. J Clin Psychiatry 78(9):1344–1350, 2017 29141124

Fagiolini A, Rocca P, De Giorgi S, et al: Clinical trial methodology to assess the efficacy/effectiveness of long-acting antipsychotics: randomized controlled trials vs naturalistic studies. Psychiatry Res 247:257–264, 2017 27936437

Falkenberg I, Benetti S, Raffin M, et al: Clinical utility of magnetic resonance imaging in first-episode psychosis. Br J Psychiatry 211(4):231–237, 2017 28473319

Fanapt (iloperidone) [prescribing information]. Washington, DC, Vanda Pharmaceuticals, February 2017

Fann WE, Lake CR: Amantadine versus trihexyphenidyl in the treatment of neuroleptic-induced parkinsonism. Am J Psychiatry 133(8):940–943, 1976 782262

Farooq S, Choudry A, Cohen D, et al: Barriers to using clozapine in treatment-resistant schizophrenia: systematic review. BJPsych Bull 43(1):8–16, 2019 30261942

Farreny A, Aguado J, Ochoa S, et al: REPYFLEC cognitive remediation group training in schizophrenia: looking for an integrative approach. Schizophr Res 142(1–3):137–144, 2012 23017827

FazaClo (clozapine) [prescribing information]. Palo Alto, CA, Jazz Pharmaceuticals, February 2017

Fazel S, Gulati G, Linsell L, et al: Schizophrenia and violence: systematic review and meta-analysis. PLoS Med 6(8):e1000120, 2009a 19668362

Fazel S, Långström N, Hjern A, et al: Schizophrenia, substance abuse, and violent crime. JAMA 301(19):2016–2023, 2009b 19454640

Fazel S, Wolf A, Palm C, Lichtenstein P: Violent crime, suicide, and premature mortality in patients with schizophrenia and related disorders: a 38-year total population study in Sweden. Lancet Psychiatry 1(1):44–54, 2014 25110636

Fenton WS: Evolving perspectives on individual psychotherapy for schizophrenia. Schizophr Bull 26(1):47–72, 2000 10755669

Fenton WS, Blyler CR, Wyatt RJ, McGlashan TH: Prevalence of spontaneous dyskinesia in schizophrenic and non-schizophrenic psychiatric patients. Br J Psychiatry 171:265–268, 1997 9337982

Fernandes-Taylor S, Harris AH: Comparing alternative specifications of quality measures: access to pharmacotherapy for alcohol use disorders. J Subst Abuse Treat 42(1):102–107, 2012 21839604

Fernandez HH, Factor SA, Hauser RA, et al: Randomized controlled trial of deutetrabenazine for tardive dyskinesia: the ARM-TD study. Neurology 88(21):2003–2010, 2017 28446646

Ferrando SJ, Owen JA, Levenson JL: Psychopharmacology, in The American Psychiatric Publishing Textbook of Psychiatry, 6th Edition. Edited by Hales RE, Yudofsky SC, Roberts LW. Washington, DC, American Psychiatric Publishing, 2014, pp 929–1003

Fink M: Rediscovering catatonia: the biography of a treatable syndrome. Acta Psychiatr Scand Suppl 441:1–47, 2013 23215963

Firth J, Cotter J, Elliott R, et al: A systematic review and meta-analysis of exercise interventions in schizophrenia patients. Psychol Med 45(7):1343–1361, 2015 25650668

Firth J, Stubbs B, Rosenbaum S, et al: Aerobic exercise improves cognitive functioning in people with schizophrenia: a systematic review and meta-analysis. Schizophr Bull 43(3):546–556, 2017 27521348

Firth J, Siddiqi N, Koyanagi A, et al: The Lancet Psychiatry Commission: a blueprint for protecting physical health in people with mental illness. Lancet Psychiatry 6(8):675–712, 2019 31324560

Fleischhacker WW, Kane JM, Geier J et al: Completed and attempted suicides among 18,154 subjects with schizophrenia included in a large simple trial. J Clin Psychiatry 75(3):e184–190, 2014 24717389

Fluphenazine decanoate injection [prescribing information]. Chestnut Ridge, NY, Par Pharmaceutical, April 2018

Fluphenazine hydrochloride elixir [prescribing information]. Greenville, SC, Pharmaceutical Associates, December 2016

Fluphenazine hydrochloride injection [prescribing information]. Schaumburg, IL, APP Pharmaceuticals, September 2010

Fluphenazine hydrochloride solution, concentrate [prescribing information]. Greenville, SC, PAI, August 2010

Fluphenazine hydrochloride tablets [prescribing information]. Morgantown, WV, Mylan, November 2016

Foglia E, Schoeler T, Klamerus E, et al: Cannabis use and adherence to antipsychotic medication: a systematic review and meta-analysis. Psychol Med 47(10):1691–1705, 2017 28179039

Fond G, Berna F, Boyer L, et al; FACE-SZ (FondaMental Academic Centers of Expertise for Schizophrenia) group: Benzodiazepine long-term administration is associated with impaired attention/working memory in schizophrenia: results from the national multicentre FACE-SZ data set. Eur Arch Psychiatry Clin Neurosci 268(1):17–26, 2018 28349247

Fontanella CA, Campo JV, Phillips GS, et al: Benzodiazepine use and risk of mortality among patients with schizophrenia: a retrospective longitudinal study. J Clin Psychiatry 77(5):661–667, 2016 27249075

Forbes M, Stefler D, Velakoulis D, et al: The clinical utility of structural neuroimaging in first-episode psychosis: a systematic review. Aust N Z J Psychiatry 53(11):1093–1104, 2019 31113237 Epub ahead of print

Fortney JC, Unützer J, Wrenn G, et al: A tipping point for measurement-based care. Psychiatr Serv 68(2):179–188, 2017 27582237

Frank JD, Frank JB: Persuasion and Healing: A Comparative Study of Psychotherapy, 3rd Edition. Baltimore, MD, Johns Hopkins University Press, 1991

Frederick DE, VanderWeele TJ: Supported employment: meta-analysis and review of randomized controlled trials of individual placement and support. PLoS One 14(2):e0212208, 2019 30785954

Frei K, Truong DD, Fahn S, et al: The nosology of tardive syndromes. J Neurol Sci 389:10–16, 2018 29433810

Freudenreich O, Francis A, Fricchione GL: Psychosis, mania, and catatonia, in The American Psychiatric Association Publishing Textbook of Psychosomatic Medicine and Consultation-Liaison Psychiatry, 3rd Edition. Edited by Levenson JL. Washington, DC, American Psychiatric Association Publishing, 2019, pp 249–279

Fries BE, Schmorrow A, Lang SW, et al: Symptoms and treatment of mental illness among prisoners: a study of Michigan state prisons. Int J Law Psychiatry 36(3–4):316–325, 2013 23688801

Froes Brandao D, Strasser-Weippl K, Goss PE: Prolactin and breast cancer: the need to avoid undertreatment of serious psychiatric illnesses in breast cancer patients: a review. Cancer 122(2):184–188, 2016 26457577

Fung WL, Butcher NJ, Costain G, et al: Practical guidelines for managing adults with 22q11.2 deletion syndrome. Genet Med 17(8):599–609, 2015 25569435

Funk MC, Beach SR, Bostwick JR, et al: Resource document on QTc prolongation and psychotropic medications. APA Resource Document. Washington, DC, American Psychiatric Association, 2018. Available at: www.psychiatry.org/File%20Library/Psychiatrists/Directories/Library-and-Archive/resource_documents/Resource-Document-2018-QTc-Prolongation-and-Psychotropic-Med.pdf. Accessed December 7, 2018.

Fusar-Poli P, Cappucciati M, Borgwardt S, et al: Heterogeneity of psychosis risk within individuals at clinical high risk: a meta-analytical stratification. JAMA Psychiatry 73(2):113–120, 2016 26719911

Gabbard GO: Techniques of psychodynamic psychotherapy, in Textbook of Psychotherapeutic Treatments. Edited by Gabbard GO. Washington, DC, American Psychiatric Publishing, 2009, pp 43–67

Gaebel W, Riesbeck M, von Wilmsdorff M, et al; EUFEST Study Group: Drug attitude as predictor for effectiveness in first-episode schizophrenia: results of an open randomized trial (EUFEST). Eur Neuropsychopharmacol 20(5):310–316, 2010 20202800

Gaedigk A, Sangkuhl K, Whirl-Carrillo M, et al: Prediction of CYP2D6 phenotype from genotype across world populations. Genet Med 19(1):69–76, 2017 27388693

Gaedigk A, Ingelman-Sundberg M, Miller NA, et al; PharmVar Steering Committee:Tthe Pharmacogene Variation (PharmVar) Consortium: incorporation of the Human Cytochrome P450 (CYP) Allele Nomenclature Database. Clin Pharmacol Ther 103(3):399–401, 2018 29134625

Galletly C, Castle D, Dark F, et al: Royal Australian and New Zealand College of Psychiatrists clinical practice guidelines for the management of schizophrenia and related disorders. Aust N Z J Psychiatry 50(5):410–472, 2016 27106681

Galling B, Roldán A, Hagi K, et al: Antipsychotic augmentation vs. monotherapy in schizophrenia: systematic review, meta-analysis and meta-regression analysis. World Psychiatry 16(1):77–89, 2017 28127934

Ganesh M, Jabbar U, Iskander FH: Acute laryngeal dystonia with novel antipsychotics: a case report and review of literature. J Clin Psychopharmacol 35(5):613–615, 2015 26252439

Gao K, Fang F, Wang Z, Calabrese JR: Subjective versus objective weight gain during acute treatment with second-generation antipsychotics in schizophrenia and bipolar disorder. J Clin Psychopharmacol 36(6):637–642, 2016 27753728

García S, Martínez-Cengotitabengoa M, López-Zurbano S, et al: Adherence to antipsychotic medication in bipolar disorder and schizophrenic patients: a systematic review. J Clin Psychopharmacol 36(4):355–371, 2016 27307187

Garety PA, Fowler DG, Freeman D, et al: Cognitive-behavioural therapy and family intervention for relapse prevention and symptom reduction in psychosis: randomised controlled trial. Br J Psychiatry 192(6):412–423, 2008 18515890

Gaynes BN, Brown C, Lux LJ, et al: Management Strategies to Reduce Psychiatric Readmissions (Technical Brief No 21, AHRQ Publ No 15-EHC018-EF). Rockville, MD, Agency for Healthcare Research and Quality, May 2015. Available at: www.effectivehealthcare.ahrq.gov/reports/final.cfm. Accessed October 3, 2019.

GBD 2017 Disease and Injury Incidence and Prevalence Collaborators: Global, regional, and national incidence, prevalence, and years lived with disability for 354 diseases and injuries for 195 countries and territories, 1990–2017: a systematic analysis for the Global Burden of Disease Study 2017. Lancet 392(10159):1789–1858, 2018 30496104

Gee SH, Shergill SS, Taylor DM: Patient attitudes to clozapine initiation. Int Clin Psychopharmacol 32(6):337–342, 2017 28704228

Geodon (ziprasidone) [prescribing information]. New York, Pfizer, November 2018

Gertner AK, Grabert B, Domino ME, et al: The effect of referral to expedited Medicaid on substance use treatment utilization among people with serious mental illness released from prison. J Subst Abuse Treat 99:9–15, 2019 30797401

Ghany MG, Hoofnagle JH: Approach to the patient with liver disease, in Harrison's Principles of Internal Medicine, 20th Edition. Edited by Jameson J, Fauci AS, Kasper DL, et al. New York, McGraw-Hill, 2018. Available at: https://accessmedicine.mhmedical.com/content.aspx?bookid=2129&sectionid=192283281. Accessed May 6, 2020.

Gibson LM, Paul L, Chappell FM, et al: Potentially serious incidental findings on brain and body magnetic resonance imaging of apparently asymptomatic adults: systematic review and meta-analysis. BMJ 363:k4577, 2018 30467245

Gierisch JM, Nieuwsma JA, Bradford DW, et al: Pharmacologic and behavioral interventions to improve cardiovascular risk factors in adults with serious mental illness: a systematic review and meta-analysis. J Clin Psychiatry 75(5):e424–e440, 2014 24922495

Glowa-Kollisch S, Kaba F, Waters A, et al: From punishment to treatment: the "Clinical Alternative to Punitive Segregation" (CAPS) program in New York City jails. Int J Environ Res Public Health 13(2):182, 2016 26848667

Glynn SM, Marder SR, Liberman RP, et al: Supplementing clinic-based skills training with manual-based community support sessions: effects on social adjustment of patients with schizophrenia. Am J Psychiatry 159(5):829–837, 2002 11986138

Glynn SM, Cather C, Gingerich S, et al: NAVIGATE Family Education Program, April 1, 2014. Available at: http://www.navigateconsultants.org/wp-content/uploads/2017/05/FE-Manual.pdf. Accessed October 9, 2019.

Godwin-Austen RB, Clark T: Persistent phenothiazine dyskinesia treated with tetrabenazine. Br Med J 4(5778):25–26, 1971 4938245

Goff DC, Arana GW, Greenblatt DJ, et al: The effect of benztropine on haloperidol-induced dystonia, clinical efficacy and pharmacokinetics: a prospective, double-blind trial. J Clin Psychopharmacol 11(2):106–112, 1991 2056136

Goff DC, Falkai P, Fleischhacker WW, et al: The long-term effects of antipsychotic medication on clinical course in schizophrenia. Am J Psychiatry 74(9):840–849, 2017 28472900

Goldberg RW, Dickerson F, Lucksted A, et al: Living Well: an intervention to improve self-management of medical illness for individuals with serious mental illness. Psychiatr Serv 64(1):51–57, 2013 23070062

Gomar JJ, Valls E, Radua J, et al; Cognitive Rehabilitation Study Group: A multisite, randomized controlled clinical trial of computerized cognitive remediation therapy for schizophrenia. Schizophr Bull 41(6):1387–1396, 2015 26006264

Grady PA, Gough LL: Self-management: a comprehensive approach to management of chronic conditions. Am J Public Health 104(8):e25–e31, 2014 24922170

Granholm EL, McQuaid JR, Holden JL: Cognitive-Behavioral Social Skills Training for Schizophrenia: A Practical Treatment Guide. New York, Guilford, 2016

Graus F, Titulaer MJ, Balu R, et al: A clinical approach to diagnosis of autoimmune encephalitis. Lancet Neurol 15(4):391–404, 2016 26906964

Gray GE, Pi EH: Ethnicity and medication-induced movement disorders. J. Practical Psychiatry 4(5):259–264, 1998

Green MF: Impact of cognitive and social cognitive impairment on functional outcomes in patients with schizophrenia. J Clin Psychiatry 77 (suppl 2):8–11, 2016 26919052

Greenblatt DJ, DiMascio A, Harmatz JS, et al: Pharmacokinetics and clinical effects of amantadine in drug-induced extrapyramidal symptoms. J Clin Pharmacol 17(11–12):704–708, 1977 336651

Greenhalgh AM, Gonzalez-Blanco L, Garcia-Rizo C, et al: Meta-analysis of glucose tolerance, insulin, and insulin resistance in antipsychotic-naïve patients with nonaffective psychosis. Schizophr Res 179:57–63, 2017 27743650

Greenhalgh T, Robert G, Macfarlane F, et al: Diffusion of innovations in service organizations: systematic review and recommendations. Milbank Q 82(4):581–629, 2004 15595944

Gregory A, Mallikarjun P, Upthegrove R: Treatment of depression in schizophrenia: systematic review and meta-analysis. Br J Psychiatry 211(4):198–204, 2017 28882827

Grigg J, Worsley R, Thew C, et al: Antipsychotic-induced hyperprolactinemia: synthesis of world-wide guidelines and integrated recommendations for assessment, management and future research. Psychopharmacology (Berl) 234(22):3279–3297, 2017 28889207

Grover S, Hazari N, Kate N: Combined use of clozapine and ECT: a review. Acta Neuropsychiatr 27(3):131–142, 2015 25697225

Grundy SM, Stone NJ, Bailey AL, et al: 2018 AHA/ACC/AACVPR/AAPA/ABC/ACPM/ADA/AGS/APhA/ASPC/NLA/PCNA Guideline on the Management of Blood Cholesterol: a report of the American College of Cardiology/American Heart Association Task Force on Clinical Practice Guidelines. J Am Coll Cardiol 73(24):e285–e350, 2018 30423393

Guenette MD, Hahn M, Cohn TA, et al: Atypical antipsychotics and diabetic ketoacidosis: a review. Psychopharmacology (Berl) 226(1):1–12, 2013 23344556

Gurrera RJ, Caroff SN, Cohen A, et al: An international consensus study of neuroleptic malignant syndrome diagnostic criteria using the Delphi method. J Clin Psychiatry 72(9):1222–1228, 2011 21733489

Gurrera RJ, Mortillaro G, Velamoor V, Caroff SN: A validation study of the international consensus diagnostic criteria for neuroleptic malignant syndrome. J Clin Psychopharmacol 37(1):67–71, 2017 28027111

Guy W (ed): ECDEU Assessment Manual for Psychopharmacology (Publ ADM 76-338.) Washington, DC, Center for Quality Assessment and Improvement in Mental Health, U.S. Department of Health, Education, and Welfare, 1976

Guyatt G, Gutterman D, Baumann MH, et al: Grading strength of recommendations and quality of evidence in clinical guidelines: report from an American College of Chest Physicians Task Force. Chest 129(1):174–181, 2006 16424429

Guyatt GH, Oxman AD, Kunz R, et al; GRADE Working Group: Going from evidence to recommendations. BMJ 336(7652):1049–1051, 2008 18467413

Guyatt G, Eikelboom JW, Akl EA, et al: A guide to GRADE guidelines for the readers of JTH. J Thromb Haemost 11(8):1603–1608, 2013 23773710

Haddad PM, Brain C, Scott J: Nonadherence with antipsychotic medication in schizophrenia: challenges and management strategies. Patient Relat Outcome Meas 5:43–62, 2014 25061342

Haldol decanoate injection (haloperidol) [prescribing information]. Titusville, NJ, Janssen Pharmaceuticals, March 2019

Haldol lactate injection (haloperidol) [prescribing information]. Titusville, NJ, Janssen Pharmaceuticals, March 2019

Hall D, Lee LW, Manseau MW, et al: Major mental illness as a risk factor for incarceration. Psychiatr Serv 70(12):1088–1093, 2019 31480926

Haloperidol [prescribing information]. Princeton, NJ, Sandoz, September 2008

Haloperidol lactate [prescribing information]. Greenville, SC, Pharmaceutical Associates, December 2008

Haloperidol lactate injection [prescribing information]. Schaumburg, IL, Sagent Pharmaceuticals, August 2011

Haloperidol lactate oral solution [prescribing information]. Greenville, SC, Pharmaceutical Associates, November 2016

Haloperidol tablets [prescribing information]. Princeton, NJ, Sandoz, July 2015

Hamann GL, Egan TM, Wells BG, Grimmig JE: Injection site reactions after intramuscular administration of haloperidol decanoate 100 mg/mL. J Clin Psychiatry 51(12):502–504, 1990 1979555

Hamann J, Heres S: Why and how family caregivers should participate in shared decision making in mental health. Psychiatr Serv 70(5):418–421, 2019 30784381

Hamann J, Mendel R, Heres S, et al: How much more effective do depot antipsychotics have to be compared to oral antipsychotics before they are prescribed? Eur Neuropsychopharmacol 20(4):276–279, 2010 20133108

Hamann J, Kissling W, Heres S: Checking the plausibility of psychiatrists? Arguments for not prescribing depot medication. Eur Neuropsychopharmacol 24(9):1506–1510, 2014 25037772

Harding KJ, Rush AJ, Arbuckle M, et al: Measurement-based care in psychiatric practice: a policy framework for implementation. J Clin Psychiatry 72(8):1136–1143, 2011 21295000

Hardy K: Cognitive behavioral therapy for psychosis (CBTp). Alexandria, VA, National Association of State Mental Health Program Directors, 2019. Available at: www.nasmhpd.org/sites/default/files/DH-CBTp_Fact_Sheet.pdf. Accessed April 12, 2019.

Harkavy-Friedman JM, Kimhy D, Nelson EA, et al: Suicide attempts in schizophrenia: the role of command auditory hallucinations for suicide. J Clin Psychiatry 64(8):871–874, 2003 12927000

Harris A, Chen W, Jones S, et al: Community treatment orders increase community care and delay readmission while in force: results from a large population-based study. Aust N Z J Psychiatry 53(3):228–235, 2019 29485289

Hartung D, Low A, Jindai K, et al: Interventions to improve pharmacological adherence among adults with psychotic spectrum disorders and bipolar disorder: a systematic review. Psychosomatics 58(2):101–112, 2017 28139249

Hartz SM, Pato CN, Medeiros H, et al; Genomic Psychiatry Cohort Consortium: Comorbidity of severe psychotic disorders with measures of substance use. JAMA Psychiatry 71(3):248–254, 2014 24382686

Harvey PD: Assessment of everyday functioning in schizophrenia. Innov Clin Neurosci 8(5):21–24, 2011 21686144

Harvey PD, McGurk SR, Mahncke H, Wykes T: Controversies in computerized cognitive training. Biol Psychiatry Cogn Neurosci Neuroimaging 3(11):907–915, 2018 30197048

Hasan A, Falkai P, Wobrock T, et al; World Federation of Societies of Biological Psychiatry (WFSBP) Task Force on Treatment Guidelines for Schizophrenia: World Federation of Societies of Biological Psychiatry (WFSBP) guidelines for biological treatment of schizophrenia, part 1: update 2012 on the acute treatment of schizophrenia and the management of treatment resistance. World J Biol Psychiatry 13(5):318–378, 2012 22834451

Hasan A, Falkai P, Wobrock T, et al; WFSBP Task Force on Treatment Guidelines for Schizophrenia: World Federation of Societies of Biological Psychiatry (WFSBP) guidelines for biological treatment of schizophrenia, part 2: update 2012 on the long-term treatment of schizophrenia and management of antipsychotic-induced side effects. World J Biol Psychiatry 14(1):2–44, 2013 23216388

Hasan A, Falkai P, Wobrock T, et al; WFSBP Task Force on Treatment Guidelines for Schizophrenia: World Federation of Societies of Biological Psychiatry (WFSBP) guidelines for biological treatment of schizophrenia, part 3: update 2015 management of special circumstances: depression, suicidality, substance use disorders and pregnancy and lactation. World J Biol Psychiatry 16(3):142–170, 2015 25822804

Hasson-Ohayon I, Roe D, Kravetz S: A randomized controlled trial of the effectiveness of the Illness Management and Recovery Program. Psychiatr Serv 58(11):1461–1466, 2007 17978257

Hatch A, Docherty JP, Carpenter D, et al: Expert consensus survey on medication adherence in psychiatric patients and use of a digital medicine system. J Clin Psychiatry 78(7):e803–e812, 2017 28541648

Hatcher-Martin JM, Armstrong KA, Scorr LM, Factor SA: Propranolol therapy for tardive dyskinesia: a retrospective examination. Parkinsonism Relat Disord 32:124–126, 2016 27622970

Hauser P, Kern S: Psychiatric and substance use disorders co-morbidities and hepatitis C: diagnostic and treatment implications. World J Hepatol 7(15):1921–1935, 2015 26244067

Hauser RA, Factor SA, Marder SR, et al: KINECT 3: a phase 3 randomized, double-blind, placebo-controlled trial of valbenazine for tardive dyskinesia. Am J Psychiatry 174(5):476–484, 2017 28320223

Hauser RA, Fernandez HH, Stamler D, et al: 45 Long-term treatment with deutetrabenazine is associated with continued improvement in tardive dyskinesia: results from an open-label extension study. CNS Spectr 24(1):200–201, 2019 30859973

Hawton K, Sutton L, Haw C, et al: Schizophrenia and suicide: systematic review of risk factors. Br J Psychiatry 187:9–20, 2005 15994566

Hayes JF, Marston L, Walters K, et al: Mortality gap for people with bipolar disorder and schizophrenia: UK-based cohort study 2000–2014. Br J Psychiatry 211(3):175–181, 2017 28684403

Hazlehurst JM, Armstrong MJ, Sherlock M, et al: A comparative quality assessment of evidence-based clinical guidelines in endocrinology. Clin Endocrinol (Oxf) 78(2):183–190, 2013 22624723

He H, Lu J, Yang L, et al: Repetitive transcranial magnetic stimulation for treating the symptoms of schizophrenia: a PRISMA compliant meta-analysis. Clin Neurophysiol 128(5):716–724, 2017 28315614

He M, Deng C, Huang XF: The role of hypothalamic H1 receptor antagonism in antipsychotic-induced weight gain. CNS Drugs 27(6):423–434, 2013 23640535

Heilä H, Haukka J, Suvisaari J, Lönnqvist J: Mortality among patients with schizophrenia and reduced psychiatric hospital care. Psychol Med 35(5):725–732, 2005 15918349

Helfer B, Samara MT, Huhn M, et al: Efficacy and safety of antidepressants added to antipsychotics for schizophrenia: a systematic review and meta-analysis. Am J Psychiatry 173(9):876–886, 2016 27282362

Helle S, Ringen PA, Melle I, et al: Cannabis use is associated with 3years earlier onset of schizophrenia spectrum disorder in a naturalistic, multi-site sample (N=1119). Schizophr Res 170(1):217–221, 2016 26682958

Henderson DC, Vincenzi B, Andrea NV, et al: Pathophysiological mechanisms of increased cardiometabolic risk in people with schizophrenia and other severe mental illnesses. Lancet Psychiatry 2(5):452–464, 2015 26360288

Heres S, Hamann J, Kissling W, Leucht S: Attitudes of psychiatrists toward antipsychotic depot medication. J Clin Psychiatry 67(12):1948–1953, 2006 17194274

Heres S, Schmitz FS, Leucht S, Pajonk FG: The attitude of patients towards antipsychotic depot treatment. Int Clin Psychopharmacol 22(5):275–282, 2007 17690596

Heres S, Frobose T, Hamann J, et al: Patients' acceptance of the deltoid application of risperidone long-acting injection. Eur Neuropsychopharmacol 22(12):897–901, 2012 22578781

Hiemke C, Dragicevic A, Gründer G, et al: Therapeutic monitoring of new antipsychotic drugs. Ther Drug Monit 26(2):156–160, 2004 15228157

Hiemke C, Bergemann N, Clement HW, et al: Consensus guidelines for therapeutic drug monitoring in neuropsychopharmacology: update 2017. Pharmacopsychiatry 51(1-02):9–62, 2018 28910830

Higashi K, Medic G, Littlewood KJ, et al: Medication adherence in schizophrenia: factors influencing adherence and consequences of nonadherence, a systematic literature review. Ther Adv Psychopharmacol 3(4):200–218, 2013 24167693

Higgins JM, San C, Lagnado G, et al: Incidence and management of clozapine-induced myocarditis in a large tertiary hospital. Can J Psychiatry 64(8):561–567, 2019 30599763

Hirsch L, Yang J, Bresee L, et al: Second-generation antipsychotics and metabolic side effects: a systematic review of population-based studies. Drug Saf 40(9):771–781, 2017 28585153

Hirschtritt ME, Delucchi KL, Olfson M: Outpatient, combined use of opioid and benzodiazepine medications in the United States, 1993–2014. Prev Med Rep 9:49–54, 2017 29340270

Hjorthøj C, Stürup AE, McGrath JJ, Nordentoft M: Years of potential life lost and life expectancy in schizophrenia: a systematic review and meta-analysis. Lancet Psychiatry 4(4):295–301, 2017 28237639

Hobkirk AL, Towe SL, Lion R, Meade CS: Primary and secondary HIV prevention among persons with severe mental illness: recent findings. Curr HIV/AIDS Rep 12(4):406–412, 2015 26428958

Hoffmann H, Jäckel D, Glauser S, et al: Long-term effectiveness of supported employment: 5-year follow-up of a randomized controlled trial. Am J Psychiatry 171(11):1183–1190, 2014 25124692

Hogarty GE, Kornblith SJ, Greenwald D, DiBarry AL, et al: Three-year trials of personal therapy among schizophrenic patients living with or independent of family, I: description of study and effects on relapse rates. Am J Psychiatry 154(11):1504–1513, 1997 9356557

Holt RI, Mitchell AJ: Diabetes mellitus and severe mental illness: mechanisms and clinical implications. Nat Rev Endocrinol 11(2):79–89, 2015 25445848

Honigfeld G, Arellano F, Sethi J, et al: Reducing clozapine-related morbidity and mortality: 5 years of experience with the Clozaril National Registry. J Clin Psychiatry 59 (suppl 3):3–7, 1998 9541331

Hor K, Taylor M: Suicide and schizophrenia: a systematic review of rates and risk factors. J Psychopharmacol 24(4) (suppl):81–90, 2010 20923923

Horvitz-Lennon M, Donohue JM, Domino ME, Normand SL: Improving quality and diffusing best practices: the case of schizophrenia. Health Aff (Millwood) 28(3):701–712, 2009 19414878

Horvitz-Lennon M, Mattke S, Predmore Z, Howes OD: The role of antipsychotic plasma levels in the treatment of schizophrenia. Am J Psychiatry 174(5):421–426, 2017 28457153

Howard R, Rabins PV, Seeman MV, Jeste DV: Late-onset schizophrenia and very-late-onset schizophrenia-like psychosis: an international consensus: the International Late-Onset Schizophrenia Group. Am J Psychiatry 157(2):172–178, 2000 10671383

Howells FM, Kingdon DG, Baldwin DS: Current and potential pharmacological and psychosocial interventions for anxiety symptoms and disorders in patients with schizophrenia: structured review. Hum Psychopharmacol 32(5), 2017 28812313

Howes OD, McCutcheon R, Agid O, et al: Treatment-resistant schizophrenia: Treatment Response and Resistance in Psychosis (TRRIP) Working Group consensus guidelines on diagnosis and terminology. Am J Psychiatry 174(3):216–229, 2017 27919182

Hughes E, Bassi S, Gilbody S, et al: Prevalence of HIV, hepatitis B, and hepatitis C in people with severe mental illness: a systematic review and meta-analysis. Lancet Psychiatry 3(1):40–48, 2016 26620388

Huhn M, Nikolakopoulou A, Schneider-Thoma J, et al: Comparative efficacy and tolerability of 32 oral antipsychotics for the acute treatment of adults with multi-episode schizophrenia: a systematic review and network meta-analysis. Lancet 394(10202):939–951, 2019 31303314 [Erratum Lancet 394(10202):918, 2019 31526735]

Huhtaniska S, Jääskeläinen E, Hirvonen N, et al: Long-term antipsychotic use and brain changes in schizophrenia—a systematic review and meta-analysis. Hum Psychopharmacol 32(2), 2017 28370309

Hui CLM, Honer WG, Lee EHM, et al: Long-term effects of discontinuation from antipsychotic maintenance following first-episode schizophrenia and related disorders: a 10 year follow-up of a randomised, double-blind trial. Lancet Psychiatry 5(5):432–442, 2018 29551618

Hunt GE, Siegfried N, Morley K, et al: Psychosocial interventions for people with both severe mental illness and substance misuse. Cochrane Database Syst Rev Oct 3(10):CD001088, 2013 24092525

Hunt GE, Large MM, Cleary M, et al: Prevalence of comorbid substance use in schizophrenia spectrum disorders in community and clinical settings, 1990–2017: systematic review and meta-analysis. Drug Alcohol Depend 191:234–258, 2018 30153606

Hynes C, Keating D, McWilliams S, et al: Glasgow Antipsychotic Side-effects Scale for clozapine: development and validation of a clozapine-specific side-effects scale. Schizophr Res 168(1–2):505–513, 2015 26276305

Ince P, Haddock G, Tai S: A systematic review of the implementation of recommended psychological interventions for schizophrenia: rates, barriers, and improvement strategies. Psychol Psychother 89(3):324–350, 2016 26537838

Ingrezza (valbenazine) [prescribing information]. San Diego, CA, Neurocrine Biosciences, July 2019

Inskip HM, Harris EC, Barraclough B: Lifetime risk of suicide for affective disorder, alcoholism and schizophrenia. Br J Psychiatry 172:35–37, 1998 9534829

Institute of Medicine: Improving the Quality of Health Care for Mental and Substance-Use Conditions. Washington, DC, National Academies Press, 2006. Available at: https://doi.org/10.17226/11470. Accessed October 3, 2019.

Institute of Medicine: Clinical Practice Guidelines We Can Trust. Washington, DC, National Academies Press, 2011

Institute of Medicine Committee on Quality of Health Care in America: Crossing the Quality Chasm: A New Health System for the 21st Century. Washington, DC, National Academies Press, 2001. Available at: www.ncbi.nlm.nih.gov/books/NBK222274. Accessed March 28, 2017.

Invega (paliperidone) [product monograph]. Toronto, ON, Canada, Janssen, September 2018

Invega (paliperidone) [prescribing information]. Titusville, NJ, Janssen Pharmaceuticals, January 2019

Invega Sustenna (paliperidone) [prescribing information]. Titusville, NJ, Janssen Pharmaceuticals, July 2018a

Invega Sustenna (paliperidone) [product monograph]. Toronto, ON, Canada, Janssen, September 2018b

Invega Trinza (paliperidone) [prescribing information]. Titusville, NJ, Janssen Pharmaceuticals, July 2018a

Invega Trinza (paliperidone) [product monograph]. Toronto, ON, Canada, Janssen, September 2018b

Iorfino F, Scott EM, Carpenter JS, et al: Clinical stage transitions in persons aged 12 to 25 years presenting to early intervention mental health services with anxiety, mood, and psychotic disorders. JAMA Psychiatry Aug 28, 2019 31461129 Epub ahead of print

Ismail Z, Wessels AM, Uchida H, et al: Age and sex impact clozapine plasma concentrations in inpatients and outpatients with schizophrenia. Am J Geriatr Psychiatry 20(1):53–60, 2012 21422906

Iyer S, Banks N, Roy MA, et al: A qualitative study of experiences with and perceptions regarding long-acting injectable antipsychotics, part I: patient perspectives. Can J Psychiatry 58(5 suppl 1):14S–22S, 2013 23945063

Iyer SP, Spaeth-Rublee B, Pincus HA: Challenges in the operationalization of mental health quality measures: an assessment of alternatives. Psychiatr Serv 67(10):1057–1059, 2016 27301768

Jahshan C, Vinogradov S, Wynn JK, et al: A randomized controlled trial comparing a "bottom-up" and "top-down" approach to cognitive training in schizophrenia. J Psychiatr Res 109:118–125, 2019 30529836

Jann MW, Ereshefsky L, Saklad SR: Clinical pharmacokinetics of the depot antipsychotics. Clin Pharmacokinet 10(4):315–333, 1985 2864156

Janssen EM, McGinty EE, Azrin ST, et al: Review of the evidence: prevalence of medical conditions in the United States population with serious mental illness. Gen Hosp Psychiatry 37(3):199–222, 2015 25881768

Jauhar S, McKenna PJ, Radua J, et al: Cognitive-behavioural therapy for the symptoms of schizophrenia: systematic review and meta-analysis with examination of potential bias. Br J Psychiatry 204(1):20–29, 2014 24385461

Jehan S, Myers AK, Zizi F, et al: Obesity, obstructive sleep apnea and type 2 diabetes mellitus: epidemiology and pathophysiologic insights. Sleep Med Disord 2(3):52–58, 2018 30167574

Jensen KG, Correll CU, Rudå D, et al: Cardiometabolic adverse effects and its predictors in children and adolescents with first-episode psychosis during treatment with quetiapine-extended release versus aripiprazole: 12-week results from the Tolerance and Effect of Antipsychotics in Children and Adolescents With Psychosis (TEA) trial. J Am Acad Child Adolesc Psychiatry 58(11):1062–1078, 2019 30858012

Jin H, Mosweu I: The societal cost of schizophrenia: a systematic review. Pharmacoeconomics 35(1):25–42, 2017 27557994

Jinnah HA, Factor SA: Diagnosis and treatment of dystonia. Neurol Clin 33(1):77–100, 2015 25432724

Jordan G, Lutgens D, Joober R, et al: The relative contribution of cognition and symptomatic remission to functional outcome following treatment of a first episode of psychosis. J Clin Psychiatry 75(6):e566–e572, 2014 25004197

Josiassen RC, Kane JM, Liang GS, et al: Long-term safety and tolerability of valbenazine (NBI-98854) in subjects with tardive dyskinesia and a diagnosis of schizophrenia or mood disorder. Psychopharmacol Bull 47(3):61–68, 2017 28839341

Juncal-Ruiz M, Ramirez-Bonilla M, Gomez-Arnau J, et al: Incidence and risk factors of acute akathisia in 493 individuals with first episode non-affective psychosis: a 6-week randomised study of antipsychotic treatment. Psychopharmacology (Berl) 234(17):2563–2570, 2017 28567698

Kaba F, Lewis A, Glowa-Kollisch S, et al: Solitary confinement and risk of self-harm among jail inmates. Am J Public Health 104(3):442–447, 2014 24521238

Kahn RS, Winter van Rossum I, Leucht S, et al; OPTiMiSE study group: Amisulpride and olanzapine followed by open-label treatment with clozapine in first-episode schizophrenia and schizophreniform disorder (OPTiMiSE): a three-phase switching study. Lancet Psychiatry 5(10):797–807, 2018 30115598

Kaiser RM: Physiological and clinical considerations of geriatric patient care, in The American Psychiatric Publishing Textbook of Geriatric Psychiatry, 5th Edition. Edited by Steffens DC, Blazer DG, Thakur ME. Arlington, VA, American Psychiatric Publishing, 2015, pp 33–59

Kalachnik JE, Sprague RL: The Dyskinesia Identification System Condensed User Scale (DISCUS): reliability, validity, and a total score cut-off for mentally ill and mentally retarded populations. J Clin Psychol 49(2):177–189, 1993 8098048

Kane JM, Marder SR, Schooler NR, et al: Clozapine and haloperidol in moderately refractory schizophrenia: a 6-month randomized and double-blind comparison. Arch Gen Psychiatry 58(10):965–972, 2001 11576036

Kane JM, Kishimoto T, Correll CU: Non-adherence to medication in patients with psychotic disorders: epidemiology, contributing factors and management strategies. World Psychiatry 12(3):216–226, 2013 24096780

Kane JM, Correll CU, Liang GS, et al: Efficacy of valbenazine (NBI-98854) in treating subjects with tardive dyskinesia and schizophrenia or schizoaffective disorder. Psychopharmacol Bull 47(3):69–76, 2017 28839342

Kane JM, Schooler NR, Marcy P, et al: Patients with early-phase schizophrenia will accept treatment with sustained-release medication (long-acting injectable antipsychotics): results from the recruitment phase of the PRELAPSE trial. J Clin Psychiatry 80(3):18m12546, 2019 31050233

Kang UJ, Burke RE, Fahn S: Natural history and treatment of tardive dystonia. Mov Disord 1(3):193–208, 1986 2904118

Kaplan J, Schwartz AC, Ward MC: Clozapine-associated aspiration pneumonia: case series and review of the literature. Psychosomatics 59(2):199–203, 2018 28992957

Kapoor R, Trestman R: Mental health effects of restrictive housing, in Restrictive Housing in the U.S.: Issues, Challenges, and Future Directions. Washington, DC, National Institute of Justice, 2016, pp 199–232. Available at www.ncjrs.gov/pdffiles1/nij/250315.pdf. Accessed October 4, 2019.

Kates J, Rockland LH: Supportive psychotherapy of the schizophrenic patient. Am J Psychother 48(4):543–561, 1994 7872417

Kato Y, Umetsu R, Abe J, et al: Hyperglycemic adverse events following antipsychotic drug administration in spontaneous adverse event reports. J Pharm Health Care Sci 1:15, 2015 26819726

Kay SR, Fiszbein A, Opler LA: The Positive and Negative Syndrome Scale (PANSS) for schizophrenia. Schizophr Bull 13(2):261–276, 1987 3616518

Kazamatsuri H, Chien C, Cole JO: Treatment of tardive dyskinesia, I: clinical efficacy of a dopamine-depleting agent, tetrabenazine. Arch Gen Psychiatry 27(1):95–99, 1972 4555831

Keck PEJr, Pope HG Jr, Cohen BM, et al: Risk factors for neuroleptic malignant syndrome: a case-control study. Arch Gen Psychiatry 46(10):914–918, 1989 2572206

Keefe RS, Vinogradov S, Medalia A, et al: Feasibility and pilot efficacy results from the multisite Cognitive Remediation in the Schizophrenia Trials Network (CRSTN) randomized controlled trial. J Clin Psychiatry 73(7):1016–1022, 2012 22687548

Keers R, Ullrich S, Destavola BL, Coid JW: Association of violence with emergence of persecutory delusions in untreated schizophrenia. Am J Psychiatry 171(3):332–339, 2014 24220644

Keller A, McGarvey EL, Clayton AH: Reliability and construct validity of the Changes in Sexual Functioning Questionnaire short-form (CSFQ-14). J Sex Marital Ther 32(1):43–52, 2006 16234225

Keller WR, Fischer BA, McMahon R, et al: Community adherence to schizophrenia treatment and safety monitoring guidelines. J Nerv Ment Dis 202(1):6–12, 2014 24375205

Kelley ME, Wan CR, Broussard B, et al: Marijuana use in the immediate 5-year premorbid period is associated with increased risk of onset of schizophrenia and related psychotic disorders. Schizophr Res 171(1–3):62–67, 2016 26785806

Kelly DL, Freudenreich O, Sayer MA, Love RC: Addressing barriers to clozapine underutilization: a national effort. Psychiatr Serv 69(2):224–227, 2018 29032704

Kelly DL, Love RC: Psychiatric pharmacist's role in overcoming barriers to clozapine use and improving management. Ment Health Clin 9(2):64–69, 2019 30842912

Kelly JT, Zimmermann RL, Abuzzahab FS, Schiele BC: A double-blind study of amantadine hydrochloride versus benztropine mesylate in drug-induced parkinsonism. Pharmacology 12(2):65–73, 1974 4610599

Kemp K, Zelle H, Bonnie RJ: Embedding advance directives in routine care for persons with serious mental illness: implementation challenges. Psychiatr Serv 66(1):10–14, 2015 25554232

Kennedy JL, Altar CA, Taylor DL, et al: The social and economic burden of treatment-resistant schizophrenia: a systematic literature review. Int Clin Psychopharmacol 29(2):63–76, 2014 23995856

Khan AA, Ashraf A, Baker D, et al: Clozapine and incidence of myocarditis and sudden death—long term Australian experience. Int J Cardiol 238:136–139, 2017 28343762

Kidney Disease: Improving Global Outcomes (KDIGO) CKD Work Group: KDIGO 2012 Clinical Practice Guideline for the Evaluation and Management of Chronic Kidney Disease. Kidney Int Suppl 3(1):1–150, 2013

Kingdon D, Turkington D: CBT for psychosis: approaches families can use. Arlington, VA, National Alliance on Mental Illness, April 15, 2019. Available at: https://nami.org/Blogs/NAMI-Blog/April-2019/CBT-for-Psychosis-Approaches-Families-Can-Use. Accessed April 21, 2019.

Kinon BJ, Gilmore JA, Liu H, Halbreich UM: Prevalence of hyperprolactinemia in schizophrenic patients treated with conventional antipsychotic medications or risperidone. Psychoneuroendocrinology 28 (suppl s):55–68, 2003 12650681

Kinoshita Y, Furukawa TA, Kinoshita K, et al: Supported employment for adults with severe mental illness. Cochrane Database Syst Rev Sep 13(9):CD008297, 2013 24030739

Kiriakakis V, Bhatia KP, Quinn NP, Marsden CD: The natural history of tardive dystonia: a long-term follow-up study of 107 cases. Brain 121 (Pt 11):2053–2066, 1998 9827766

Kirino E: Serum prolactin levels and sexual dysfunction in patients with schizophrenia treated with antipsychotics: comparison between aripiprazole and other atypical antipsychotics. Ann Gen Psychiatry 16:43, 2017 29209406

Kirschner M, Theodoridou A, Fusar-Poli P, et al: Patients' and clinicians' attitude towards long-acting depot antipsychotics in subjects with a first episode of psychosis. Ther Adv Psychopharmacol 3(2):89–99, 2013 24167680

Kirsh B: Client, contextual and program elements influencing supported employment: a literature review. Community Ment Health J 52(7):809–820, 2016 27055809

Kisely S, Smith M, Lawrence D, et al: Inequitable access for mentally ill patients to some medically necessary procedures. CMAJ 176(6):779–784, 2007 17353530

Kisely S, Crowe E, Lawrence D: Cancer-related mortality in people with mental illness. JAMA Psychiatry 70(2):209–217, 2013 23247556

Kisely S, Baghaie H, Lalloo R, et al: A systematic review and meta-analysis of the association between poor oral health and severe mental illness. Psychosom Med 77(1):83–92, 2015 25526527

Kishi T, Matsunaga S, Iwata N: Mortality risk associated with long-acting injectable antipsychotics: a systematic review and meta-analyses of randomized controlled trials. Schizophr Bull 42(6):1438–1445, 2016a 27086079

Kishi T, Oya K, Iwata N: Long-acting injectable antipsychotics for the prevention of relapse in patients with recent-onset psychotic disorders: a systematic review and meta-analysis of randomized controlled trials. Psychiatry Res 246:750–755, 2016b 27863801

Kishi T, Ikuta T, Matsui Y, et al: Effect of discontinuation v. maintenance of antipsychotic medication on relapse rates in patients with remitted/stable first-episode psychosis: a meta-analysis. Psychol Med 49(5):772–779, 2019 29909790

Kishimoto T, Nitta M, Borenstein M, et al: Long-acting injectable versus oral antipsychotics in schizophrenia: a systematic review and meta-analysis of mirror-image studies. J Clin Psychiatry 74(10):957–965, 2013 24229745

Kishimoto T, Robenzadeh A, Leucht C, et al: Long-acting injectable vs oral antipsychotics for relapse prevention in schizophrenia: a meta-analysis of randomized trials. Schizophr Bull 40(1):192–213, 2014 23256986

Kishimoto T, Hagi K, Nitta M, et al: Effectiveness of long-acting injectable vs oral antipsychotics in patients with schizophrenia: a meta-analysis of prospective and retrospective cohort studies. Schizophr Bull 44(3):603–619, 2018 29868849

Kiviniemi M, Suvisaari J, Koivumaa-Honkanen H, et al: Antipsychotics and mortality in first-onset schizophrenia: prospective Finnish register study with 5-year follow-up. Schizophr Res 150(1):274–280, 2013 23953217

Klil-Drori AJ, Yin H, Abenhaim HA, et al: Prolactin-elevating antipsychotics and the risk of endometrial cancer. J Clin Psychiatry 78(6):714–719, 2017 28199787

Knegtering H, van den Bosch R, Castelein S, et al: Are sexual side effects of prolactin-raising antipsychotics reducible to serum prolactin? Psychoneuroendocrinology 33(6):711–717, 2008 18395353

Knoph KN, Morgan RJ III, Palmer BA, et al: Clozapine-induced cardiomyopathy and myocarditis monitoring: a systematic review. Schizophr Res 199:17–30, 2018 29548760

Koek RJ, Pi EH: Acute laryngeal dystonic reactions to neuroleptics. Psychosomatics 30(4):359–364, 1989 2572029

König P, Chwatal K, Havelec L, et al: Amantadine versus biperiden: a double-blind study of treatment efficacy in neuroleptic extrapyramidal movement disorders. Neuropsychobiology 33(2):80–84, 1996 8927233

Koopmans AB, Vinkers DJ, Poulina IT, et al: No effect of dose adjustment to the CYP2D6 genotype in patients with severe mental illness. Front Psychiatry 9:349, 2018 30131727

Kopelovich SL, Hughes M, Monroe-DeVita MB, et al: Statewide implementation of cognitive behavioral therapy for psychosis through a learning collaborative model. Cognit Behav Pract 26(3):439–452, 2019a

Kopelovich SL, Strachan E, Sivec H, Kreider V: Stepped care as an implementation and service delivery model for cognitive behavioral therapy for psychosis. Community Ment Health J 55(5):755–767, 2019b 30623294

Kopelowicz A, Liberman RP, Zarate R: Recent advances in social skills training for schizophrenia. Schizophr Bull 32 (suppl 1):S12–S23, 2006 16885207

Kopelowicz A, Zarate R, Wallace CJ, et al: The ability of multifamily groups to improve treatment adherence in Mexican Americans with schizophrenia. Arch Gen Psychiatry 69(3):265–273, 2012 22393219

Koskinen J, Löhönen J, Koponen H, et al: Rate of cannabis use disorders in clinical samples of patients with schizophrenia: a meta-analysis. Schizophr Bull 36(6):1115–1130, 2010 19386576

Kotin J, Wilbert DE, Verburg D, Soldinger SM: Thioridazine and sexual dysfunction. Am J Psychiatry 133(1):82–85, 1976 1247127

Koytchev R, Alken RG, McKay G, Katzarov T: Absolute bioavailability of oral immediate and slow release fluphenazine in healthy volunteers. Eur J Clin Pharmacol 51(2):183–187, 1996 8911886

Krakowski MI, Czobor P, Citrome L, et al: Atypical antipsychotic agents in the treatment of violent patients with schizophrenia and schizoaffective disorder. Arch Gen Psychiatry 63(6):622–629, 2006 16754835

Krakowski MI, Czobor P, Nolan KA: Atypical antipsychotics, neurocognitive deficits, and aggression in schizophrenic patients. J Clin Psychopharmacol 28(5):485–493, 2008 18794642

Krelstein MS: The role of mental health in the inmate disciplinary process: a national survey. J Am Acad Psychiatry Law 30(4):488–496, 2002 12539901

Kreyenbuhl J, Buchanan RW, Dickerson FB, Dixon LB; Schizophrenia Patient Outcomes Research Team (PORT): The Schizophrenia Patient Outcomes Research Team (PORT): updated treatment recommendations 2009. Schizophr Bull 36(1):94–103, 2010 19955388

Kreyenbuhl J, Record EJ, Palmer-Bacon J: A review of behavioral tailoring strategies for improving medication adherence in serious mental illness. Dialogues Clin Neurosci 18(2):191–201, 2016 27489459

Kroeze WK, Hufeisen SJ, Popadak BA, et al: H1-histamine receptor affinity predicts short-term weight gain for typical and atypical antipsychotic drugs. Neuropsychopharmacology 28(3):519–526, 2003 12629531

Kroon LA: Drug interactions with smoking. Am J Health Syst Pharm 64(18):1917–1921, 2007 17823102

Kugathasan P, Horsdal HT, Aagaard J, et al: Association of secondary preventive cardiovascular treatment after myocardial infarction with mortality among patients with schizophrenia. JAMA Psychiatry 75(12):1234–1240, 2018 30422158

Kuhnigk O, Slawik L, Meyer J, et al: Valuation and attainment of treatment goals in schizophrenia: perspectives of patients, relatives, physicians, and payers. J Psychiatr Pract 18(5):321–328, 2012 22995959

Kukla M, Bell MD, Lysaker PH: A randomized controlled trial examining a cognitive behavioral therapy intervention enhanced with cognitive remediation to improve work and neurocognition outcomes among persons with schizophrenia spectrum disorders. Schizophr Res 197:400–406, 2018 29422299

Lachkar Y, Bouassida W: Drug-induced acute angle closure glaucoma. Curr Opin Ophthalmol 18(2):129–133, 2007 17301614

Lagishetty CV, Deng J, Lesko LJ, et al: How informative are drug-drug interactions of gene-drug interactions? J Clin Pharmacol 56(10):1221–1231, 2016 27040602

La Grenade L, Graham D, Trontell A: Myocarditis and cardiomyopathy associated with clozapine use in the United States. N Engl J Med 345(3):224–225, 2001 11463031

Lally J, Docherty MJ, MacCabe JH: Pharmacological interventions for clozapine-induced sinus tachycardia. Cochrane Database Syst Rev Jun 9(6):CD011566, 2016a 27277334

Lally J, Tully J, Robertson D, et al: Augmentation of clozapine with electroconvulsive therapy in treatment resistant schizophrenia: a systematic review and meta-analysis. Schizophr Res 171(1–3):215–224, 2016b 26827129

Lally J, Ajnakina O, Stubbs B, et al: Hyperprolactinaemia in first episode psychosis: a longitudinal assessment. Schizophr Res 189:117–125, 2017a 28755878

Lally J, Malik S, Krivoy A, et al: The use of granulocyte colony-stimulating factor in clozapine rechallenge: a systematic review. J Clin Psychopharmacol 37(5):600–604, 2017b 28817489

Lally J, Malik S, Whiskey E, et al: Clozapine-associated agranulocytosis treatment with granulocyte colony-stimulating factor/granulocyte-macrophage colony-stimulating factor: a systematic review. J Clin Psychopharmacol 37(4):441–446, 2017c 28437295

Land R, Siskind D, McArdle P, et al: The impact of clozapine on hospital use: a systematic review and meta-analysis. Acta Psychiatr Scand 135(4):296–309, 2017 28155220

Landa Y: Cognitive behavioral therapy for psychosis (CBTp): an introductory manual for clinicians. New York, MIRECC VISN 2, 2019. Available at: www.mirecc.va.gov/visn2/docs/CBTp_Manual_VA_Yulia_Landa_2017.pdf. Accessed April 1, 2019.

Large MM, Nielssen O: Violence in first-episode psychosis: a systematic review and meta-analysis. Schizophr Res 125(2–3):209–220, 2011 21208783

Large M, Sharma S, Compton MT, et al: Cannabis use and earlier onset of psychosis: a systematic meta-analysis. Arch Gen Psychiatry 68(6):555–561, 2011 21300939

Large M, Mullin K, Gupta P, et al: Systematic meta-analysis of outcomes associated with psychosis and co-morbid substance use. Aust N Z J Psychiatry 48(5):418–432, 2014 24589980

Lariscy JT, Hummer RA, Rogers RG: Cigarette smoking and all-cause and cause-specific adult mortality in the United States. Demography 55(5):1855–1885, 2018 30232778

Laties AM, Flach AJ, Baldycheva I, et al: Cataractogenic potential of quetiapine versus risperidone in the long-term treatment of patients with schizophrenia or schizoaffective disorder: a randomized, open-label, ophthalmologist-masked, flexible-dose, non-inferiority trial. J Psychopharmacol 29(1):69–79, 2015 25315830

Latimer E, Wynant W, Clark R, et al: Underprescribing of clozapine and unexplained variation in use across hospitals and regions in the Canadian province of Québec. Clin Schizophr Relat Psychoses 7(1):33–41, 2013 23367500

La Torre A, Conca A, Duffy D, et al: Sexual dysfunction related to psychotropic drugs: a critical review, part II: antipsychotics. Pharmacopsychiatry 46(6):201–208, 2013 23737244

Latuda (lurasidone) [prescribing information]. Marlborough, MA, Sunovion Pharmaceuticals, March 2018

Lauby-Secretan B, Scoccianti C, Loomis D, et al; International Agency for Research on Cancer Handbook Working Group: Body fatness and cancer: viewpoint of the IARC Working Group. N Engl J Med 375(8):794–798, 2016 27557308

Laursen TM, Wahlbeck K, Hällgren J, et al: Life expectancy and death by diseases of the circulatory system in patients with bipolar disorder or schizophrenia in the Nordic countries. PLoS One 8(6):e67133, 2013 23826212

Laursen TM, Nordentoft M, Mortensen PB: Excess early mortality in schizophrenia. Annu Rev Clin Psychol 10:425–448, 2014 24313570

Lawrence D, Kisely S, Pais J: The epidemiology of excess mortality in people with mental illness. Can J Psychiatry 55(12):752–760, 2010 21172095

Lawson W, Johnston S, Karson C, et al: Racial differences in antipsychotic use: claims database analysis of Medicaid-insured patients with schizophrenia. Ann Clin Psychiatry 27(4):242–252, 2015 26554365

Lean M, Fornells-Ambrojo M, Milton A, et al: Self-management interventions for people with severe mental illness: systematic review and meta-analysis. Br J Psychiatry 214(5):260–268, 2019 30898177

Le Boutillier C, Leamy M, Bird VJ, et al: What does recovery mean in practice? A qualitative analysis of international recovery-oriented practice guidance. Psychiatr Serv 62(12):1470–1476, 2011 22193795

Lecomte T, Leclerc C, Wykes T: Group CBT for Psychosis: A Guidebook for Clinicians. New York, Oxford University Press, 2016, p 296

Lee EE, Liu J, Tu X, et al: A widening longevity gap between people with schizophrenia and general population: a literature review and call for action. Schizophr Res 196:9–13, 2018 28964652

Lee WM, Stravitz RT, Larson AM: AASLD position paper: the management of acute liver failure: update 2011. Alexandria, VA, American Association for the Study of Liver Diseases, 2011. Available at: www.aasld.org/sites/default/files/2019-06/AcuteLiverFailureUpdate201journalformat1.pdf. Accessed March 31, 2017.

Legge SE, Hamshere ML, Ripke S, et al: Genome-wide common and rare variant analysis provides novel insights into clozapine-associated neutropenia. Mol Psychiatry 22(10):1502–1508, 2017 27400856

Leucht S, Kane JM, Kissling W, et al: Clinical implications of Brief Psychiatric Rating Scale scores. Br J Psychiatry 187:366–371, 2005 16199797

Leucht S, Tardy M, Komossa K, et al: Antipsychotic drugs versus placebo for relapse prevention in schizophrenia: a systematic review and meta-analysis. Lancet 379(9831):2063–2071, 2012 22560607

Leucht S, Cipriani A, Spineli L, et al: Comparative efficacy and tolerability of 15 antipsychotic drugs in schizophrenia: a multiple-treatments meta-analysis. Lancet 382(9896):951–962, 2013 23810019

Leucht S, Samara M, Heres S, et al: Dose equivalents for second-generation antipsychotics: the minimum effective dose method. Schizophr Bull 40(2):314–326, 2014 24493852

Leucht S, Samara M, Heres S, et al: Dose equivalents for second-generation antipsychotic drugs: the classical mean dose method. Schizophr Bull 41(6):1397–1402, 2015 25841041

Leucht S, Leucht C, Huhn M, et al: Sixty years of placebo-controlled antipsychotic drug trials in acute schizophrenia: systematic review, Bayesian meta-analysis, and meta-regression of efficacy predictors. Am J Psychiatry 174(10):927–942, 2017 28541090

Leung JG, Breden EL: Tetrabenazine for the treatment of tardive dyskinesia. Ann Pharmacother 45(4):525–531, 2011 21487088

Leung JG, Hasassri ME, Barreto JN, et al: Characterization of admission types in medically hospitalized patients prescribed clozapine. Psychosomatics 58(2):164–172, 2017 28153339

Leung JG, Cusimano J, Gannon JM, et al: Addressing clozapine under-prescribing and barriers to initiation: a psychiatrist, advanced practice provider, and trainee survey. Int Clin Psychopharmacol 34(5):247–256, 2019 31107831

Levitan B, Markowitz M, Mohamed AF, et al: Patients' preferences related to benefits, risks, and formulations of schizophrenia treatment. Psychiatr Serv 66(7):719–726, 2015 25772762

Levounis P, Arnaout B, Marienfeld C: Motivational Interviewing for Clinical Practice. Arlington, VA, American Psychiatric Association Publishing, 2017

Lewis CC, Boyd M, Puspitasari A, et al: Implementing measurement-based care in behavioral health: a review. JAMA Psychiatry 76(3):324–335, 2019 30566197

Lewis-Fernández R, Aggarwal NK, Hinton L, et al (eds): DSM-5® Handbook on the Cultural Formulation Interview. Arlington, VA, American Psychiatric Association Publishing, 2016

Lexicomp: Lexicomp database. Riverwoods IL, Wolters Kluwer Health, 2019. Available at: http://online.lexi.com. Accessed January 4, 2019.

Liang CS, Ho PS, Shen LJ, et al: Comparison of the efficacy and impact on cognition of glycopyrrolate and biperiden for clozapine-induced sialorrhea in schizophrenic patients: a randomized, double-blind, crossover study. Schizophr Res 119(1–3):138–144, 2010 20299191

Liao TV, Phan SV: Acute hyperglycemia associated with short-term use of atypical antipsychotic medications. Drugs 74(2):183–194, 2014 24399515

Lieberman JA, First MB: Psychotic disorders. N Engl J Med 379(3):270–280, 2018 30021088

Lieberman JA, Saltz BL, Johns CA, et al: The effects of clozapine on tardive dyskinesia. Br J Psychiatry 158:503–510, 1991 1675900

Lima AR, Soares-Weiser K, Bacaltchuk J, Barnes TR: Benzodiazepines for neuroleptic-induced acute akathisia. Cochrane Database Syst Rev (1):CD001950, 2002 11869614

Lima AR, Bacalcthuk J, Barnes TR, Soares-Weiser K: Central action beta-blockers versus placebo for neuroleptic-induced acute akathisia. Cochrane Database Syst Rev Oct 18(4):CD001946, 2004 15495022

Lindenmayer JP: Long-acting injectable antipsychotics: focus on olanzapine pamoate. Neuropsychiatr Dis Treat 6:261–267, 2010 20628628

Lindström E, Lewander T, Malm U, et al: Patient-rated versus clinician-rated side effects of drug treatment in schizophrenia: clinical validation of a self-rating version of the UKU Side Effect Rating Scale (UKU-SERS-Pat). Nord J Psychiatry 55 (suppl 44):5–69, 2001 11860666

Lingjaerde O, Ahlfors UG, Bech P, et al: The UKU Side Effect Rating Scale: a new comprehensive rating scale for psychotropic drugs and a cross-sectional study of side effects in neuroleptic-treated patients. Acta Psychiatr Scand Suppl 334:1–100, 1987 2887090

Lopez LV, Kane JM: Plasma levels of second-generation antipsychotics and clinical response in acute psychosis: a review of the literature. Schizophr Res 147(2–3):368–374, 2013 23664462

Lopez LV, Shaikh A, Merson J, et al: Accuracy of clinician assessments of medication status in the emergency setting: a comparison of clinician assessment of antipsychotic usage and plasma level determination. J Clin Psychopharmacol 37(3):310–314, 2017 28353490

López-Moríñigo JD, Ramos-Ríos R, David AS, Dutta R: Insight in schizophrenia and risk of suicide: a systematic update. Compr Psychiatry 53(4):313–322, 2012 21821236

Lopez-Morinigo JD, Fernandes AC, Chang CK, et al: Suicide completion in secondary mental healthcare: a comparison study between schizophrenia spectrum disorders and all other diagnoses. BMC Psychiatry 14:213, 2014 25085220

Lowe CM, Grube RR, Scates AC: Characterization and clinical management of clozapine-induced fever. Ann Pharmacother 41(10):1700–1704, 2007 17785616

Loxapac (loxapine hydrochloride) [product monograph]. Boucherville, QC, Canada, Sandoz Canada, July 2014

Loxitane (loxapine) [prescribing information]. Corona, CA, Watson Pharma, February 2017

Luciano A, Bond GR, Drake RE: Does employment alter the course and outcome of schizophrenia and other severe mental illnesses? A systematic review of longitudinal research. Schizophr Res 159(2–3):312–321, 2014 25278105

Lucksted A, Medoff D, Burland J, et al: Sustained outcomes of a peer-taught family education program on mental illness. Acta Psychiatr Scand 127(4):279–286, 2013 22804103

Lum A, Skelton E, Wynne O, Bonevski B: A systematic review of psychosocial barriers and facilitators to smoking cessation in people living with schizophrenia. Front Psychiatry 9:565, 2018 30459658

MacEwan JP, Forma FM, Shafrin J, et al: Patterns of adherence to oral atypical antipsychotics among patients diagnosed with schizophrenia. J Manag Care Spec Pharm 22(11):1349–1361, 2016a 27783548

MacEwan JP, Kamat SA, Duffy RA, et al: Hospital readmission rates among patients with schizophrenia treated with long-acting injectables or oral antipsychotics. Psychiatr Serv 67(11):1183–1188, 2016b 27417897

MacKinnon R, Michels R, Buckley P: The Psychiatric Interview in Clinical Practice, 3rd Edition. Arlington, VA, American Psychiatric Association Publishing, 2016

Maeda K, Sugino H, Akazawa H, et al: In vitro and in vivo characterization of a novel serotonin-dopamine activity modulator. J Pharmacol Exp Ther 350(3):589–604, 2014 24947465

Maher S, Cunningham A, O'Callaghan N, et al: Clozapine-induced hypersalivation: an estimate of prevalence, severity and impact on quality of life. Ther Adv Psychopharmacol 6(3):178–184, 2016 27354906

Mahmood S, Booker I, Huang J, Coleman CI: Effect of topiramate on weight gain in patients receiving atypical antipsychotic agents. J Clin Psychopharmacol 33(1):90–94, 2013 23277264

Malla A, McGorry P: Early intervention in psychosis in young people: a population and public health perspective. Am J Public Health 109(S3):S181–S184, 2019 31242015

Man WH, Colen-de Koning JC, Schulte PF, et al: The effect of glycopyrrolate on nocturnal sialorrhea in patients using clozapine: a randomized, crossover, double-blind, placebo-controlled trial. J Clin Psychopharmacol 37(2):155–161, 2017 28129312

Mangurian C, Newcomer JW, Modlin C, Schillinger D: Diabetes and cardiovascular care among people with severe mental illness: a literature review. J Gen Intern Med 31(9):1083–1091, 2016 27149967

Manu P, Dima L, Shulman M, et al: Weight gain and obesity in schizophrenia: epidemiology, pathobiology, and management. Acta Psychiatr Scand 132(2):97–108, 2015 26016380

Manu P, Lapitskaya Y, Shaikh A, Nielsen J: Clozapine rechallenge after major adverse effects: clinical guidelines based on 259 cases. Am J Ther 25(2):e218–e223, 2018 29505490

Mar PL, Raj SR: Orthostatic hypotension for the cardiologist. Curr Opin Cardiol 33(1):66–72, 2018 28984649

Marcus SM, Medoff D, Fang LJ, et al: Generalizability in the Family-to-Family education program randomized waitlist-control trial. Psychiatr Serv 64(8):754–763, 2013 23633161

Marino LA, Dixon LB: An update on supported employment for people with severe mental illness. Curr Opin Psychiatry 27(3):210–215, 2014 24613982

Marques TR, Smith S, Bonaccorso S, et al: Sexual dysfunction in people with prodromal or first-episode psychosis. Br J Psychiatry 201:131–136, 2012 22700081

Marshall M, Lockwood A: Assertive community treatment for people with severe mental disorders. Cochrane Database Syst Rev (2):CD001089, 2000 10796415

Marshall M, Rathbone J: Early intervention for psychosis. Cochrane Database Syst Rev Jun 15(6):CD004718, 2011 21678345

Marshall T, Goldberg RW, Braude L, et al: Supported employment: assessing the evidence. Psychiatr Serv 65(1):16–23, 2014 24247197

Martin-Latry K, Goumy MP, Latry P, et al: Psychotropic drugs use and risk of heat-related hospitalisation. Eur Psychiatry 22(6):335–338, 2007 17513091

Martino D, Karnik V, Osland S, et al: Movement disorders associated with antipsychotic medication in people with schizophrenia: an overview of Cochrane reviews and meta-analysis. Can J Psychiatry 63(11):706743718777392, 2018 29758999 Epub ahead of print

Mason M, Cates CJ, Smith I: Effects of opioid, hypnotic and sedating medications on sleep-disordered breathing in adults with obstructive sleep apnoea. Cochrane Database Syst Rev Jul 14(7):CD011090, 2015 26171909

Matsuo M, Sano I, Ikeda Y, et al: Intraoperative floppy-iris syndrome associated with use of antipsychotic drugs. Can J Ophthalmol 51(4):294–296, 2016 27521670

Maust DT, Lin LA, Blow FC: Benzodiazepine use and misuse among adults in the United States. Psychiatr Serv 70(2):97–106, 2019 30554562

Mayoral F, Berrozpe A, de la Higuera J, et al: Efficacy of a family intervention program for prevention of hospitalization in patients with schizophrenia: a naturalistic multicenter controlled and randomized study in Spain. Rev Psiquiatr Salud Ment 8(2):83–91, 2015 25017624

McCrary KJ, Weiden PJ, Gever MP: Schizophrenia: understanding your illness. Jacksonville, Florida Self-Directed Care Program District 4, 2019. Available at: www.floridasdc4.com/01_understanding.pdf. Accessed March 30, 2019.

McCutcheon R, Beck K, D'Ambrosio E, et al: Antipsychotic plasma levels in the assessment of poor treatment response in schizophrenia. Acta Psychiatr Scand 137(1):39–46, 2018 29072776

McDonagh MS, Dana T, Selph S, et al: Treatments for adults with schizophrenia: a systematic review [Comparative Effectiveness Review No 198, AHRQ Publ No 17(18)-EHC031-EF]. Rockville, MD, Agency for Healthcare Research and Quality, October 2017. Available at: https://effectivehealthcare.ahrq.gov/topics/schizophrenia-adult/research-2017. Accessed May 10, 2019.

McDonald-McGinn DM, Sullivan KE, Marino B, et al: 22q11.2 deletion syndrome. Nat Rev Dis Primers 1:15071, 2015 27189754

McDowell C, Fossey E: Workplace accommodations for people with mental illness: a scoping review. J Occup Rehabil 25(1):197–206, 2015 24841728

McEvoy JP: A double-blind crossover comparison of antiparkinson drug therapy: amantadine versus anticholinergics in 90 normal volunteers, with an emphasis on differential effects on memory function. J Clin Psychiatry 48 (suppl):20–23, 1987 2887553

McEvoy JP, McCue M, Freter S: Replacement of chronically administered anticholinergic drugs by amantadine in outpatient management of chronic schizophrenia. Clin Ther 9(4):429–433, 1987 2886223

McEvoy JP, Lieberman JA, Stroup TS, et al; CATIE Investigators: Effectiveness of clozapine versus olanzapine, quetiapine, and risperidone in patients with chronic schizophrenia who did not respond to prior atypical antipsychotic treatment. Am J Psychiatry 163(4):600–610, 2006 16585434

McEvoy J, Gandhi SK, Rizio AA, et al: Effect of tardive dyskinesia on quality of life in patients with bipolar disorder, major depressive disorder, and schizophrenia. Qual Life Res 28(12):3303–3312, 2019 31435866

McFarlane WR: Family interventions for schizophrenia and the psychoses: a review. Fam Process 55(3):460–482, 2016 27411376

McGinty EE, Baller J, Azrin ST, et al: Interventions to address medical conditions and health-risk behaviors among persons with serious mental illness: a comprehensive review. Schizophr Bull 42(1):96–124, 2016 26221050

McGrath J, Saha S, Chant D, Welham J: Schizophrenia: a concise overview of incidence, prevalence, and mortality. Epidemiol Rev 30:67–76, 2008 18480098

McGurk SR, Twamley EW, Sitzer DI, et al: A meta-analysis of cognitive remediation in schizophrenia. Am J Psychiatry 164(12):1791–1802, 2007 18056233

McGurk SR, Mueser KT, Xie H, et al: Cognitive enhancement treatment for people with mental illness who do not respond to supported employment: a randomized controlled trial. Am J Psychiatry 172(9):852–861, 2015 25998278

McGurk SR, Mueser KT, Xie H, et al: Cognitive remediation for vocational rehabilitation nonresponders. Schizophr Res 175(1–3):48–56, 2016 27209526

McNiel DE, Eisner JP, Binder RL: The relationship between command hallucinations and violence. Psychiatr Serv 51(10):1288–1292, 2000 11013329

Medalia A: Seven common questions about cognitive remediation. New York, Lieber Recovery Clinic, 2019. Available at: www.lieberclinic.com/cognitive-remediation. Accessed April 12, 2019.

Medalia A, Herlands T, Saperstein A, Revheim N: Cognitive Remediation for Psychological Disorders: Therapist Guide (Treatments That Work), 2nd Edition. New York, Oxford University Press, 2018

Medalia A, Erlich MD, Soumet-Leman C, Saperstein AM: Translating cognitive behavioral interventions from bench to bedside: the feasibility and acceptability of cognitive remediation in research as compared to clinical settings. Schizophr Res 203:49–54, 2019 28768601

Mehta SH, Morgan JC, Sethi KD: Drug-induced movement disorders. Neurol Clin 33(1):153–174, 2015 25432728

Meldrum ML, Kelly EL, Calderon R, et al: Implementation status of assisted outpatient treatment programs: a national survey. Psychiatr Serv 67(6):630–635, 2016 26828396

Melkote R, Singh A, Vermeulen A, et al: Relationship between antipsychotic blood levels and treatment failure during the Clinical Antipsychotic Trials of Intervention Effectiveness (CATIE) study. Schizophr Res 201:324–328, 2018 29804929

Meltzer HY, Alphs L, Green AI, et al; International Suicide Prevention Trial Study Group: Clozapine treatment for suicidality in schizophrenia: International Suicide Prevention Trial (InterSePT). Arch Gen Psychiatry 60(1):82–91, 2003 12511175

Melzer-Ribeiro DL, Rigonatti SP, Kayo M, et al: Efficacy of electroconvulsive therapy augmentation for partial response to clozapine: a pilot randomized ECT–sham controlled trial. Archives of Clinical Psychiatry (São Paulo) 44(2):45–50, 2017

Mental Health America: Mental Health America. Alexandria, VA, Mental Health America, 2019. Available at: www.mhanational.org. Accessed September 29, 2019.

Mentzel TQ, Lieverse R, Bloemen O, et al; Genetic Risk and Outcome of Psychosis (GROUP) Investigators: High incidence and prevalence of drug-related movement disorders in young patients with psychotic disorders. J Clin Psychopharmacol 37(2):231–238, 2017 28141621

Mentzel TQ, van der Snoek R, Lieverse R, et al: Clozapine monotherapy as a treatment for antipsychotic-induced tardive dyskinesia: a meta-analysis. J Clin Psychiatry 79(6):17r11852, 2018 30257080

Metcalfe JD, Drake RE, Bond GR: Economic, labor, and regulatory moderators of the effect of individual placement and support among people with severe mental illness: a systematic review and meta-analysis. Schizophr Bull 44(1):22–31, 2018 29036727

Metzner JL: Class action litigation in correctional psychiatry. J Am Acad Psychiatry Law 30(1):19–29, discussion 30–32, 2002 11931366

Metzner JL: Mental health considerations for segregated inmates, in Standards for Health Services in Prisons. Chicago, IL, National Commission on Correctional Healthcare, 2003, pp 241–254

Metzner JL, Fellner J: Solitary confinement and mental illness in U.S. prisons: a challenge for medical ethics. J Am Acad Psychiatry Law 38(1):104–108, 2010 20305083

Meyer JM: Understanding depot antipsychotics: an illustrated guide to kinetics. CNS Spectr 18 (suppl 1):58–67, quiz 68, 2013 24345710

Meyer JM: Converting oral to long-acting injectable antipsychotics: a guide for the perplexed. CNS Spectr 22(S1):14–28, 2017 29350127

Meyer JM, Koro CE: The effects of antipsychotic therapy on serum lipids: a comprehensive review. Schizophr Res 70(1):1–17, 2004 15246458

MGH Center for Women's Mental Health: National pregnancy registry for atypical antipsychotics. Boston, MA, MGH Center for Women's Mental Health, 2019. Available at: https://womensmentalhealth.org/research/pregnancyregistry/atypicalantipsychotic. Accessed September 21, 2019.

Michl J, Scharinger C, Zauner M, et al: A multivariate approach linking reported side effects of clinical antidepressant and antipsychotic trials to in vitro binding affinities. Eur Neuropsychopharmacol 24(9):1463–1474, 2014 25044049

Micromedex: IBM Micromedex® Web Applications Access. Greenwood Village, CO, IBM Watson Health, 2019. Available at: www.micromedexsolutions.com. Accessed January 4, 2019.

Miller DD, McEvoy JP, Davis SM, et al: Clinical correlates of tardive dyskinesia in schizophrenia: baseline data from the CATIE schizophrenia trial. Schizophr Res 80(1):33–43, 2005 16171976

Miller DD, Caroff SN, Davis SM, et al; Clinical Antipsychotic Trials of Intervention Effectiveness (CATIE) Investigators: Extrapyramidal side-effects of antipsychotics in a randomised trial. Br J Psychiatry 193(4):279–288, 2008 18827289

Miller DT, Adam MP, Aradhya S, et al: Consensus statement: chromosomal microarray is a first-tier clinical diagnostic test for individuals with developmental disabilities or congenital anomalies. Am J Hum Genet 86(5):749–764, 2010 20466091

Mindham RH, Gaind R, Anstee BH, Rimmer L: Comparison of amantadine, orphenadrine, and placebo in the control of phenothiazine-induced parkinsonism. Psychol Med 2(4):406–413, 1972 4571143

Mintz AR, Dobson KS, Romney DM: Insight in schizophrenia: a meta-analysis. Schizophr Res 61(1):75–88, 2003 12648738

Misiak B, Stanczykiewicz B, Laczmanski L, Frydecka D: Lipid profile disturbances in antipsychotic-naive patients with first-episode non-affective psychosis: a systematic review and meta-analysis. Schizophr Res 190:18–27, 2017 28325572

Mitchell AJ, Delaffon V, Vancampfort D, et al: Guideline concordant monitoring of metabolic risk in people treated with antipsychotic medication: systematic review and meta-analysis of screening practices. Psychol Med 42(1):125–147, 2012 21846426

Mitchell AJ, Vancampfort D, De Herdt A, et al: Is the prevalence of metabolic syndrome and metabolic abnormalities increased in early schizophrenia? A comparative meta-analysis of first episode, untreated and treated patients. Schizophr Bull 39(2):295–305, 2013a 22927670

Mitchell AJ, Vancampfort D, Sweers K, et al: Prevalence of metabolic syndrome and metabolic abnormalities in schizophrenia and related disorders: a systematic review and meta-analysis. Schizophr Bull 39(2):306–318, 2013b 22207632

Mizuno Y, Suzuki T, Nakagawa A, et al: Pharmacological strategies to counteract antipsychotic-induced weight gain and metabolic adverse effects in schizophrenia: a systematic review and meta-analysis. Schizophr Bull 40(6):1385–1403, 2014 24636967

Moban (molindone) [prescribing information]. Malvern, PA, Endo Pharmaceuticals, February 2017

Moberg PJ, Richman MJ, Roalf DR, et al: Neurocognitive functioning in patients with 22q11.2 deletion syndrome: a meta-analytic review. Behav Genet 48(4):259–270, 2018 29922984

Modini M, Tan L, Brinchmann B, et al: Supported employment for people with severe mental illness: systematic review and meta-analysis of the international evidence. Br J Psychiatry 209(1):14–22, 2016 27103678

Mohamed S, Rosenheck R, McEvoy J, et al: Cross-sectional and longitudinal relationships between insight and attitudes toward medication and clinical outcomes in chronic schizophrenia. Schizophr Bull 35(2):336–346, 2009 18586692

Molindone hydrochloride tablets [prescribing information]. Middlesex, NJ, CorePharma, August 2014

Molindone hydrochloride tablets [prescribing information]. Laurelton, NY, Epic Pharma, April 2018

Moncrieff J, Steingard S: A critical analysis of recent data on the long-term outcome of antipsychotic treatment. Psychol Med 49(5):750–753, 2019 30563582

Monroe-DeVita M, Morse G, Bond GR: Program fidelity and beyond: multiple strategies and criteria for ensuring quality of assertive community treatment. Psychiatr Serv 63(8):743–750, 2012 22508406

Monuteaux MC, Lee LK, Hemenway D, et al: Firearm ownership and violent crime in the U.S.: an ecologic study. Am J Prev Med 49(2):207–214, 2015 26091930

Moons T, de Roo M, Claes S, Dom G: Relationship between P-glycoprotein and second-generation antipsychotics. Pharmacogenomics 12(8):1193–1211, 2011 21843066

Moore S, Shiers D, Daly B, et al: Promoting physical health for people with schizophrenia by reducing disparities in medical and dental care. Acta Psychiatr Scand 132(2):109–121, 2015 25958971

Moreno-Küstner B, Martín C, Pastor L: Prevalence of psychotic disorders and its association with methodological issues: a systematic review and meta-analyses. PLoS One 13(4):e0195687, 2018 29649252

Morgan VA, Morgan F, Galletly C, et al: Sociodemographic, clinical and childhood correlates of adult violent victimisation in a large, national survey sample of people with psychotic disorders. Soc Psychiatry Psychiatr Epidemiol 51(2):269–279, 2016 26581211

Moriarty DG, Zack MM, Kobau R: The Centers for Disease Control and Prevention's Healthy Days Measures: population tracking of perceived physical and mental health over time. Health Qual Life Outcomes 1:37, 2003 14498988

Morosini PL, Magliano L, Brambilla L, et al: Development, reliability and acceptability of a new version of the DSM-IV Social and Occupational Functioning Assessment Scale (SOFAS) to assess routine social functioning. Acta Psychiatr Scand 101(4):323–329, 2000 10782554

Morrato EH, Newcomer JW, Kamat S, et al: Metabolic screening after the American Diabetes Association's consensus statement on antipsychotic drugs and diabetes. Diabetes Care 32(6):1037–1042, 2009 19244091

Morrison AP: A manualised treatment protocol to guide delivery of evidence-based cognitive therapy for people with distressing psychosis: learning from clinical trials. Psychosis 9(3):271–281, 2017

Morrison AP, Pyle M, Gumley A, et al; FOCUS trial group: Cognitive behavioural therapy in clozapine-resistant schizophrenia (FOCUS): an assessor-blinded, randomised controlled trial. Lancet Psychiatry 5(8):633–643, 2018 30001930

Morrissey JP, Domino ME, Cuddeback GS: Expedited Medicaid enrollment, mental health service use, and criminal recidivism among released prisoners with severe mental illness. Psychiatr Serv 67(8):842–849, 2016 26975522

Morse G, Glass AM, Monroe-DeVita M: ACT and recovery: what we know about their compatibility. Adm Policy Ment Health 43(2):219–230, 2016 25638223

Mościcki EK, Clarke DE, Kuramoto SJ, et al: Testing DSM-5 in routine clinical practice settings: feasibility and clinical utility. Psychiatr Serv 64(10):952–960, 2013 23852272

Mosheva M, Korotkin L, Gur RE, et al: Effectiveness and side effects of psychopharmacotherapy in individuals with 22q11.2 deletion syndrome with comorbid psychiatric disorders: a systematic review. Eur Child Adolesc Psychiatry Apr 4, 2019 30949827 Epub ahead of print

Mountjoy CQ, Baldacchino AM, Stubbs JH: British experience with high-dose olanzapine for treatment-refractory schizophrenia. Am J Psychiatry 156(1):158–159, 1999 9892320

Mueller DR, Schmidt SJ, Roder V: One-year randomized controlled trial and follow-up of integrated neurocognitive therapy for schizophrenia outpatients. Schizophr Bull 41(3):604–616, 2015 25713462

Mueser KT, Corrigan PW, Hilton DW, et al: Illness management and recovery: a review of the research. Psychiatr Serv 53(10):1272–1284, 2002 12364675

Mueser KT, Clark RE, Haines M, et al: The Hartford study of supported employment for persons with severe mental illness. J Consult Clin Psychol 72(3):479–490, 2004 15279531

Mueser KT, Pratt SI, Bartels SJ, et al: Randomized trial of social rehabilitation and integrated health care for older people with severe mental illness. J Consult Clin Psychol 78(4):561–573, 2010 20658812

Mueser KT, Deavers F, Penn DL, Cassisi JE: Psychosocial treatments for schizophrenia. Annu Rev Clin Psychol 9:465–497, 2013 23330939

Mueser KT, Penn DL, Addington J, et al: The NAVIGATE program for first-episode psychosis: rationale, overview, and description of psychosocial components. Psychiatr Serv 66(7):680–690, 2015 25772766

Mukundan A, Faulkner G, Cohn T, Remington G: Antipsychotic switching for people with schizophrenia who have neuroleptic-induced weight or metabolic problems. Cochrane Database Syst Rev Dec 8(12):CD006629, 2010 21154372

Munetz MR, Benjamin S: How to examine patients using the Abnormal Involuntary Movement Scale. Hosp Community Psychiatry 39(11):1172–1177, 1988 2906320

Muralidharan A, Brown CH, Peer JE, et al: Living Well: an intervention to improve medical illness self-management among individuals with serious mental illness. Psychiatr Serv 70(1):19–25, 2019 30353790

Murray H, Wortzel HS: Psychiatric advance directives: origins, benefits, challenges, and future directions. J Psychiatr Pract 25(4):303–307, 2019 31291211

Myles H, Myles N, Antic NA, et al: Obstructive sleep apnea and schizophrenia: a systematic review to inform clinical practice. Schizophr Res 170(1):222–225, 2016 26621003

Myles N, Newall HD, Curtis J, et al: Tobacco use before, at, and after first-episode psychosis: a systematic meta-analysis. J Clin Psychiatry 73(4):468–475, 2012 22579146

Myles N, Myles H, Clark SR, et al: Use of granulocyte-colony stimulating factor to prevent recurrent clozapine-induced neutropenia on drug rechallenge: a systematic review of the literature and clinical recommendations. Aust N Z J Psychiatry 51(10):980–989, 2017 28747065

Myles N, Myles H, Xia S, et al: Meta-analysis examining the epidemiology of clozapine-associated neutropenia. Acta Psychiatr Scand 138(2):101–109, 2018 29786829

Myles N, Myles H, Xia S, et al: A meta-analysis of controlled studies comparing the association between clozapine and other antipsychotic medications and the development of neutropenia. Aust N Z J Psychiatry 53(5):403–412, 2019 30864459

Naber D, Leppig M, Grohmann R, Hippius H: Efficacy and adverse effects of clozapine in the treatment of schizophrenia and tardive dyskinesia: a retrospective study of 387 patients. Psychopharmacology (Berl) 99(suppl):S73–S76, 1989 2813668

Narrow WE, Clarke DE, Kuramoto SJ, et al: DSM-5 field trials in the United States and Canada, part III: development and reliability testing of a cross-cutting symptom assessment for DSM-5. Am J Psychiatry 170(1):71–82, 2013 23111499

Naslund JA, Aschbrenner KA, Scherer EA, et al: Lifestyle intervention for people with severe obesity and serious mental illness. Am J Prev Med 50(2):145–153, 2016 26385164

Nasrallah HA, Tandon R: Classic antipsychotic medications, in The American Psychiatric Association Publishing Textbook of Psychopharmacology, 5th Edition. Edited by Schatzberg AF, Nemeroff CB. Arlington, VA, American Psychiatric Association Publishing, 2017, pp 603–621

Nasser AF, Henderson DC, Fava M, et al: Efficacy, safety, and tolerability of RBP-7000 once-monthly risperidone for the treatment of acute schizophrenia. J Clin Psychopharmacol 36(2):130–140, 2016 26862829

National Alliance on Mental Illness: NAMI Family & Friends. Arlington, VA, National Alliance on Mental Illness, 2019a. Available at: www.nami.org/find-support/nami-programs/nami-family-friends. Accessed September 29, 2019.

National Alliance on Mental Illness: NAMI Family-to-Family. Arlington, VA, National Alliance on Mental Illness, 2019b. Available at: www.nami.org/Find-Support/NAMI-Programs/NAMI-Family-to-Family. Accessed April 11, 2019.

National Cancer Institute: Quit smoking. Bethesda, MD, National Cancer Institute, 2019. Available at: https://smokefree.gov/quit-smoking. Accessed December 31, 2018.

National Commission on Correctional Health Care: Position statement: solitary confinement (isolation). J Correct Health Care 22(3):257–263, 2016 27302711

National Institute for Health and Care Excellence: Psychosis and schizophrenia in adults: prevention and management: updated edition 2014. London, National Collaborating Centre for Mental Health, 2014. Available at: www.nice.org.uk/guidance/cg178. Accessed May 7, 2019.

National Institute of Mental Health: What is RAISE? Bethesda, MD, National Institute of Mental Health, 2019a. Available at: www.nimh.nih.gov/health/topics/schizophrenia/raise/what-is-raise.shtml. Accessed October 1, 2019.

National Institute of Mental Health: Recovery After an Initial Schizophrenia Episode (RAISE): State Health Administrators and Clinics. Bethesda, MD, National Institute of Mental Health, 2019b. Available at: www.nimh.nih.gov/health/topics/schizophrenia/raise/state-health-administrators-and-clinics.shtml. Accessed on March 31, 2019.

Navane (thiothixene) [prescribing information]. New York, Pfizer, December 2010

NAVIGATE: NAVIGATE. Philadelphia, PA, NAVIGATE, 2019. Available at: http://navigateconsultants.org/manuals. Accessed May 6, 2020.

Nesvåg R, Knudsen GP, Bakken IJ, et al: Substance use disorders in schizophrenia, bipolar disorder, and depressive illness: a registry-based study. Soc Psychiatry Psychiatr Epidemiol 50(8):1267–1276, 2015 25680837

Newcomer JW, Weiden PJ, Buchanan RW: Switching antipsychotic medications to reduce adverse event burden in schizophrenia: establishing evidence-based practice. J Clin Psychiatry 74(11):1108–1120, 2013 24330898

Nielsen SM, Toftdahl NG, Nordentoft M, Hjorthøj C: Association between alcohol, cannabis, and other illicit substance abuse and risk of developing schizophrenia: a nationwide population based register study. Psychol Med 47(9):1668–1677, 2017 28166863

Niskanen P, Achté K, Jaskari M, et al: Results of a comparative double-blind study with clozapine and chlorpromazine in the treatment of schizophrenic patients. Psychiatria Fennica 307–313, 1974

Nordentoft M, Jeppesen P, Abel M, et al: OPUS study: suicidal behaviour, suicidal ideation and hopelessness among patients with first-episode psychosis: one-year follow-up of a randomised controlled trial. Br J Psychiatry Suppl 43:s98–s106, 2002 12271808

Nordentoft M, Mortensen PB, Pedersen CB: Absolute risk of suicide after first hospital contact in mental disorder. Arch Gen Psychiatry 68(10):1058–1064, 2011 21969462

Norman R, Lecomte T, Addington D, Anderson E: Canadian treatment guidelines on psychosocial treatment of schizophrenia in adults. Can J Psychiatry 62(9):617–623, 2017 28703017

Novalis PN, Rojcewicz SJ, Peele R: Clinical Manual of Supportive Psychotherapy. Washington, DC, American Psychiatric Press, 1993, p 384

Nuplazid (10 and 34 mg pimavanserin) [prescribing information]. San Diego, CA, Acadia Pharmaceuticals, June 2018

Nuplazid (17 mg pimavanserin) [prescribing information]. San Diego, CA, Acadia Pharmaceuticals, June 2018

Oakley P, Kisely S, Baxter A, et al: Increased mortality among people with schizophrenia and other non-affective psychotic disorders in the community: a systematic review and meta-analysis. J Psychiatr Res 102:245–253, 2018 29723811

O'Brien A: Comparing the risk of tardive dyskinesia in older adults with first-generation and second-generation antipsychotics: a systematic review and meta-analysis. Int J Geriatr Psychiatry 31(7):683–693, 2016 26679687

O'Brien CF, Jimenez R, Hauser RA, et al: NBI-98854, a selective monoamine transport inhibitor for the treatment of tardive dyskinesia: a randomized, double-blind, placebo-controlled study. Mov Disord 30(12):1681–1687, 2015 26346941

Office for Civil Rights: Health information privacy: information related to mental and behavioral health, including opioid overdose. Washington, DC, U.S. Department of Health and Human Services, December 19, 2017a. Available at: www.hhs.gov/hipaa/for-professionals/special-topics/mental-health/index.html. Accessed November 18, 2018.

Office for Civil Rights: HIPAA privacy rule and sharing information related to mental health. Washington, DC, U.S. Department of Health and Human Services, December 19, 2017b. Available at: www.hhs.gov/sites/default/files/hipaa-privacy-rule-and-sharing-info-related-to-mental-health.pdf. Accessed November 18, 2018.

O'Keefe ML, Klebe KJ, Metzner J, et al: A longitudinal study of administrative segregation. J Am Acad Psychiatry Law 41(1):49–60, 2013 23503176

Olbert CM, Nagendra A, Buck B: Meta-analysis of black vs. white racial disparity in schizophrenia diagnosis in the United States: do structured assessments attenuate racial disparities? J Abnorm Psychol 127(1):104–115, 2018 29094963

Olfson M, Gerhard T, Huang C, et al: Premature mortality among adults with schizophrenia in the United States. JAMA Psychiatry 72(12):1172–1181, 2015 26509694

Olfson M, Gerhard T, Crystal S, Stroup TS: Clozapine for schizophrenia: state variation in evidence-based practice. Psychiatr Serv 67(2):152, 2016 26522679

Olten B, Bloch MH: Meta regression: relationship between antipsychotic receptor binding profiles and side-effects. Prog Neuropsychopharmacol Biol Psychiatry 84 (Pt A):272–281, 2018 29410000

Oluwoye O, Monroe-DeVita M, Burduli E, et al: Impact of tobacco, alcohol and cannabis use on treatment outcomes among patients experiencing first episode psychosis: data from the national RAISE-ETP study. Early Interv Psychiatry 13(1):142–146, 2018 29356438

Ondo WG, Hanna PA, Jankovic J: Tetrabenazine treatment for tardive dyskinesia: assessment by randomized videotape protocol. Am J Psychiatry 156(8):1279–1281, 1999 10450276

OnTrackNY: Resources. New York, OnTrackNY, 2019. Available at: https://ontrackny.org/Resources. Accessed March 31, 2019.

Opler MGA, Yavorsky C, Daniel DG: Positive and Negative Syndrome Scale (PANSS) training: challenges, solutions, and future directions. Innov Clin Neurosci 14(11–12):77–81, 2017 29410941

Opoka SM, Lincoln TM: The effect of cognitive behavioral interventions on depression and anxiety symptoms in patients with schizophrenia spectrum disorders: a systematic review. Psychiatr Clin North Am 40(4):641–659, 2017 29080591

Orap (pimozide) [prescribing information]. Sellersville, PA, Teva Pharmaceuticals, March 2014

Orap (pimozide) [prescribing information]. Horsham, PA, Teva Select Brands, April 2018

Orap (pimozide) [product monograph]. Vaughan, ON, Canada, AA Pharma, February 2019

Ortiz-Orendain J, Castiello-de Obeso S, Colunga-Lozano LE, et al: Antipsychotic combinations for schizophrenia. Cochrane Database Syst Rev Jun 28 6(6):CD009005, 2017 28658515

Østergaard MLD, Nordentoft M, Hjorthøj C: Associations between substance use disorders and suicide or suicide attempts in people with mental illness: a Danish nation-wide, prospective, register-based study of patients diagnosed with schizophrenia, bipolar disorder, unipolar depression or personality disorder. Addiction 112(7):1250–1259, 2017 28192643

Østergaard SD, Foldager L, Mors O, et al: The validity and sensitivity of PANSS-6 in the Clinical Antipsychotic Trials of Intervention Effectiveness (CATIE) study. Schizophr Bull 44(2):453–462, 2018a 28575321

Østergaard SD, Foldager L, Mors O, et al: The validity and sensitivity of PANSS-6 in treatment-resistant schizophrenia. Acta Psychiatr Scand 138(5):420–431, 2018b 30168131

Ostuzzi G, Bighelli I, So R, et al: Does formulation matter? A systematic review and meta-analysis of oral versus long-acting antipsychotic studies. Schizophr Res 183:10–21, 2017 27866695

Ouzzine M, Gulberti S, Ramalanjaona N, et al: The UDP-glucuronosyltransferases of the blood-brain barrier: their role in drug metabolism and detoxication. Front Cell Neurosci 8:349, 2014 25389387

Overall JE, Gorham DR: The Brief Psychiatric Rating Scale. Psychol Rep 10:799–812, 1962

Ozbilen M, Adams CE: Systematic overview of Cochrane reviews for anticholinergic effects of antipsychotic drugs. J Clin Psychopharmacol 29(2):141–146, 2009 19512975

Pakzad-Vaezi KL, Etminan M, Mikelberg FS: The association between cataract surgery and atypical antipsychotic use: a nested case-control study. Am J Ophthalmol 156(6):1141–1146.e1, 2013 24075430

Palmer BA, Pankratz VS, Bostwick JM: The lifetime risk of suicide in schizophrenia: a reexamination. Arch Gen Psychiatry 62(3):247–253, 2005 15753237

Palmer SE, McLean RM, Ellis PM, Harrison-Woolrych M: Life-threatening clozapine-induced gastrointestinal hypomotility: an analysis of 102 cases. J Clin Psychiatry 69(5):759–768, 2008 18452342

Palmier-Claus JE, Ainsworth J, Machin M, et al: The feasibility and validity of ambulatory self-report of psychotic symptoms using a smartphone software application. BMC Psychiatry 12:172, 2012 23075387

Pappa S, Tsouli S, Apostolou G, et al: Effects of amantadine on tardive dyskinesia: a randomized, double-blind, placebo-controlled study. Clin Neuropharmacol 33(6):271–275, 2010 21121175

Paschen S, Deuschl G: Patient evaluation and selection for movement disorders surgery: the changing spectrum of indications. Prog Neurol Surg 33:80–93, 2018 29332075

Patel MM, Brown JD, Croake S, et al: The current state of behavioral health quality measures: where are the gaps? Psychiatr Serv 66(8):865–871, 2015 26073415

Patel MX, De Zoysa N, Bernadt M, David A: Depot and oral antipsychotics: patient preferences and attitudes are not the same thing. J Psychopharmacol 23(7):789–796, 2009 18583438

Patel MX, de Zoysa N, Bernadt M, et al: Are depot antipsychotics more coercive than tablets? The patient's perspective. J Psychopharmacol 24(10):1483–1489, 2010a 19304865

Patel MX, Haddad PM, Chaudhry IB, et al: Psychiatrists' use, knowledge and attitudes to first- and second-generation antipsychotic long-acting injections: comparisons over 5 years. J Psychopharmacol 24(10):1473–1482, 2010b 19477883

Patterson-Lomba O, Ayyagari R, Carroll B: Risk assessment and prediction of TD incidence in psychiatric patients taking concomitant antipsychotics: a retrospective data analysis. BMC Neurol 19(1):174, 2019 31325958

PDSP: PDSP K$_i$ database: Chapel Hill, NC, PDSP, 2019. Available at: https://pdsp.unc.edu/databases/kidb.php. Accessed January 16, 2019.

Pearsall R, Smith DJ, Pelosi A, Geddes J: Exercise therapy in adults with serious mental illness: a systematic review and meta-analysis. BMC Psychiatry 14:117, 2014 24751159

Pekkala E, Merinder L: Psychoeducation for schizophrenia. Cochrane Database Syst Rev (2):CD002831, 2002 12076455

Pelzer AC, van der Heijden FM, den Boer E: Systematic review of catatonia treatment. Neuropsychiatr Dis Treat 14:317–326, 2018 29398916

Pendopharm: ^{Pr}pdp-benztropine prescribing information. Montreal, QC, Canada, Pendopharm, February 2, 2015. Available at: https://pdf.hres.ca/dpd_pm/00029138.PDF. Accessed April 22, 2019.

Pentaraki A, Utoblo B, Kokkoli EM: Cognitive remediation therapy plus standard care versus standard care for people with schizophrenia. Cochrane Database Syst Rev (11):CD012865, 2017

Penttilä M, Jääskeläinen E, Hirvonen N, et al: Duration of untreated psychosis as predictor of long-term outcome in schizophrenia: systematic review and meta-analysis. Br J Psychiatry 205(2):88–94, 2014 25252316

Perphenazine [prescribing information]. Atlanta, GA, Wilshire Pharmaceuticals, November 2016

Perphenazine [prescribing information]. Morgantown, WV, Mylan Pharmaceuticals, March 2017

Perry BI, McIntosh G, Weich S, et al: The association between first-episode psychosis and abnormal glycaemic control: systematic review and meta-analysis. Lancet Psychiatry 3(11):1049–1058, 2016 27720402

Perry LA, Ramson D, Stricklin S: Mirtazapine adjunct for people with schizophrenia. Cochrane Database Syst Rev May 26 5(5):CD011943, 2018 29802811

Perseris (risperidone) [prescribing information]. North Chesterfield, VA, Indivior, July 2018

Petrides G, Malur C, Braga RJ, et al: Electroconvulsive therapy augmentation in clozapine-resistant schizophrenia: a prospective, randomized study. Am J Psychiatry 172(1):52–58, 2015 25157964

Pharoah F, Mari J, Rathbone J, Wong W: Family intervention for schizophrenia. Cochrane Database Syst Rev Dec 8(12):CD000088, 2010 21154340

Phillips IR, Shephard EA: Drug metabolism by flavin-containing monooxygenases of human and mouse. Expert Opin Drug Metab Toxicol 13(2):167–181, 2017 27678284

Pileggi DJ, Cook AM: Neuroleptic malignant syndrome. Ann Pharmacother 50(11):973–981, 2016 27423483

Pillinger T, Beck K, Gobjila C, et al: Impaired glucose homeostasis in first-episode schizophrenia: a systematic review and meta-analysis. JAMA Psychiatry 74(3):261–269, 2017a 28097367

Pillinger T, Beck K, Stubbs B, Howes OD: Cholesterol and triglyceride levels in first-episode psychosis: systematic review and meta-analysis. Br J Psychiatry 211(6):339–349, 2017b 28982658

Pincus HA, Scholle SH, Spaeth-Rublee B, et al: Quality measures for mental health and substance use: gaps, opportunities, and challenges. Health Aff (Millwood) 35(6):1000–1008, 2016 27269015

Pinninti NR, Faden J, Adityanjee A: Are second-generation antipsychotics useful in tardive dystonia? Clin Neuropharmacol 38(5):183–197, 2015 26366970

Pisani F, Oteri G, Costa C, et al: Effects of psychotropic drugs on seizure threshold. Drug Saf 25(2):91–110, 2002 11888352

Pisciotta AV: Agranulocytosis induced by certain phenothiazine derivatives. JAMA 208(10):1862–1868, 1969 4890332

Plana-Ripoll O, Pedersen CB, Holtz Y, et al: Exploring comorbidity within mental disorders among a Danish national population. JAMA Psychiatry 76(3):259–270, 2019 30649197

Poewe W, Djamshidian-Tehrani A: Movement disorders in systemic diseases. Neurol Clin 33(1):269–297, 2015 25432733

Polcwiartek C, Vang T, Bruhn CH, et al: Diabetic ketoacidosis in patients exposed to antipsychotics: a systematic literature review and analysis of Danish adverse drug event reports. Psychopharmacology (Berl) 233(21–22):3663–3672, 2016 27592232

Pompili M, Amador XF, Girardi P, et al: Suicide risk in schizophrenia: learning from the past to change the future. Ann Gen Psychiatry 6:10, 2007 17367524

Pompili M, Lester D, Dominici G, et al: Indications for electroconvulsive treatment in schizophrenia: a systematic review. Schizophr Res 146(1-3):1–9, 2013 23499244

Popovic D, Benabarre A, Crespo JM, et al: Risk factors for suicide in schizophrenia: systematic review and clinical recommendations. Acta Psychiatr Scand 130(6):418–426, 2014 25230813

Pottegård A, Lash TL, Cronin-Fenton D, et al: Use of antipsychotics and risk of breast cancer: a Danish nationwide case-control study. Br J Clin Pharmacol 84(9):2152–2161, 2018 29858518

Poyurovsky M, Weizman A: Very low-dose mirtazapine (7.5 mg) in treatment of acute antipsychotic-associated akathisia. J Clin Psychopharmacol 38(6):609–611, 2018 30300293

Praharaj SK, Kongasseri S, Behere RV, Sharma PS: Mirtazapine for antipsychotic-induced acute akathisia: a systematic review and meta-analysis of randomized placebo-controlled trials. Ther Adv Psychopharmacol 5(5):307–313, 2015 26557987

Predmore Z, Mattke S, Horvitz-Lennon M: Potential benefits to patients and payers from increased measurement of antipsychotic plasma levels in the management of schizophrenia. Psychiatr Serv 69(1):12–14, 2018 29191139

Preskorn S, Flynn A, Macaluso M: Determining whether a definitive causal relationship exists between aripiprazole and tardive dyskinesia and/or dystonia in patients with major depressive disorder, part 1. J Psychiatr Pract 21(5):359–369, 2015 26348804

Pringsheim T, Kelly M, Urness D, et al: Physical health and drug safety in individuals with schizophrenia. Can J Psychiatry 62(9):673–683, 2017 28718324

Pringsheim T, Gardner D, Addington D, et al: The assessment and treatment of antipsychotic-induced akathisia. Can J Psychiatry Jan 1:706743718760288, 2018 29685069 Epub ahead of print

Procyshyn RM, Bezchlibnyk-Butler KZ, Jeffries JJ (eds): Clinical Handbook of Psychotropic Drugs, 23rd Edition. Boston, MA, Göttingen Hogrefe, 2019. Available at: https://chpd.hogrefe.com. Accessed January 4, 2019.

Pugh RN, Murray-Lyon IM, Dawson JL, et al: Transection of the oesophagus for bleeding oesophageal varices. Br J Surg 60(8):646–649, 1973 4541913

Pui-yin Chung J, Shiu-yin Chong C, Lai-wah Dunn E, et al: The incidence and characteristics of clozapine-induced fever in a local psychiatric unit in Hong Kong. Can J Psychiatry 53(12):857–862, 2008 19087484

Pyne JM, Fischer EP, Gilmore L, et al: Development of a patient-centered antipsychotic medication adherence intervention. Health Educ Behav 41(3):315–324, 2014 24369177

Quetiapine (Seroquel) and QT-interval prolongation. Med Lett Drugs Ther 53(1374):79–80, 2011 21959358

Rabinowitz J, Levine SZ, Garibaldi G, et al: Negative symptoms have greater impact on functioning than positive symptoms in schizophrenia: analysis of CATIE data. Schizophr Res 137(1–3):147–150, 2012 22316568

Ranasinghe I, Sin J: A systematic review of evidence-based treatment for individuals with treatment-resistant schizophrenia and a suboptimal response to clozapine monotherapy. Psychosis 6(3):253–265, 2014

Randall JR, Walld R, Finlayson G, et al: Acute risk of suicide and suicide attempts associated with recent diagnosis of mental disorders: a population-based, propensity score-matched analysis. Can J Psychiatry 59(10):531–538, 2014 25565686

Ratey JJ, Leveroni C, Kilmer D, et al: The effects of clozapine on severely aggressive psychiatric inpatients in a state hospital. J Clin Psychiatry 54(6):219–223, 1993 8331090

Rathbone J, Soares-Weiser K: Anticholinergics for neuroleptic-induced acute akathisia. Cochrane Database Syst Rev Oct 18(4):CD003727, 2006 17054182

Rautaharju PM, Surawicz B, Gettes LS, et al; American Heart Association Electrocardiography and Arrhythmias Committee, Council on Clinical Cardiology; American College of Cardiology Foundation; Heart Rhythm Society: AHA/ACCF/HRS recommendations for the standardization and interpretation of the electrocardiogram, part IV: the ST segment, T and U waves, and the QT interval: a scientific statement from the American Heart Association Electrocardiography and Arrhythmias Committee, Council on Clinical Cardiology; the American College of Cardiology Foundation; and the Heart Rhythm Society. Endorsed by the International Society for Computerized Electrocardiology. J Am Coll Cardiol 53(11):982–991, 2009 19281931

Reagu S, Jones R, Kumari V, Taylor PJ: Angry affect and violence in the context of a psychotic illness: a systematic review and meta-analysis of the literature. Schizophr Res 146(1–3):46–52, 2013 23452505

Rebok GW, Ball K, Guey LT, et al; ACTIVE Study Group: Ten-year effects of the Advanced Cognitive Training for Independent and Vital Elderly cognitive training trial on cognition and everyday functioning in older adults. J Am Geriatr Soc 62(1):16–24, 2014 24417410

Reeder C, Pile V, Crawford P, et al: The feasibility and acceptability to service users of CIRCuiTS, a computerized cognitive remediation therapy programme for schizophrenia. Behav Cogn Psychother 44(3):288–305, 2016 26004421

Reeder C, Huddy V, Cella M, et al: A new generation computerised metacognitive cognitive remediation programme for schizophrenia (CIRCuiTS): a randomised controlled trial. Psychol Med 1–11, 2017 28866988

Register-Brown K, Hong LE: Reliability and validity of methods for measuring the duration of untreated psychosis: a quantitative review and meta-analysis. Schizophr Res 160(1–3):20–26, 2014 25464915

Reingle Gonzalez JM, Connell NM: Mental health of prisoners: identifying barriers to mental health treatment and medication continuity. Am J Public Health 104(12):2328–2333, 2014 25322306

Relling MV, Klein TE: CPIC: Clinical Pharmacogenetics Implementation Consortium of the Pharmacogenomics Research Network. Clin Pharmacol Ther 89(3):464–467, 2011 21270786

Remington G, Agid O, Foussias G, et al: Clozapine and therapeutic drug monitoring: is there sufficient evidence for an upper threshold? Psychopharmacology (Berl) 225(3):505–518, 2013 23179967

Remington G, Addington D, Honer W, et al: Guidelines for the pharmacotherapy of schizophrenia in adults. Can J Psychiatry 62(9):604–616, 2017 28703015

Reser MP, Slikboer R, Rossell SL: A systematic review of factors that influence the efficacy of cognitive remediation therapy in schizophrenia. Aust N Z J Psychiatry 53(7):624–641, 2019 31177813

Revell ER, Neill JC, Harte M, et al: A systematic review and meta-analysis of cognitive remediation in early schizophrenia. Schizophr Res 168(1–2):213–222, 2015 26305063

Rexulti (brexpiprazole) [prescribing information]. Rockville, MD, Otsuka America Pharmaceutical, May 2019

Reynolds RJ, Day SM, Shafer A, Becker E: Mortality rates and excess death rates for the seriously mentally ill. J Insur Med 47(4):212–219, 2018 30653378

Rezansoff SN, Moniruzzaman A, Fazel S, et al: Housing first improves adherence to antipsychotic medication among formerly homeless adults with schizophrenia: results of a randomized controlled trial. Schizophr Bull 43(4):852–861, 2017 27665002

Richter D, Hoffmann H: Effectiveness of supported employment in non-trial routine implementation: systematic review and meta-analysis. Soc Psychiatry Psychiatr Epidemiol 54(5):525–531, 2019 30078035

Risperdal Consta (risperidone) [prescribing information]. Titusville, NJ, Janssen Pharmaceuticals, January 2019

Risperdal (risperidone) [prescribing information]. Titusville, NJ, Janssen Pharmaceuticals, January 2019

Risperidone orally disintegrating tablets (risperidone) [prescribing information]. Princeton, NJ, Sandoz, February 2019

Roché MW, Boyle DJ, Cheng CC, et al: Prevalence and risk of violent ideation and behavior in serious mental illnesses: an analysis of 63,572 patient records. J Interpers Violence Mar 1: 886260518759976, 2018 29534632 Epub ahead of print

Røge R, Møller BK, Andersen CR, et al: Immunomodulatory effects of clozapine and their clinical implications: what have we learned so far? Schizophr Res 140(1–3):204–213, 2012 22831769

Rogers HL, Bhattaram A, Zineh I, et al: CYP2D6 genotype information to guide pimozide treatment in adult and pediatric patients: basis for the U.S. Food and Drug Administration's new dosing recommendations. J Clin Psychiatry 73(9):1187–1190, 2012 23059146

Rohde C, Polcwiartek C, Kragholm K, et al: Adverse cardiac events in out-patients initiating clozapine treatment: a nationwide register-based study. Acta Psychiatr Scand 137(1):47–53, 2018 29064084

Ronaldson KJ, Fitzgerald PB, McNeil JJ: Clozapine-induced myocarditis, a widely overlooked adverse reaction. Acta Psychiatr Scand 132(4):231–240, 2015 25865238

Rosebush P, Stewart T: A prospective analysis of 24 episodes of neuroleptic malignant syndrome. Am J Psychiatry 146(6):717–725, 1989 2567121

Rosenheck RA, Davis S, Covell N, et al: Does switching to a new antipsychotic improve outcomes? Data from the CATIE trial. Schizophr Res 107(1):22–29, 2009 18993031

Rostack J: FDA to require diabetes warning on antipsychotics. Psychiatric News 30(20), Oct 17, 2003

Roth BL, Kroeze WK, Patel WK, Lopez E: The multiplicity of serotonin receptors: uselessly diverse molecules or an embarrasment of riches? Neuroscientist 6(4):252–262, 2000

Rothe PH, Heres S, Leucht S: Dose equivalents for second generation long-acting injectable antipsychotics: the minimum effective dose method. Schizophr Res 193:23–28, 2018 28735640

Rouillon F, Eriksson L, Burba B, et al: Functional recovery results from the risperidone long-acting injectable versus quetiapine relapse prevention trial (ConstaTRE). Acta Neuropsychiatr 25(5):297–306, 2013 25287730

Rowland A, Miners JO, Mackenzie PI: The UDP-glucuronosyltransferases: their role in drug metabolism and detoxification. Int J Biochem Cell Biol 45(6):1121–1132, 2013 23500526

Roy L, Crocker AG, Nicholls TL, et al: Criminal behavior and victimization among homeless individuals with severe mental illness: a systematic review. Psychiatr Serv 65(6):739–750, 2014 24535245

Rubio-Abadal E, Del Cacho N, Saenz-Navarrete G, et al; PROLACT Group: How hyperprolactinemia affects sexual function in patients under antipsychotic treatment. J Clin Psychopharmacol 36(5):422–428, 2016 27433851

Rush AJ, First MB, Blacker D (eds): Handbook of Psychiatric Measures, 2nd Edition. Washington, DC, American Psychiatric Publishing, 2008

Sachdev P, Mason C, Hadzi-Pavlovic D: Case-control study of neuroleptic malignant syndrome. Am J Psychiatry 154(8):1156–1158, 1997 9247408

Sachs HC; Committee on Drugs: The transfer of drugs and therapeutics into human breast milk: an update on selected topics. Pediatrics 132(3):e796–e809, 2013 23979084

Saha S, Chant D, McGrath J: A systematic review of mortality in schizophrenia: is the differential mortality gap worsening over time? Arch Gen Psychiatry 64(10):1123–1131, 2007 17909124

Saklad SR: Paliperidone palmitate: adjusting dosing intervals and measuring serum concentrations. Curr Psychiatr 17(8):45–47, 55, 2018

Saks ER: Some thoughts on denial of mental illness. Am J Psychiatry 166(9):972–973, 2009 19723794

Salahudeen MS, Duffull SB, Nishtala PS: Anticholinergic burden quantified by anticholinergic risk scales and adverse outcomes in older people: a systematic review. BMC Geriatr 15:31, 2015 25879993

Saltz BL, Woerner MG, Kane JM, et al: Prospective study of tardive dyskinesia incidence in the elderly. JAMA 266(17):2402–2406, 1991 1681122

Samara M, Leucht S: Clozapine in treatment-resistant schizophrenia. Br J Psychiatry 210(4):299, 2017 28373226

Samara MT, Leucht C, Leeflang MM, et al: Early improvement as a predictor of later response to antipsychotics in schizophrenia: a diagnostic test review. Am J Psychiatry 172(7):617–629, 2015 26046338

Samara MT, Dold M, Gianatsi M, et al: Efficacy, acceptability, and tolerability of antipsychotics in treatment-resistant schizophrenia: a network meta-analysis. JAMA Psychiatry 73(3):199–210, 2016 26842482

Samara MT, Klupp E, Helfer B, et al: Increasing antipsychotic dose for non response in schizophrenia. Cochrane Database Syst Rev May 11 5(5):CD0011883, 2018 29750432

SAMHSA-HRSA Center of Excellence for Integrated Health Solutions: Tobacco cessation. Rockville, MD, SAMHSA-HRSA Center for Integrated Health Solutions, 2018. Available at: www.integration.samhsa.gov/health-wellness/wellness-strategies/tobacco-cessation-2. Accessed December 31, 2018.

SAMHSA-HRSA Center of Excellence for Integrated Health Solutions: SBIRT: Screening, brief intervention, and referral to treatment. Rockville, MD, SAMHSA-HRSA Center for Integrated Health Solutions, 2019. Available at: www.integration.samhsa.gov/clinical-practice/sbirt. Accessed September 22, 2019.

Santesteban-Echarri O, Paino M, Rice S, et al: Predictors of functional recovery in first-episode psychosis: a systematic review and meta-analysis of longitudinal studies. Clin Psychol Rev 58:59–75, 2017 29042139

Saperstein AM, Medalia A: The empirical basis for the practice of cognitive remediation for schizophrenia. Neuropsychiatry (London) 2(2):101–109, 2012

Saphris (asenapine) [prescribing information]. Irvine, CA, Allergan USA, February 2017

Sara GE, Burgess PM, Malhi GS, et al: Stimulant and other substance use disorders in schizophrenia: prevalence, correlates and impacts in a population sample. Aust N Z J Psychiatry 48(11):1036–1047, 2014 24819935

Sariaslan A, Lichtenstein P, Larsson H, Fazel S: Triggers for violent criminality in patients with psychotic disorders. JAMA Psychiatry 73(8):796–803, 2016 27410165

Satterthwaite TD, Wolf DH, Rosenheck RA, et al: A meta-analysis of the risk of acute extrapyramidal symptoms with intramuscular antipsychotics for the treatment of agitation. J Clin Psychiatry 69(12):1869–1879, 2008 19192477

Schalinski I, Breinlinger S, Hirt V, et al: Environmental adversities and psychotic symptoms: the impact of timing of trauma, abuse, and neglect. Schizophr Res 205:4–9, 2019 29141785

Scherf-Clavel M, Samanski L, Hommers LG, et al: Analysis of smoking behavior on the pharmacokinetics of antidepressants and antipsychotics: evidence for the role of alternative pathways apart from CYP1A2. Int Clin Psychopharmacol 34(2):93–100, 2019 30557209

Schneider M, Regente J, Greiner T, et al: Neuroleptic malignant syndrome: evaluation of drug safety data from the AMSP program during 1993–2015. Eur Arch Psychiatry Clin Neurosci Nov 30, 2018 30506147 Epub ahead of print

Schoenbaum M, Sutherland JM, Chappel A, et al: Twelve-month health care use and mortality in commercially insured young people with incident psychosis in the United States. Schizophr Bull 43(6):1262–1272, 2017 28398566

Schwartz RC, Blankenship DM: Racial disparities in psychotic disorder diagnosis: a review of empirical literature. World J Psychiatry 4(4):133–140, 2014 25540728

Scott D, Platania-Phung C, Happell B: Quality of care for cardiovascular disease and diabetes amongst individuals with serious mental illness and those using antipsychotic medications. J Healthc Qual 34(5):15–21, 2012 22092725

Scottish Intercollegiate Guidelines Network (SIGN): Management of schizophrenia. Edinburgh, SIGN, May 2013. Available at: www.sign.ac.uk/assets/sign131.pdf. Accessed April 26, 2019.

Secher RG, Hjorthøj CR, Austin SF, et al: Ten-year follow-up of the OPUS specialized early intervention trial for patients with a first episode of psychosis. Schizophr Bull 41(3):617–626, 2015 25381449

Segal SP, Hayes SL, Rimes L: The utility of outpatient commitment I: a need for treatment and a least restrictive alternative to psychiatric hospitalization. Psychiatr Serv 68(12):1247–1254, 2017a Epub Aug 1 2017 28760100

Segal SP, Hayes SL, Rimes L: The utility of outpatient commitment II: mortality risk and protecting health, safety, and quality of life. Psychiatr Serv 68(12):1255–1261, 2017b 28760099

Sellwood W, Barrowclough C, Tarrier N, et al: Needs-based cognitive-behavioural family intervention for carers of patients suffering from schizophrenia: 12-month follow-up. Acta Psychiatr Scand 104(5):346–355, 2001 11722315

Sellwood W, Wittkowski A, Tarrier N, Barrowclough C: Needs-based cognitive-behavioural family intervention for patients suffering from schizophrenia: 5-year follow-up of a randomized controlled effectiveness trial. Acta Psychiatr Scand 116(6):447–452, 2007 17961200

Semenza DC, Grosholz JM: Mental and physical health in prison: how co-occurring conditions influence inmate misconduct. Health Justice 7(1):1, 2019 30612284

Seroquel (quetiapine) [prescribing information]. Wilmington, DE, AstraZeneca Pharmaceuticals, August 2019

Seroquel XR (quetiapine) [prescribing information]. Wilmington, DE, AstraZeneca Pharmaceuticals, August 2019

Serretti A, Chiesa A: A meta-analysis of sexual dysfunction in psychiatric patients taking antipsychotics. Int Clin Psychopharmacol 26(3):130–140, 2011 21191308

Shafrin J, Schwartz TT, Lakdawalla DN, Forma FM: Estimating the value of new technologies that provide more accurate drug adherence information to providers for their patients with schizophrenia. J Manag Care Spec Pharm 22(11):1285–1291, 2016 27783545

Sharma R, Alla K, Pfeffer D, et al: An appraisal of practice guidelines for smoking cessation in people with severe mental illness. Aust N Z J Psychiatry 51(11):1106–1120, 2017 28859486

Shen V, Clarence-Smith K, Hunter C, Jankovic J: Safety and efficacy of tetrabenazine and use of concomitant medications during long-term, open-label treatment of chorea associated with Huntington's and other diseases. Tremor Other Hyperkinet Mov (NY) 3:tre-03-191-4337-1, 2013 24255799

Shen WK, Sheldon RS, Benditt DG, et al: 2017 ACC/AHA/HRS guideline for the evaluation and management of patients with syncope: a report of the American College of Cardiology/American Heart Association Task Force on clinical practice guidelines and the Heart Rhythm Society. J Am Coll Cardiol 70(5):e39–e110, 2017 28286221

Sherman LJ, Lynch SE, Teich J, Hudock WJ: Availability of supported employment in specialty mental health treatment facilities and facility characteristics: 2014. The CBHSQ Report. Rockville, MD, Substance Abuse and Mental Health Services Administration, 2017 28749638

Shields LS, Pathare S, van der Ham AJ, Bunders J: A review of barriers to using psychiatric advance directives in clinical practice. Adm Policy Ment Health 41(6):753–766, 2014 24248818

Short T, Thomas S, Mullen P, Ogloff JR: Comparing violence in schizophrenia patients with and without comorbid substance-use disorders to community controls. Acta Psychiatr Scand 128(4):306–313, 2013 23379839

Siegel M, Rothman EF: Firearm ownership and suicide rates among US men and women, 1981–2013. Am J Public Health 106(7):1316–1322, 2016 27196643

Silberstein J, Harvey PD: Impaired introspective accuracy in schizophrenia: an independent predictor of functional outcomes. Cogn Neuropsychiatry 24(1):28–39, 2019 30477401

Silver H, Geraisy N, Schwartz M: No difference in the effect of biperiden and amantadine on parkinsonian- and tardive dyskinesia-type involuntary movements: a double-blind crossover, placebo-controlled study in medicated chronic schizophrenic patients. J Clin Psychiatry 56(4):167–170, 1995 7713856

Sin J, Gillard S, Spain D, et al: Effectiveness of psychoeducational interventions for family carers of people with psychosis: a systematic review and meta-analysis. Clin Psychol Rev 56:13–24, 2017a 28578249

Sin J, Spain D, Furuta M, et al: Psychological interventions for post-traumatic stress disorder (PTSD) in people with severe mental illness. Cochrane Database Syst Rev Jan 24 1(1):CD011464, 2017b 28116752

Sinclair D, Adams CE: Treatment resistant schizophrenia: a comprehensive survey of randomised controlled trials. BMC Psychiatry 14:253, 2014 25227719

Sinclair DJ, Zhao S, Qi F, et al: Electroconvulsive therapy for treatment-resistant schizophrenia. Cochrane Database Syst Rev Mar 19 3(3):CD011847, 2019 30888709

Singh JP, Grann M, Lichtenstein P, et al: A novel approach to determining violence risk in schizophrenia: developing a stepped strategy in 13,806 discharged patients. PLoS One 7(2):e31727, 2012 22359622

Singh ML, Papas A: Oral implications of polypharmacy in the elderly. Dent Clin North Am 58(4):783–796, 2014 25201542

Siskind DJ, Leung J, Russell AW, et al: Metformin for clozapine associated obesity: a systematic review and meta-analysis. PLoS One 11(6):e0156208, 2016a 27304831

Siskind D, McCartney L, Goldschlager R, Kisely S: Clozapine v. first- and second-generation antipsychotics in treatment-refractory schizophrenia: systematic review and meta-analysis. Br J Psychiatry 209(5):385–392, 2016b 27388573

Siskind DJ, Harris M, Phillipou A, et al: Clozapine users in Australia: their characteristics and experiences of care based on data from the 2010 National Survey of High Impact Psychosis. Epidemiol Psychiatr Sci 26(3):325–337, 2017a 27426892

Siskind D, Siskind V, Kisely S: Clozapine response rates among people with treatment-resistant schizophrenia: data from a systematic review and meta-analysis. Can J Psychiatry 62(11):772–777, 2017b 28655284

Siskind DJ, Lee M, Ravindran A, et al: Augmentation strategies for clozapine refractory schizophrenia: a systematic review and meta-analysis. Aust N Z J Psychiatry 52(8):751–767, 2018 29732913

Siskind D, Hahn M, Correll CU, et al: Glucagon-like peptide-1 receptor agonists for antipsychotic-associated cardio-metabolic risk factors: a systematic review and individual participant data meta-analysis. Diabetes Obes Metab 21(2):293–302, 2019 30187620

Siu AL; U.S. Preventive Services Task Force: Behavioral and pharmacotherapy interventions for tobacco smoking cessation in adults, including pregnant women: U.S. Preventive Services Task Force recommendation statement. Ann Intern Med 163(8):622–634, 2015 26389730

Skevington SM, Lotfy M, O'Connell KA; WHOQOL Group: The World Health Organization's WHOQOL-BREF quality of life assessment: psychometric properties and results of the international field trial. A report from the WHOQOL Group. Qual Life Res 13(2):299–310, 2004 15085902

SMI Adviser: How do I establish tolerability before starting a long acting injectable antipsychotic medication (LAI), and how do I ensure the patient will not have side effects? Washington, DC, American Psychiatric Association, September 4, 2019. Available at: https://smiadviser.org/knowledge_post/how-do-i-establishing-tolerability-before-starting-a-long-acting-injectable-antipsychotic-medication-lai-and-how-do-i-ensure-the-patient-will-not-have-side-effects. Accessed October 9, 2019.

Smith FA, Levenson JL, Stern TA: Psychiatric assessment and consultation, in The American Psychiatric Association Publishing Textbook of Psychosomatic Medicine and Consultation-Liaison Psychiatry, 3rd Edition. Edited by Levenson JL. Washington, DC, American Psychiatric Association Publishing, 2019, pp 3–24

Smith PH, Mazure CM, McKee SA: Smoking and mental illness in the U.S. population. Tob Control 23(e2):e147–e153, 2014 24727731

Soares-Weiser K, Rathbone J: Calcium channel blockers for neuroleptic-induced tardive dyskinesia. Cochrane Database Syst Rev (11):CD000206, 2011 14973950

Soares-Weiser K, Maayan N, Bergman H: Vitamin E for antipsychotic-induced tardive dyskinesia. Cochrane Database Syst Rev Jan 17 1(1):CD000209, 2018a 29341067

Soares-Weiser K, Rathbone J, Ogawa Y, et al: Miscellaneous treatments for antipsychotic-induced tardive dyskinesia. Cochrane Database Syst Rev Mar 19 3(3):CD000208, 2018b 29552749

Solmi M, Pigato G, Kane JM, Correll CU: Clinical risk factors for the development of tardive dyskinesia. J Neurol Sci 389:21–27, 2018a 29439776

Solmi M, Pigato G, Kane JM, Correll CU: Treatment of tardive dyskinesia with VMAT-2 inhibitors: a systematic review and meta-analysis of randomized controlled trials. Drug Des Devel Ther 12:1215–1238, 2018b 29795977

Solmi M, Fornaro M, Toyoshima K, et al: Systematic review and exploratory meta-analysis of the efficacy, safety, and biological effects of psychostimulants and atomoxetine in patients with schizophrenia or schizoaffective disorder. CNS Spectr 24(5):479–495, 2019 30460884

Sood S, James W, Bailon MJ: Priapism associated with atypical antipsychotic medications: a review. Int Clin Psychopharmacol 23(1):9–17, 2008 18090503

Souza JS, Kayo M, Tassell I, et al: Efficacy of olanzapine in comparison with clozapine for treatment-resistant schizophrenia: evidence from a systematic review and meta-analyses. CNS Spectr 18(2):82–89, 2013 23253621

Sparshatt A, Taylor D, Patel MX, Kapur S: A systematic review of aripiprazole: dose, plasma concentration, receptor occupancy, and response: implications for therapeutic drug monitoring. J Clin Psychiatry 71(11):1447–1456, 2010 20584524

Spina E, Sturiale V, Valvo S, et al: Prevalence of acute dystonic reactions associated with neuroleptic treatment with and without anticholinergic prophylaxis. Int Clin Psychopharmacol 8(1):21–24, 1993 8097213

Spina E, Avenoso A, Facciolà G, et al: Relationship between plasma concentrations of clozapine and norclozapine and therapeutic response in patients with schizophrenia resistant to conventional neuroleptics. Psychopharmacology (Berl) 148(1):83–89, 2000 10663421

Spitz A, Studerus E, Koranyi S, et al: Correlations between self-rating and observer-rating of psychopathology in at-risk mental state and first-episode psychosis patients: influence of disease stage and gender. Early Interv Psychiatry 11(6):461–470, 2017 26376725

Stanilla JK, Simpson GM: Drugs to treat extrapyramidal side effects, in The American Psychiatric Association Publishing Textbook of Psychopharmacology, 5th Edition. Edited by Schatzberg AF, Nemeroff CB. Arlington, VA, American Psychiatric Association Publishing, 2017, pp 855–885

Stanley B, Brown GK: Safety planning intervention: a brief intervention to mitigate suicide risk. Cognit Behav Pract 19(2):256–264, 2012

Stanley B, Brown GK: About safety planning. Safety Planning Intervention 2019. Available at: http://suicidesafetyplan.com/About_Safety_Planning.html. Accessed December 28, 2018.

Stanley B, Brown GK, Brenner LA, et al: Comparison of the safety planning intervention with follow-up vs usual care of suicidal patients treated in the emergency department. JAMA Psychiatry 75(9):894–900, 2018 29998307

Stanton AH, Gunderson JG, Knapp PH, et al: Effects of psychotherapy in schizophrenia I: design and implementation of a controlled study. Schizophr Bull 10(4):520–563, 1984 6151245

Stark A, Scott J: A review of the use of clozapine levels to guide treatment and determine cause of death. Aust N Z J Psychiatry 46(9):816–825, 2012 22327098

Steadman HJ, Osher FC, Robbins PC, et al: Prevalence of serious mental illness among jail inmates. Psychiatr Serv 60(6):761–765, 2009 19487344

Stirman SW, Spokas M, Creed TA, et al: Training and consultation in evidence-based psychosocial treatments in public mental health settings: the ACCESS model. Prof Psychol Res Pr 41(1):48–56, 2010 22872783

Stoecker ZR, George WT, O'Brien JB, et al: Clozapine usage increases the incidence of pneumonia compared with risperidone and the general population: a retrospective comparison of clozapine, risperidone, and the general population in a single hospital over 25 months. Int Clin Psychopharmacol 32(3):155–160, 2017 28059928

Strawn JR, Keck PE Jr, Caroff SN: Neuroleptic malignant syndrome. Am J Psychiatry 164(6):870–876, 2007 17541044

Streck JM, Weinberger AH, Pacek LR, et al: Cigarette smoking quit rates among persons with serious psychological distress in the United States from 2008 to 2016: are mental health disparities in cigarette use increasing? Nicotine Tob Res 22(1):130–134, 2020 30351429

Stringhini S, Carmeli C, Jokela M, et al; LIFEPATH consortium: Socioeconomic status and the 25×25 risk factors as determinants of premature mortality: a multicohort study and meta-analysis of 1·7 million men and women. Lancet 389(10075):1229–1237, 2017 28159391

Stroup TS, Lieberman JA, McEvoy JP, et al; CATIE Investigators: Effectiveness of olanzapine, quetiapine, and risperidone in patients with chronic schizophrenia after discontinuing perphenazine: a CATIE study. Am J Psychiatry 164(3):415–427, 2007 17329466

Stroup TS, Lieberman JA, McEvoy JP, et al; CATIE Investigators: Results of phase 3 of the CATIE schizophrenia trial. Schizophr Res 107(1):1–12, 2009 19027269

Stroup TS, McEvoy JP, Ring KD, et al; Schizophrenia Trials Network: A randomized trial examining the effectiveness of switching from olanzapine, quetiapine, or risperidone to aripiprazole to reduce metabolic risk: comparison of antipsychotics for metabolic problems (CAMP). Am J Psychiatry 168(9):947–956, 2011 21768610

Stroup TS, Byerly MJ, Nasrallah HA, et al: Effects of switching from olanzapine, quetiapine, and risperidone to aripiprazole on 10-year coronary heart disease risk and metabolic syndrome status: results from a randomized controlled trial. Schizophr Res 146(1–3):190–195, 2013 23434503

Stroup TS, Gerhard T, Crystal S, et al: Geographic and clinical variation in clozapine use in the United States. Psychiatr Serv 65(2):186–192, 2014 24233347

Stroup TS, Gerhard T, Crystal S, et al: Comparative effectiveness of adjunctive psychotropic medications in patients with schizophrenia. JAMA Psychiatry 76(5):508–515, 2019 30785609

Strub RL, Black FW: The Mental Status Examination in Neurology. Philadelphia, PA, FA Davis, 2000

Stubbs B, De Hert M, Sepehry AA, et al: A meta-analysis of prevalence estimates and moderators of low bone mass in people with schizophrenia. Acta Psychiatr Scand 130(6):470–486, 2014 25041606

Stubbs B, Gaughran F, Mitchell AJ, et al: Schizophrenia and the risk of fractures: a systematic review and comparative meta-analysis. Gen Hosp Psychiatry 37(2):126–133, 2015 25666994

Stubbs B, Firth J, Berry A, et al: How much physical activity do people with schizophrenia engage in? A systematic review, comparative meta-analysis and meta-regression. Schizophr Res 176(2-3):431–440, 2016a 27261419

Stubbs B, Vancampfort D, Veronese N, et al: The prevalence and predictors of obstructive sleep apnea in major depressive disorder, bipolar disorder and schizophrenia: a systematic review and meta-analysis. J Affect Disord 197:259–267, 2016b 26999550

Stübner S, Rustenbeck E, Grohmann R, et al: Severe and uncommon involuntary movement disorders due to psychotropic drugs. Pharmacopsychiatry 37 (suppl 1):S54–S64, 2004 15052515

Subotnik KL, Casaus LR, Ventura J, et al: Long-acting injectable risperidone for relapse prevention and control of breakthrough symptoms after a recent first episode of schizophrenia: a randomized clinical trial. JAMA Psychiatry 72(8):822–829, 2015 26107752

Substance Abuse and Mental Health Services Administration: Assertive Community Treatment (ACT) Evidence-Based Practices (EBP) KIT. Rockville, MD, Substance Abuse and Mental Health Services Administration, October 2008. Available at: https://store.samhsa.gov/product/Assertive-Community-Treatment-ACT-Evidence-Based-Practices-EBP-KIT/sma08-4345. Accessed March 31, 2019.

Substance Abuse and Mental Health Services Administration: Family Psychoeducation Evidence-Based Practices (EBP) KIT (HHS Publ No SMA-09-4422). Rockville, MD, Substance Abuse and Mental Health Services Administration, 2009. Available at: https://store.samhsa.gov/product/Family-Psychoeducation-Evidence-Based-Practices-EBP-KIT/sma09-4422. Accessed October 1, 2019.

Substance Abuse and Mental Health Services Administration: Illness Management and Recovery Evidence-Based Practices (EBP) KIT. Rockville, MD, Substance Abuse and Mental Health Services Administration, March 2010a. Available at: https://store.samhsa.gov/product/Illness-Management-and-Recovery-Evidence-Based-Practices-EBP-KIT/sma09-4463. Accessed April 6, 2019.

Substance Abuse and Mental Health Services Administration: Supported Employment Evidence-Based Practices (EBP) KIT. Rockville, MD, Substance Abuse and Mental Health Services Administration, February 2010b. Available at: https://store.samhsa.gov/product/Supported-Employment-Evidence-Based-Practices-EBP-Kit/SMA08-4364. Accessed July 24, 2020.

Substance Abuse and Mental Health Services Administration: SAMHSA's working definition of recovery: 10 guiding principles of recovery. Rockville, MD, Substance Abuse and Mental Health Services Administration, 2012a. Available at: https://store.samhsa.gov/system/files/pep12-recdef.pdf. Accessed August 3, 2019.

Substance Abuse and Mental Health Services Administration: Supported Education Evidence-Based Practices (EBP) KIT. Rockville, MD, Substance Abuse and Mental Health Services Administration, August 2012b. Available at: https://store.samhsa.gov/product/Supported-Education-Evidence-Based-Practices-EBP-KIT/SMA11-4654CD-ROM. Accessed August 19, 2019.

Suijkerbuijk YB, Schaafsma FG, van Mechelen JC, et al: Interventions for obtaining and maintaining employment in adults with severe mental illness, a network meta-analysis. Cochrane Database Syst Rev Sep 12 9(9):CD011867, 2017 28898402

Sultana J, Hurtado I, Bejarano-Quisoboni D, et al: Antipsychotic utilization patterns among patients with schizophrenic disorder: a cross-national analysis in four countries. Eur J Clin Pharmacol 75(7):1005–1015, 2019 30824947

Susman VL, Addonizio G: Recurrence of neuroleptic malignant syndrome. J Nerv Ment Dis 176(4):234–241, 1988 2895164

Suzuki T, Uchida H, Watanabe K, Kashima H: Factors associated with response to clozapine in schizophrenia: a review. Psychopharmacol Bull 44(1):32–60, 2011 22506438

Swanson CL, Trestman RL: Rural assertive community treatment and telepsychiatry. J Psychiatr Pract 24(4):269–273, 2018 30427810

Swanson JW, Swartz MS, Van Dorn RA, et al: A national study of violent behavior in persons with schizophrenia. Arch Gen Psychiatry 63(5):490–499, 2006 16651506

Swanson SJ, Becker DR, Bond GR: Job development guidelines in supported employment. Psychiatr Rehabil J 36(2):122–123, 2013 23750766

Swartz MS, Wagner HR, Swanson JW, et al: Substance use in persons with schizophrenia: baseline prevalence and correlates from the NIMH CATIE study. J Nerv Ment Dis 194(3):164–172, 2006 16534433

Swartz MS, Bhattacharya S, Robertson AG, Swanson JW: Involuntary outpatient commitment and the elusive pursuit of violence prevention. Can J Psychiatry 62(2):102–108, 2017 27777274

Swillen A, McDonald-McGinn D: Developmental trajectories in 22q11.2 deletion. Am J Med Genet C Semin Med Genet 169(2):172–181, 2015 25989227

Sytema S, Wunderink L, Bloemers W, et al: Assertive community treatment in the Netherlands: a randomized controlled trial. Acta Psychiatr Scand 116(2):105–112, 2007 17650271

Taipale H, Mehtälä J, Tanskanen A, Tiihonen J: Comparative effectiveness of antipsychotic drugs for rehospitalization in schizophrenia: a nationwide study with 20-year follow-up. Schizophr Bull 44(6):1381–1387, 2018a 29272458

Taipale H, Mittendorfer-Rutz E, Alexanderson K, et al: Antipsychotics and mortality in a nationwide cohort of 29,823 patients with schizophrenia. Schizophr Res 197:274–280, 2018b 29274734

Takeuchi H, Powell V, Geisler S, et al: Clozapine administration in clinical practice: once-daily versus divided dosing. Acta Psychiatr Scand 134(3):234–240, 2016 27182769

Takeuchi H, Kantor N, Uchida H, et al: Immediate vs gradual discontinuation in antipsychotic switching: a systematic review and meta-analysis. Schizophr Bull 43(4):862–871, 2017a 28044008

Takeuchi H, Thiyanavadivel S, Agid O, Remington G: Gradual vs. wait-and-gradual discontinuation in antipsychotic switching: a meta-analysis. Schizophr Res 189:4–8, 2017b 28242107

Takeuchi H, Siu C, Remington G, et al: Does relapse contribute to treatment resistance? Antipsychotic response in first- vs. second-episode schizophrenia. Neuropsychopharmacology 44(6):1036–1042, 2019 30514883

Tam J, Warner KE, Meza R: Smoking and the reduced life expectancy of individuals with serious mental illness. Am J Prev Med 51(6):958–966, 2016 27522471

Tamburello A, Metzner J, Fergusen E, et al: The American Academy of Psychiatry and the Law practice resource for prescribing in corrections. J Am Acad Psychiatry Law 46(2):242–243, 2018 30026404

Tammenmaa-Aho I, Asher R, Soares-Weiser K, Bergman H: Cholinergic medication for antipsychotic-induced tardive dyskinesia. Cochrane Database Syst Rev Mar 19 3(3):CD000207, 2018 29553158

Tang Y, Horvitz-Lennon M, Gellad WF, et al: Prescribing of clozapine and antipsychotic polypharmacy for schizophrenia in a large Medicaid program. Psychiatr Serv 68(6):579–586, 2017 28196460

Tanskanen A, Tiihonen J, Taipale H: Mortality in schizophrenia: 30-year nationwide follow-up study. Acta Psychiatr Scand 138(6):492-499, 2018 29900527

Tarsy D, Baldessarini RJ: Epidemiology of tardive dyskinesia: is risk declining with modern antipsychotics? Mov Disord 21(5):589–598, 2006 16532448

Tauber R, Wallace CJ, Lecomte T: Enlisting indigenous community supporters in skills training programs for persons with severe mental illness. Psychiatr Serv 51(11):1428–1432, 2000 11058191

Teasdale SB, Samaras K, Wade T, et al: A review of the nutritional challenges experienced by people living with severe mental illness: a role for dietitians in addressing physical health gaps. J Hum Nutr Diet 30(5):545–553, 2017 28419586

Thioridazine hydrochloride [prescribing information]. Morgantown, WV, Mylan Pharmaceuticals, November 2016

Thomas EC, Despeaux KE, Drapalski AL, Bennett M: Person-oriented recovery of individuals with serious mental illnesses: a review and meta-analysis of longitudinal findings. Psychiatr Serv 69(3):259–267, 2018 29191141

Thompson A, Winsper C, Marwaha S, et al: Maintenance antipsychotic treatment versus discontinuation strategies following remission from first episode psychosis: systematic review. BJPsych Open 4(4):215–225, 2018 29988997

Thorning H, Marino L, Jean-Noel P, et al: Adoption of a blended training curriculum for ACT in New York State. Psychiatr Serv 67(9):940–942, 2016 27181739

Tiihonen J, Haukka J, Taylor M, et al: A nationwide cohort study of oral and depot antipsychotics after first hospitalization for schizophrenia. Am J Psychiatry 168(6):603–609, 2011 21362741

Tiihonen J, Mittendorfer-Rutz E, Torniainen M, et al: Mortality and cumulative exposure to antipsychotics, antidepressants, and benzodiazepines in patients with schizophrenia: an observational follow-up study. Am J Psychiatry 173(6):600–606, 2016 26651392

Tiihonen J, Mittendorfer-Rutz E, Majak M, et al: Real-world effectiveness of antipsychotic treatments in a nationwide cohort of 29 823 patients with schizophrenia. JAMA Psychiatry 74(7):686–693, 2017 28593216

Tiihonen J, Tanskanen A, Taipale H: 20-year nationwide follow-up study on discontinuation of antipsychotic treatment in first-episode schizophrenia. Am J Psychiatry 75(8):765–773, 2018 29621900

Tiihonen J, Taipale H, Mehtälä J, et al: Association of antipsychotic polypharmacy vs monotherapy with psychiatric rehospitalization among adults with schizophrenia. JAMA Psychiatry 76(5):499–507, 2019 30785608

Toftdahl NG, Nordentoft M, Hjorthøj C: Prevalence of substance use disorders in psychiatric patients: a nationwide Danish population-based study. Soc Psychiatry Psychiatr Epidemiol 51(1):129–140, 2016 26260950

Toohey MJ, Muralidharan A, Medoff D, et al: Caregiver positive and negative appraisals: effects of the National Alliance on Mental Illness Family-to-Family intervention. J Nerv Ment Dis 204(2):156–159, 2016 26825266

Tosato S, Albert U, Tomassi S, et al: A systematized review of atypical antipsychotics in pregnant women: balancing between risks of untreated illness and risks of drug-related adverse effects. J Clin Psychiatry 78(5):e477–e489, 2017 28297592

Trifluoperazine [prescribing information]. Princeton, NJ, Sandoz, October 2017

Trihexyphenidyl hydrochloride oral solution [prescribing information]. Greenville, SC, Pai Pharmaceutical Associates, October 2010

Trihexyphenidyl hydrochloride tablets [prescribing information]. Buffalo Grove, IL, Pack Pharmaceuticals, June 2015

Trotta A, Murray RM, Fisher HL: The impact of childhood adversity on the persistence of psychotic symptoms: a systematic review and meta-analysis. Psychol Med 45(12):2481–2498, 2015 25903153

Tseng PT, Chen YW, Yeh PY, et al: Bone mineral density in schizophrenia: an update of current meta-analysis and literature review under guideline of PRISMA. Medicine (Baltimore), 94(47):e1967, 2015 26632691

Tsuboi T, Bies RR, Suzuki T, et al: Hyperprolactinemia and estimated dopamine D2 receptor occupancy in patients with schizophrenia: analysis of the CATIE data. Prog Neuropsychopharmacol Biol Psychiatry 45:178–182, 2013 23727135

Turkington D, Spencer HM: Back to Life, Back to Normality, Vol 2: CBT Informed Recovery for Families With Relatives With Schizophrenia and Other Psychosis. Cambridge, UK, Cambridge University Press, 2019

Turkington D, Kingdon D, Weiden PJ: Cognitive behavior therapy for schizophrenia. Am J Psychiatry 163(3):365–373, 2006 16513854

Turner DT, McGlanaghy E, Cuijpers P, et al: A meta-analysis of social skills training and related interventions for psychosis. Schizophr Bull 44(3):475–491, 2018 29140460

Twamley EW, Vella L, Burton CZ, et al: Compensatory cognitive training for psychosis: effects in a randomized controlled trial. J Clin Psychiatry 73(9):1212–1219, 2012 22939029

Uchida H, Suzuki T, Takeuchi H, et al: Low dose vs standard dose of antipsychotics for relapse prevention in schizophrenia: meta-analysis. Schizophr Bull 37(4):788–799, 2011a 19946012

Uchida H, Takeuchi H, Graff-Guerrero A, et al: Predicting dopamine D2 receptor occupancy from plasma levels of antipsychotic drugs: a systematic review and pooled analysis. J Clin Psychopharmacol 31(3):318–325, 2011b 21508857

Unal A, Altindag A, Demir B, Aksoy I: The use of lorazepam and electroconvulsive therapy in the treatment of catatonia: treatment characteristics and outcomes in 60 patients. J ECT 33(4):290–293, 2017 28640169

Unützer J, Katon W, Callahan CM, et al; IMPACT Investigators. Improving Mood-Promoting Access to Collaborative Treatment: Collaborative care management of late-life depression in the primary care setting: a randomized controlled trial. JAMA 288(22):2836–2845, 2002 12472325

U.S. Department of Health and Human Services: The Health Consequences of Smoking—50 Years of Progress: A Report of the Surgeon General. Atlanta, GA, Centers for Disease Control and Prevention, 2014. Available at: www.cdc.gov/tobacco/data_statistics/sgr/50th-anniversary/index.htm. Accessed December 29, 2018.

U.S. Department of Health and Human Services; U.S. National Library of Medicine: Chlorpromazine, in LiverTox. U.S. Department of Health and Human Services, October 5, 2017a. Available at: www.ncbi.nlm.nih.gov/books/NBK548793. Accessed May 6, 2020.

U.S. Department of Health and Human Services; U.S. National Library of Medicine: Antipsychotic agents. Washington, DC, U.S. Department of Health and Human Services, July 20, 2017b. Available at: www.ncbi.nlm.nih.gov/books/NBK548317. Accessed May 6, 2020.

U.S. Food and Drug Administration: Pharmacokinetics in patients with impaired hepatic function: study design, data analysis, and impact on dosing and labeling. Silver Spring, MD, U.S. Food and Drug Administration, May 2003. Available at: www.fda.gov/downloads/drugs/guidancecomplianceregulatoryinformation/guidances/ucm072123.pdf. Accessed May 8, 2019.

U.S. Food and Drug Administration: FDA drug safety communication: antipsychotic drug labels updated on use during pregnancy and risk of abnormal muscle movements and withdrawal symptoms in newborns. Silver Spring, MD, U.S. Food and Drug Administration, February 22, 2011a. Available at: www.fda.gov/Drugs/DrugSafety/ucm243903.htm#sa. Accessed September 22, 2019.

U.S. Food and Drug Administration: Center for Drug Evaluation and Research approval package for Orap (pimozide), NDA 17-473/S046. Silver Spring, MD, U.S. Food and Drug Administration, September 27, 2011b. Available at: www.accessdata.fda.gov/drugsatfda_docs/nda/2011/017473Orig1s046.pdf. Accessed on February 1, 2019.

U.S. Food and Drug Administration: FDA approves pill with sensor that digitally tracks if patients have ingested their medication. Silver Spring, MD, U.S. Food and Drug Administration, November 13, 2017. Available at: www.fda.gov/NewsEvents/Newsroom/PressAnnouncements/ucm584933.htm. Accessed February 1, 2019.

U.S. Food and Drug Administration: Table of pharmacogenomic biomarkers in drug labeling. Silver Spring, MD, U.S. Food and Drug Administration, 2019. Available at: www.fda.gov/drugs/science-research-drugs/table-pharmacogenomic-biomarkers-drug-labeling. Accessed August 11, 2019.

U.S. National Library of Medicine: Daily Med: pimozide tablet. Bethesda, MD, National Institutes of Health, May 2018a. Available at: https://dailymed.nlm.nih.gov/dailymed/drugInfo.cfm?setid=70b079e2-a1f7-4a93-8685-d60a4d7c1280. Accessed May 7, 2020.

U.S. National Library of Medicine: Daily Med. Thioridazine Hydrochloride. Bethesda, MD, National Institutes of Health, December 21, 2018b. Available at: https://dailymed.nlm.nih.gov/dailymed/drugInfo.cfm?setid=52fea941-0b47-41c1-b00d-f88150e8ab93#boxedwarning. Accessed February 8, 2019.

Üstün TB, Kostanjsek N, Chatterji S, Rehm J: Measuring Health and Disability: Manual for WHO Disability Assessment Schedule (WHODAS 2.0). Geneva, Switzerland, World Health Organization, 2010

Valencia M, Rascon ML, Juarez F, Murow E: A psychosocial skills training approach in Mexican out-patients with schizophrenia. Psychol Med 37(10):1393–1402, 2007 17472761

Valencia M, Fresan A, Juárez F, et al: The beneficial effects of combining pharmacological and psychosocial treatment on remission and functional outcome in outpatients with schizophrenia. J Psychiatr Res 47(12):1886–1892, 2013 24112947

Valenstein M, Ganoczy D, McCarthy JF, et al: Antipsychotic adherence over time among patients receiving treatment for schizophrenia: a retrospective review. J Clin Psychiatry 67(10):1542–1550, 2006 17107245

Valenstein M, Adler DA, Berlant J, et al: Implementing standardized assessments in clinical care: now's the time. Psychiatr Serv 60(10):1372–1375, 2009 19797378

Valmaggia LR, Tabraham P, Morris E, Bouman TK: Cognitive behavioral therapy across the stages of psychosis: prodromal, first episode, and chronic schizophrenia. Cogn Behav Pract 15(2):179–193, 2008

Van L, Boot E, Bassett AS: Update on the 22q11.2 deletion syndrome and its relevance to schizophrenia. Curr Opin Psychiatry 30(3):191–196, 2017 28230630

Vancampfort D, Stubbs B, Mitchell AJ, et al: Risk of metabolic syndrome and its components in people with schizophrenia and related psychotic disorders, bipolar disorder and major depressive disorder: a systematic review and meta-analysis. World Psychiatry 14(3):339–347, 2015 26407790

Vancampfort D, Correll CU, Galling B, et al: Diabetes mellitus in people with schizophrenia, bipolar disorder and major depressive disorder: a systematic review and large scale meta-analysis. World Psychiatry 15(2):166–174, 2016a 27265707

Vancampfort D, Rosenbaum S, Schuch FB, et al: Prevalence and predictors of treatment dropout from physical activity interventions in schizophrenia: a meta-analysis. Gen Hosp Psychiatry 39:15–23, 2016b 26719106

Vancampfort D, Rosenbaum S, Schuch F, et al: Cardiorespiratory fitness in severe mental illness: a systematic review and meta-analysis. Sports Med 47(2):343–352, 2017 27299747

Vancampfort D, Firth J, Correll CU, et al: The impact of pharmacological and non-pharmacological interventions to improve physical health outcomes in people with schizophrenia: a meta-review of meta-analyses of randomized controlled trials. World Psychiatry 18(1):53–66, 2019 30600626

Van Citters AD, Pratt SI, Jue K, et al: A pilot evaluation of the In SHAPE individualized health promotion intervention for adults with mental illness. Community Ment Health J 46(6):540–552, 2010 20012197

Vandenberk B, Vandael E, Robyns T, et al: Which QT correction formulae to use for QT monitoring? J Am Heart Assoc 5(6):e003264, 2016 27317349

van der Gaag M, Stant AD, Wolters KJ, et al: Cognitive-behavioural therapy for persistent and recurrent psychosis in people with schizophrenia-spectrum disorder: cost-effectiveness analysis. Br J Psychiatry 198(1):59–65, 2011

Vanderlip ER, Henwood BF, Hrouda DR, et al: Systematic literature review of general health care interventions within programs of assertive community treatment. Psychiatr Serv 68(3):218–224, 2017 27903142

van der Werf M, Hanssen M, Köhler S, et al: Systematic review and collaborative recalculation of 133,693 incident cases of schizophrenia. Psychol Med 44(1):9–16, 2014 23244442

VanderZwaag C, McGee M, McEvoy JP, et al: Response of patients with treatment-refractory schizophrenia to clozapine within three serum level ranges. Am J Psychiatry 153(12):1579–1584, 1996 8942454

van Dijk F, de Wit I, Blankers M, et al: The Personal Antipsychotic Choice Index. Pharmacopsychiatry 51(3):89–99, 2018 28810270

van Duin D, de Winter L, Oud M, et al: The effect of rehabilitation combined with cognitive remediation on functioning in persons with severe mental illness: systematic review and meta-analysis. Psychol Med 49(9):1414–1425, 2019 30696500

van Dulmen SA, Lukersmith S, Muxlow J, et al; G-I-N Allied Health Steering Group: Supporting a person-centred approach in clinical guidelines: a position paper of the Allied Health Community—Guidelines International Network (G-I-N). Health Expect 18(5):1543–1558, 2015 24118821

van Harten PN, Hoek HW, Kahn RS: Acute dystonia induced by drug treatment. BMJ 319(7210):623–626, 1999 10473482

Van Putten T, Aravagiri M, Marder SR, et al: Plasma fluphenazine levels and clinical response in newly admitted schizophrenic patients. Psychopharmacol Bull 27(2):91–96, 1991 1924666

Van Schayck OCP, Williams S, Barchilon V, et al: Treating tobacco dependence: guidance for primary care on life-saving interventions. Position statement of the IPCRG. NPJ Prim Care Respir Med 27(1):38, 2017 28600490

van Strien AM, Keijsers CJ, Derijks HJ, van Marum RJ: Rating scales to measure side effects of antipsychotic medication: a systematic review. J Psychopharmacol 29(8):857–866, 2015 26156860

Varese F, Smeets F, Drukker M, et al: Childhood adversities increase the risk of psychosis: a meta-analysis of patient-control, prospective- and cross-sectional cohort studies. Schizophr Bull 38(4):661–671, 2012 22461484

Vaucher J, Keating BJ, Lasserre AM, et al: Cannabis use and risk of schizophrenia: a Mendelian randomization study. Mol Psychiatry 23(5):1287–1292, 2018 28115737

Veerman SR, Schulte PF, Begemann MJ, de Haan L: Non-glutamatergic clozapine augmentation strategies: a review and meta-analysis. Pharmacopsychiatry 47(7):231–238, 2014 25121994

Velligan DI, Lam YW, Glahn DC, et al: Defining and assessing adherence to oral antipsychotics: a review of the literature. Schizophr Bull 32(4):724–742, 2006 16707778

Velligan DI, Weiden PJ, Sajatovic M, et al; Expert Consensus Panel on Adherence Problems in Serious and Persistent Mental Illness: The Expert Consensus Guideline Series: adherence problems in patients with serious and persistent mental illness. J Clin Psychiatry 70 (suppl 4):1–46, 2009 19686636

Velligan DI, Weiden PJ, Sajatovic M, et al: Strategies for addressing adherence problems in patients with serious and persistent mental illness: recommendations from the expert consensus guidelines. J Psychiatr Pract 16(5):306–324, 2010 20859108

Velligan DI, Medellin E, Draper M, et al: Barriers to, and strategies for, starting a long acting injection clinic in a community mental health center. Community Ment Health J 47(6):654–659, 2011 21253830

Velligan DI, Sajatovic M, Hatch A, et al: Why do psychiatric patients stop antipsychotic medication? A systematic review of reasons for nonadherence to medication in patients with serious mental illness. Patient Prefer Adherence 11:449–468, 2017 28424542

Velthorst E, Koeter M, van der Gaag M, et al: Adapted cognitive-behavioural therapy required for targeting negative symptoms in schizophrenia: meta-analysis and meta-regression. Psychol Med 45(3):453–465, 2015 24993642

Ventura J, Green MF, Shaner A, Liberman RP: Training and quality assurance in the use of the Brief Psychiatric Rating Scale: the "drift busters." Int J Methods Psychiatr Res 3:221–244, 1993

Verbiest M, Brakema E, van der Kleij R, et al: National guidelines for smoking cessation in primary care: a literature review and evidence analysis. NPJ Prim Care Respir Med 27(1):2, 2017 28108747

Verdoux H, Quiles C, Bachmann CJ, Siskind D: Prescriber and institutional barriers and facilitators of clozapine use: a systematic review. Schizophr Res 201:10–19, 2018 29880453

Verhaeghe N, Clays E, Vereecken C, et al: Health promotion in individuals with mental disorders: a cluster preference randomized controlled trial. BMC Public Health 13:657, 2013 23855449

Vermeir M, Naessens I, Remmerie B, et al: Absorption, metabolism, and excretion of paliperidone, a new monoaminergic antagonist, in humans. Drug Metab Dispos 36(4):769–779, 2008 18227146

Vermeulen J, van Rooijen G, Doedens P, et al: Antipsychotic medication and long-term mortality risk in patients with schizophrenia: a systematic review and meta-analysis. Psychol Med 47(13):2217–2228, 2017 28397632

Vermeulen JM, van Rooijen G, van de Kerkhof MPJ, et al: Clozapine and long-term mortality risk in patients with schizophrenia: a systematic review and meta-analysis of studies lasting 1.1–12.5 years. Schizophr Bull 45(2):315–329, 2019 29697804

Victoroff J, Coburn K, Reeve A, et al: Pharmacological management of persistent hostility and aggression in persons with schizophrenia spectrum disorders: a systematic review. J Neuropsychiatry Clin Neurosci 26(4):283–312, 2014 26037853.

Viejo LF, Morales V, Puñal P, et al: Risk factors in neuroleptic malignant syndrome: a case-control study. Acta Psychiatr Scand 107(1):45–49, 2003 12558541

Viertiö S, Laitinen A, Perälä J, et al: Visual impairment in persons with psychotic disorder. Soc Psychiatry Psychiatr Epidemiol 42(11):902–908, 2007 17846698

Vinogradov S, Fisher M, Warm H, et al: The cognitive cost of anticholinergic burden: decreased response to cognitive training in schizophrenia. Am J Psychiatry 166(9):1055–1062, 2009 19570929

Vita A, De Peri L, Barlati S, et al: Effectiveness of different modalities of cognitive remediation on symptomatological, neuropsychological, and functional outcome domains in schizophrenia: a prospective study in a real-world setting. Schizophr Res 133(1–3):223–231, 2011 21907544

Volavka J, Van Dorn RA, Citrome L, et al: Hostility in schizophrenia: an integrated analysis of the combined Clinical Antipsychotic Trials of Intervention Effectiveness (CATIE) and the European First Episode Schizophrenia Trial (EUFEST) studies. Eur Psychiatry 31:13–19, 2016 26657597

Vraylar (cariprazine) [prescribing information]. Madison, NJ, Allergan USA, May 2019

Vuk A, Baretic M, Osvatic MM, et al: Treatment of diabetic ketoacidosis associated with antipsychotic medication: literature review. J Clin Psychopharmacol 37(5):584–589, 2017 28816925

Waddell L, Taylor M: A new self-rating scale for detecting atypical or second-generation antipsychotic side effects. J Psychopharmacol 22(3):238–243, 2008 18541624

Waddell L, Taylor M: Attitudes of patients and mental health staff to antipsychotic long-acting injections: systematic review. Br J Psychiatry Suppl 52:S43–S50, 2009 19880916

Wade M, Tai S, Awenat Y, Haddock G: A systematic review of service-user reasons for adherence and nonadherence to neuroleptic medication in psychosis. Clin Psychol Rev 51:75–95, 2017 27838461

Wagner E, Löhrs L, Siskind D, et al: Clozapine augmentation strategies: a systematic meta-review of available evidence: treatment options for clozapine resistance. J Psychopharmacol 33(4):423–435, 2019a 30696332

Wagner E, Wobrock T, Kunze B, et al: Efficacy of high-frequency repetitive transcranial magnetic stimulation in schizophrenia patients with treatment-resistant negative symptoms treated with clozapine. Schizophr Res 208:370–376, 2019b 30704862

Walburn J, Gray R, Gournay K, et al: Systematic review of patient and nurse attitudes to depot antipsychotic medication. Br J Psychiatry 179:300–307, 2001 11581109

Walker ER, McGee RE, Druss BG: Mortality in mental disorders and global disease burden implications: a systematic review and meta-analysis. JAMA Psychiatry 72(4):334–341, 2015 25671328

Waln O, Jankovic J: Paroxysmal movement disorders. Neurol Clin 33(1):137–152, 2015 25432727

Wampold BE: How important are the common factors in psychotherapy? An update. World Psychiatry 14(3):270–277, 2015 26407772

Wang G, Zheng W, Li XB, et al: ECT augmentation of clozapine for clozapine-resistant schizophrenia: a meta-analysis of randomized controlled trials. J Psychiatr Res 105:23–32, 2018 30144667

Wang K, Varma DS, Prosperi M: A systematic review of the effectiveness of mobile apps for monitoring and management of mental health symptoms or disorders. J Psychiatr Res 107:73–78, 2018 30347316

Wang PS, Walker AM, Tsuang MT, et al: Dopamine antagonists and the development of breast cancer. Arch Gen Psychiatry 59(12):1147–1154, 2002 12470131

Ward M, Druss B: The epidemiology of diabetes in psychotic disorders. Lancet Psychiatry 2(5):431–451, 2015 26360287

Warnez S, Alessi-Severini S: Clozapine: a review of clinical practice guidelines and prescribing trends. BMC Psychiatry 14:102, 2014 24708834

Watkins K, Horvitz-Lennon M, Caldarone LB, et al: Developing medical record-based performance indicators to measure the quality of mental healthcare. J Healthc Qual 33(1):49–66, quiz 66–67, 2011 21199073

Watkins KE, Farmer CM, De Vries D, Hepner KA: The Affordable Care Act: an opportunity for improving care for substance use disorders? Psychiatr Serv 66(3):310–312, 2015 25727120

Watkins KE, Smith B, Akincigil A, et al: The quality of medication treatment for mental disorders in the Department of Veterans Affairs and in private-sector plans. Psychiatr Serv 67(4):391–396, 2016 26567931

Way BB, Miraglia R, Sawyer DA, Beer RJ: Factors related to suicide in New York State prisons. Int J Law Psychiatry 28(3):207–221, 2005 15950281

Weaver J, Kawsky J, Corboy A: Antipsychotic use and fracture risk: an evaluation of incidence at a Veterans Affairs medical center. Ment Health Clin 9(1):6–11, 2019 30627497

Weibell MA, Hegelstad WTV, Auestad B, et al: The effect of substance use on 10-year outcome in first-episode psychosis. Schizophr Bull 43(4):843–851, 2017 28199703

Weiden PJ, Roma RS, Velligan DI, et al: The challenge of offering long-acting antipsychotic therapies: a preliminary discourse analysis of psychiatrist recommendations for injectable therapy to patients with schizophrenia. J Clin Psychiatry 76(6):684–690, 2015 25939027

Wenzlow AT, Ireys HT, Mann B, et al: Effects of a discharge planning program on Medicaid coverage of state prisoners with serious mental illness. Psychiatr Serv 62(1):73–78, 2011 21209303

West JC, Marcus SC, Wilk J, et al: Use of depot antipsychotic medications for medication nonadherence in schizophrenia. Schizophr Bull 34(5):995–1001, 2008 18093962

Whicher CA, Price HC, Holt RIG: Mechanisms in endocrinology: antipsychotic medication and type 2 diabetes and impaired glucose regulation. Eur J Endocrinol 178(6):R245–R258, 2018 29559497

Whirl-Carrillo M, McDonagh EM, Hebert JM, et al: Pharmacogenomics knowledge for personalized medicine. Clin Pharmacol Ther 92(4):414–417, 2012 22992668

WHOQOL Group: Development of the World Health Organization WHOQOL-BREF quality of life assessment. Psychol Med 28(3):551–558, 1998 9626712

Wilder CM, Elbogen EB, Moser LL, et al: Medication preferences and adherence among individuals with severe mental illness and psychiatric advance directives. Psychiatr Serv 61(4):380–385, 2010 20360277

Wilper AP, Woolhandler S, Boyd JW, et al: The health and health care of US prisoners: results of a nationwide survey. Am J Public Health 99(4):666–672, 2009 19150898

Wimberley T, MacCabe JH, Laursen TM, et al: Mortality and self-harm in association with clozapine in treatment-resistant schizophrenia. Am J Psychiatry 174(10):990–998, 2017 28750580

Winston A: Supportive psychotherapy, in The American Psychiatric Publishing Textbook of Psychiatry, 6th Edition. Edited by Hales RE, Yudofsky SC, Roberts LW. Washington, DC, American Psychiatric Publishing, 2014, pp 1161–1186

Winston A, Rosenthal RN, Pinsker H: Learning Supportive Psychotherapy: An Illustrated Guide. Washington, DC, American Psychiatric Publishing, 2012, p 211

Witt K, van Dorn R, Fazel S: Risk factors for violence in psychosis: systematic review and meta-regression analysis of 110 studies. PLoS One 8(2):e55942, 2013 23418482

Witt K, Hawton K, Fazel S: The relationship between suicide and violence in schizophrenia: analysis of the Clinical Antipsychotic Trials of Intervention Effectiveness (CATIE) dataset. Schizophr Res 154(1–3):61–67, 2014 24581550

Witt K, Lichtenstein P, Fazel S: Improving risk assessment in schizophrenia: epidemiological investigation of criminal history factors. Br J Psychiatry 206(5):424–430, 2015 25657352

Wittenauer Welsh J, Janjua AU, Garlow SJ, et al: Use of expert consultation in a complex case of neuroleptic malignant syndrome requiring electroconvulsive therapy. J Psychiatr Pract 22(6):484489, 2016 27824784

Wium-Andersen MK, Ørsted DD, Nordestgaard BG: Tobacco smoking is causally associated with antipsychotic medication use and schizophrenia, but not with antidepressant medication use or depression. Int J Epidemiol 44(2):566–577, 2015 26054357

Wojcik JD, Falk WE, Fink JS, et al: A review of 32 cases of tardive dystonia. Am J Psychiatry 148(8):1055–1059, 1991 1677236

Wong J, Delva N: Clozapine-induced seizures: recognition and treatment. Can J Psychiatry 52(7):457–463, 2007 17688010

Wong Z, Öngür D, Cohen B, et al: Command hallucinations and clinical characteristics of suicidality in patients with psychotic spectrum disorders. Compr Psychiatry 54(6):611–617, 2013 23375263

Wood L, Burke E, Morrison A: Individual cognitive behavioural therapy for psychosis (CBTp): a systematic review of qualitative literature. Behav Cogn Psychother 43(3):285–297, 2015 24308817

Woods SW, Morgenstern H, Saksa JR, et al: Incidence of tardive dyskinesia with atypical versus conventional antipsychotic medications: a prospective cohort study. J Clin Psychiatry 71(4):463–474, 2010 20156410

Woosley RL, Heise CW, Gallo T: QTdrugs List. Oro Valley, AZ, AZCERT, March 29, 2009. Available at: www.crediblemeds.org. Accessed April 23, 2019.

Woosley RL, Romero K, Heise CW, et al: Adverse Drug Event Causality Analysis (ADECA): a process for evaluating evidence and assigning drugs to risk categories for sudden death. Drug Saf 40(6):465–474, 2017 28275963

Wright JH, Turkington D, Kingdon DG, Basco MR: Cognitive-Behavior Therapy for Severe Mental Illness: An Illustrated Guide. Washington, DC, American Psychiatric Publishing, 2009

Wykes T, Steel C, Everitt B, Tarrier N: Cognitive behavior therapy for schizophrenia: effect sizes, clinical models, and methodological rigor. Schizophr Bull 34(3):523–537, 2008 17962231

Wykes T, Huddy V, Cellard C, et al: A meta-analysis of cognitive remediation for schizophrenia: methodology and effect sizes. Am J Psychiatry 168(5):472–485, 2011 21406461

Xenazine (tetrabenazine) tablets [prescribing information]. Deerfield, IL, Lundbeck, September 2018

Xia J, Merinder LB, Belgamwar MR: Psychoeducation for schizophrenia (update). Cochrane Database Syst Rev (6):CD002831, 2011 12076455

Yan H, Chen JD, Zheng XY: Potential mechanisms of atypical antipsychotic-induced hypertriglyceridemia. Psychopharmacology (Berl) 229(1):1–7, 2013 23832387

Yates K, Lång U, Cederlöf M, et al: Association of psychotic experiences with subsequent risk of suicidal ideation, suicide attempts, and suicide deaths: a systematic review and meta-analysis of longitudinal population studies. JAMA Psychiatry 76(2):180–189, 2019 30484818

Yeo V, Dowsey M, Alguera-Lara V, et al: Antipsychotic choice: understanding shared decision-making among doctors and patients. J Ment Health Jun 26:1–8, 2019 31240989 Epub ahead of print

Yoon HW, Lee JS, Park SJ, et al: Comparing the effectiveness and safety of the addition of and switching to aripiprazole for resolving antipsychotic-induced hyperprolactinemia: a multicenter, open-label, prospective study. Clin Neuropharmacol 39(6):288–294, 2016 27438182

Zanger UM, Schwab M: Cytochrome P450 enzymes in drug metabolism: regulation of gene expression, enzyme activities, and impact of genetic variation. Pharmacol Ther 138(1):103–141, 2013 23333322

Zhang JP, Gallego JA, Robinson DG, et al: Efficacy and safety of individual second-generation vs. first-generation antipsychotics in first-episode psychosis: a systematic review and meta-analysis. Int J Neuropsychopharmacol 16(6):1205–1218, 2013 23199972

Zhang Y, Liu Y, Su Y, et al: The metabolic side effects of 12 antipsychotic drugs used for the treatment of schizophrenia on glucose: a network meta-analysis. BMC Psychiatry 17(1):373, 2017 29162032

Zheng W, Li XB, Tang YL, et al: Metformin for weight gain and metabolic abnormalities associated with antipsychotic treatment: meta-analysis of randomized placebo-controlled trials. J Clin Psychopharmacol 35(5):499–509, 2015 26280837

Zheng W, Cao XL, Ungvari GS, et al: Electroconvulsive therapy added to non-clozapine antipsychotic medication for treatment resistant schizophrenia: meta-analysis of randomized controlled trials. PLoS One 11(6):e0156510, 2016 27285996

Zhou SF: Polymorphism of human cytochrome P450 2D6 and its clinical significance, part I. Clin Pharmacokinet 48(11):689–723, 2009 19817501

Zhu Y, Krause M, Huhn M, et al: Antipsychotic drugs for the acute treatment of patients with a first episode of schizophrenia: a systematic review with pairwise and network meta-analyses. Lancet Psychiatry 4(9):694–705, 2017 28736102

Zhuo C, Xu Y, Liu S, et al: Topiramate and metformin are effective add-on treatments in controlling antipsychotic-induced weight gain: a systematic review and network meta-analysis. Front Pharmacol 9:1393, 2018 30546312

Zimmer M, Duncan AV, Laitano D, et al: A twelve-week randomized controlled study of the cognitive-behavioral integrated psychological therapy program: positive effect on the social functioning of schizophrenic patients. Braz J Psychiatry 29(2):140–147, 2007 17650536

Zimmerman M, Chelminski I, Young D, Dalrymple K: Using outcome measures to promote better outcomes. Clinical Neuropsychiatry 8:28–36, 2011

Zou H, Li Z, Nolan MT, et al: Self-management education interventions for persons with schizophrenia: a meta-analysis. Int J Ment Health Nurs 22(3):256–271, 2013 22882803

Zubek JP, Bayer L, Shephard JM: Relative effects of prolonged social isolation and confinement: behavioral and EEG changes. J Abnorm Psychol 74(5):625–631, 1969 5349408

Zyprexa (olanzapine) [prescribing information]. Indianapolis, IN, Lilly USA, March 2018a

Zyprexa (olanzapine) [product monograph]. Toronto, ON, Canada, Eli Lilly Canada, April 2018b

Zyprexa Relprevv (olanzapine) [prescribing information]. Indianapolis, IN, Eli Lilly, March 2018

Disclosures

The Guideline Writing Group and Systematic Review Group reported the following disclosures during development and approval of this guideline:

Dr. Keepers is employed as Professor and Chair of the Department of Psychiatry by Oregon Health & Science University. He receives travel funds from the American Board of Psychiatry and Neurology, the American College of Psychiatry, and the Accreditation Council for Graduate Medical Education related to his activities as a member or chair of various committees. He reports no conflicts of interest with his work on this guideline.

Dr. Fochtmann is employed by Stony Brook University, where she is a Distinguished Service Professor of Psychiatry, Pharmacological Sciences, and Biomedical Informatics. She also serves as a Deputy Chief Medical Information Officer for Stony Brook Medicine. Dr. Fochtmann has received payment for grant reviews for the National Institute of Mental Health (NIMH) and is a co-investigator on a grant funded by NIMH. She consults for the American Psychiatric Association on the development of practice guidelines and has received travel funds to attend meetings related to these duties. She reports no conflicts of interest with her work on this guideline.

Dr. Anzia is employed as Professor of Psychiatry and Behavioral Sciences and Residency Program Director/Vice Chair for Education at Northwestern University/Feinberg School of Medicine. She receives part of her salary from the Medical Staff Office of Northwestern Medicine for her role as Physician Health Liaison. Dr. Anzia receives travel funds from the American Board of Psychiatry and Neurology, the American College of Psychiatry, and the Accreditation Council for Graduate Medical Education for her activities as Board Director, committee chair, and various other committees. She has no conflicts of interest with her work on this guideline.

Dr. Benjamin is employed as the Interim Chair of Psychiatry at University of Massachusetts Medical School and UMass Memorial Health Care, where he is also Director of Residency Training, Director of Neuropsychiatry, and Professor of Psychiatry and Neurology. He periodically receives honoraria for lectures, provides consultation to the Massachusetts Department of Mental Health, and serves as an expert witness on neuropsychiatric issues. He is a partner in and author for Brain Educators, LLC, a publisher of educational materials designed to improve neuropsychiatric assessment skills. Any income received is used to offset production and development costs of the materials. He reports no conflicts of interest with his work on this guideline.

Dr. Lyness is employed as Senior Associate Dean for Academic Affairs and Professor of Psychiatry and Neurology in the School of Medicine & Dentistry at the University of Rochester Medical Center. He receives compensation for his work as a Psychiatry Director of the American Board of Psychiatry and Neurology. At times he provides independent medical examinations for various attorneys. He has no other relevant financial or fiduciary interests and reports no conflicts of interest with his work on this guideline.

Dr. Mojtabai is employed as Professor of Public Health at Johns Hopkins Bloomberg School of Public Health in Baltimore, Maryland, and as a psychiatrist at Johns Hopkins Hospital. During the period of preparation of this guideline, he received royalties from UpToDate, Inc., and consulting fees from the RAND Corporation. He reports no conflicts of interest with his work on this guideline.

Dr. Servis is employed as Professor of Psychiatry and Behavioral Sciences and the Vice Dean for Medical Education at the University of California Davis School of Medicine. He consults to the Medical Board of California and serves on the Psychiatry Residency in Training Examination Editorial Board for the American College of Psychiatrists and the Interdisciplinary Review Committee for the USMLE Step 2 Examination for the National Board of Medical Examiners. He reports no conflicts of interest with his work on this guideline.

Dr. Walaszek is employed as Professor of Psychiatry at the University of Wisconsin School of Medicine and Public Health, where he is Residency Training Director and Vice Chair for Education and Faculty Development. He is past President of the American Association of Directors of Psychiatric Residency Training. He reports no conflict of interest with his work on this guideline.

Dr. Buckley is Dean of the Virginia Commonwealth University School of Medicine. He receives payment for grant reviews for the National Institute of Mental Health (NIMH) and conducts collaborative research funded by NIMH, the Stanley Foundation, and the Brain and Behavior Research Foundation. He reports no conflicts of interest with his work on this guideline.

Dr. Lenzenweger is employed as Distinguished Professor of Psychology at the State University of New York at Binghamton. He is also appointed as Adjunct Professor of Psychology in Psychiatry, Department of Psychiatry, Weill Cornell Medical College. He has received consulting fees for research consultations to the Personality Disorders Institute at Weill Cornell Medical College. He also maintains an independent clinical practice in Ithaca, New York. He reports no conflicts of interest with his work on this guideline.

Dr. Young is employed as Professor of Psychiatry at the University of California Los Angeles and as Physician at the Department of Veterans Affairs in Los Angeles, California. He served on the American Psychiatric Association's Council on Quality Care and received travel funds to attend meetings related to those duties. He reports no conflicts of interest with his work on this guideline.

Dr. Degenhardt is employed as a fifth-year resident in psychiatry by Vancouver Coastal Health at the University of British Columbia in Vancouver, British Columbia, Canada. She is a member of the APA Council of Research and APA Leadership fellowship. She is also on the board of directors of the Canadian Psychiatric Association (CPA), is Chair of the CPA Members-in-Training Executive Committee, and various other committees. She has received travel funds to attend meetings related to these duties. She reports no conflicts of interest with her work on this guideline.

Individuals and Organizations That Submitted Comments

Donald Addington, M.B.B.S.
Jonathan E. Alpert, M.D., Ph.D.
Gustavo Alva, M.D., DFAPA
Anne S. Bassett, M.D., FRCPC
Scott R. Beach, M.D.
Lora Beebe, Ph.D., PMHNP-BC, FAAN
Jeffrey Bennett, M.D., A.B.
Jolene Bostwick, Pharm.D.
Vasileios-Panteleimon Bozikas, M.D., Ph.D.
Nancy Burke, Ph.D.
Stanley N. Caroff, M.D.
Nicola Cascella, M.D.
Christopher Celano, M.D.
Michael Champion, M.D.
Hemlata Charitar, M.D., Ph.D., FAPA
Leslie Citrome, M.D., M.P.H.
Michael Davidson, M.D.
Erica Davis, Pharm.D., BCPS, BCPP
Sonia Dollfus, M.D., Ph.D.
Gail A. Edelsohn, M.D., M.S.P.H.
Michael Enenbach, M.D.
Peter Falkai, Dr. med.
Marlene Freeman, M.D.
Oliver Freudenreich, M.D., FACLP
Kenneth Fung, M.D.
Margo C. Funk, M.D., M.A.
Wolfgang Gaebel, Dr. med.
Carles Garcia-Ribera, M.D., Ph.D.
Paul Gionfriddo
Christina Girgis, M.D.
Robert M. Goisman, M.D.
Lisa W. Goldstone, M.S., Pharm.D., BCPS, BCPP
Philip D. Harvey, Ph.D.
Steven Hoge, M.D.
William G. Honer, M.D., FRCPC, FCAHS
Liwei L. Hua, M.D., Ph.D.
Nikola Ilankovic, M.D., Ph.D., DFAPA
Kelly Irwin, M.D., M.P.H.
John M. Kane, M.D.
Reena Kapoor, M.D.
Michael B. Knable, D.O.
Maju Koola, M.D.
Sarah L. Kopelovich, Ph.D.
Robert S. Laitman, M.D.
Susan N Legacy, M.D., M.S.

Raquel López-Carrilero
Paul H. Lysaker, Ph.D.
Stephen Marder, M.D.
Russell L. Margolis, M.D.
Ashley M. Schnakenberg Martin, Ph.D.
Patrick McGorry
John McGrath, M.D., Ph.D.
Alice Medalia, Ph.D.
Gaurav Mehta, CPA Lead for Obesity, M.B.B.S., DCP, M.Sc. (Psych), M.Sc. (Diabetes), FAcadMEd, FRCPC, FAPA, CISAM, CCSAM, DAM, CBE
Jeffrey L. Metzner, M.D.
Jonathan Meyer, M.D.
Linda Michaels, Psy.D.
Kim T. Mueser, Ph.D.
Janice Muhr, Ph.D.
Sachin Nagendrappa, M.D.
Anna-Greta Nylander, Ph.D., M.B.A.
Susana Ochoa
Carol A. Ott, Pharm.D., BCPP
Raymond Patterson, M.D.
Edmond Pi, M.D.
Debra Pinals, M.D.
Rajiv Radhakrishnan, M.B.B.S., M.D.
Gary Remington, M.D., Ph.D.
Arnold Robbins, M.D.
Alvin Rosenfeld, M.D.
Ada Ruiz-Ripoll, M.D., Ph.D.
Stephen R. Saklad, Pharm.D., BCPP
Elyn R. Saks, B.A., M.Litt., J.D., Ph.D., LL.D. (hon)
John P.D. Shemo, M.D.
Dan Siskind, M.B.B.S., M.P.H., Ph.D., FRANZCP
John Snook, J.D.
Amro Soliman, M.Sc., ARCPsych, M.D.
Melina Spyridaki-Dodd, M.D.
Linda Whitten Stalters, M.S.N., APRN (ret)
David M. Tobolowsky, M.D.
John Torous, M.D., M.B.I.
Robert Trestman, Ph.D., M.D.
Margaret Tuttle, M.D.
Nina Vadiei, Pharm.D., BCPP
John Waddington, Ph.D., D.Sc.
Scott Weigold, M.D.
Kazunari Yoshida, M.D., Ph.D.

Academy of Consultation-Liaison Psychiatry
Alkermes, Inc.
American Academy of Child and Adolescent Psychiatry
American Psychological Association
American Society of Clinical Psychopharmacology
APA Council on Consultation-Liaison Psychiatry Workgroup on QTc Prolongation and Psychotropic Medications
APA Council on Psychiatry and the Law, Subcommittee on Correctional Psychiatry
ATP Clinical Research
Cairo Neuropsychiatric Clinic
Canadian Psychiatric Association
College of Psychiatric & Neurologic Pharmacists
International Society for Psychological and Social Approaches to Psychosis, United States Chapter
International Society of Psychiatric Nurses
Mental Health America
National Alliance on Mental Illness
Psychotherapy Action Network
Schizophrenia and Related Disorders Alliance of America
Schizophrenia International Research Society
Treatment Advocacy Center Psychiatric Advisory Board
World Psychiatric Association Section on Schizophrenia

Appendix A.
Clinical Questions

The following key questions formed the basis of the Agency for Healthcare Research and Quality review:

1a. What are the comparative benefits and harms of pharmacological treatments for adults with schizophrenia?
1b. How do the benefits and harms of pharmacological treatments for adults with schizophrenia vary by patient characteristics?
2a. What are the benefits and harms of psychosocial and other nonpharmacological treatments for adults with schizophrenia?
2b. How do the benefits and harms of psychosocial and other nonpharmacological treatments for adults with schizophrenia vary by patient characteristics (e.g., age, sex, race, ethnicity, socioeconomic status, time since illness onset, prior treatment history, co-occurring psychiatric disorders, pregnancy)?

The following key questions formed the basis of searches related to neurological side effects of antipsychotic medications:

1. What are the comparative benefits and harms of pharmacological treatments for acute dystonia associated with antipsychotic therapy?
2. What are the comparative benefits and harms of pharmacological treatments for parkinsonism associated with antipsychotic therapy?
3. What are the comparative benefits and harms of pharmacological treatments for akathisia associated with antipsychotic therapy?
4. What are the comparative benefits and harms of pharmacological treatments for tardive syndromes associated with antipsychotic therapy?

Appendix B.
Search Strategies, Study Selection, and Search Results

AHRQ Review

The Agency for Healthcare Research and Quality's (AHRQ) systematic review *Treatments for Schizophrenia in Adults* (McDonagh et al. 2017) served as the predominant source of information for this guideline. Databases that were searched are Ovid MEDLINE® (PubMed®), the Cochrane Central Register of Controlled Trials, the Cochrane Database of Systematic Reviews, and PsycINFO®. Results were limited to English-language, adult (18 and older), and human-only studies. The search varied by key question because high-quality systematic reviews were used as a starting point for the review. For key question 1, search dates for first-generation antipsychotic medications (FGAs) versus second-generation antipsychotic medications (SGAs) began in 2011 and for SGAs versus SGAs began in 2013. Key question 2 did not restrict the start date. All searches were conducted through February 1, 2017. The search strategies used can be found in Appendix A of the AHRQ review (McDonagh et al. 2017).

The AHRQ review (McDonagh et al. 2017) adhered to the procedures outlined in the AHRQ Methods Guide for Effectiveness and Comparative Effectiveness Reviews (Agency for Healthcare Research and Quality 2014). Recent, comprehensive, good- or fair-quality systematic reviews served as a primary source of evidence, supplemented by information from randomized controlled trials (RCTs) published since the systematic reviews or when no systematic reviews were available. For assessment of harms of treatment, systematic reviews of observational trials were also included. Eligibility for inclusion and exclusion of articles adhered to preestablished criteria. Specifically, the AHRQ review included articles that had at least 12 weeks of follow-up and were conducted in outpatient settings in countries that were relevant to the United States' health care system. Articles that addressed benefits of treatment were included if at least 90% of the sample had a diagnosis of schizophrenia (or schizophreniform disorder), with a schizophrenia spectrum disorder in at least 50% of the sample (minimum sample size >50) for studies of harms of treatment. For key questions that related to antipsychotic treatment, all of the SGAs were included; for FGAs, studies on fluphenazine, haloperidol, and perphenazine were included. Only head-to-head comparison studies were included. For studies of psychosocial and other nonpharmacological interventions, studies were included if they compared usual care, standard care, treatment as usual, or a waitlist control group to active treatment with assertive community treatment, cognitive adaptive training, cognitive-behavioral therapy, cognitive remediation, early interventions for first-episode psychosis, family interventions, intensive case management, illness self-management training, interventions for co-occurring schizophrenia and substance use, psychoeducation, social skills training, supported employment, or supportive psychotherapy.

Using these criteria, titles and abstracts were reviewed by two individuals (McDonagh et al. 2017). Full-text articles were retrieved if either reviewer felt inclusion was warranted. Full-text articles were also evaluated by two reviewers, and disagreements about inclusion were resolved by consensus. Included studies are listed in Appendix B of the AHRQ review, and excluded studies (with the reason for exclusion) are listed in Appendix C of the AHRQ review (McDonagh et al. 2017). For key question 1 on antipsychotic treatment, 698 citations were identified, 519 of which were excluded on the basis of title and abstract review, yielding 179 full-text articles that were reviewed, of which 38 were included in the final AHRQ review. For key question 2 on psychosocial and other nonpharmacological interventions, 2,766 citations were identified, 1,871 of which were excluded on the basis of title and abstract review, yielding 895 full-text articles that were reviewed, of which 53 were included in the final AHRQ review. Additional summary information about the included studies is shown in Table B-1, and additional details can be found in the AHRQ review (McDonagh et al. 2017).

For included studies, abstracted information was verified for accuracy and completeness by a second individual and included citation, year, study design, setting, funding source, country, sample size, eligibility criteria, clinical characteristics, and other characteristics of the study design, population, intervention, and outcomes (McDonagh et al. 2017). In addition, individual controlled trials and systematic reviews were assessed by two team members with predefined criteria for study quality, yielding ratings of "good," "fair," or "poor," with disagreements resolved by consensus (McDonagh et al. 2017). Included systematic reviews were generally of good quality, whereas additional included studies were generally of fair quality.

Treatment of Neurological Side Effects of Antipsychotic Medications

Additional searches were undertaken to supplement the AHRQ review and to identify studies that addressed approaches to treatment of neurological side effects of antipsychotic medications. Search strategies for MEDLINE (PubMed) and Cochrane Library are shown in Tables B–2 and B–3, respectively. For each search, all available citations were identified from the inception of the database to July 29, 2018, the date when the searches were conducted. A search of MEDLINE yielded 2,980 citations, and a search of the Cochrane Library yielded 2,450. After duplicate citations were removed, titles and abstracts for 4,196 articles were screened by one reviewer (L.J.F.) to identify articles in humans, 18 years of age or older, published in English, that investigated the treatment of antipsychotic-associated dystonia, parkinsonism, akathisia, tardive syndromes, or neuroleptic malignant syndrome. Systematic reviews and meta-analyses were used as a primary source of evidence, and if multiple Cochrane reviews on a topic had been done, only the most recent review was included. For topics on which no systematic review was available, RCTs with a sample size of at least 20 subjects and observational studies with a sample of at least 50 individuals were included. Included studies had a follow-up period of at least 1 week for acute dystonia or neuroleptic malignant syndrome and 8 weeks for other side effects.

TABLE B–1. Studies used in the Agency for Healthcare Research Quality review

	Systematic reviews	Number of publications	Number of trials in systematic reviews	Number of subjects in systematic reviews	Number of additional trials	Number of publications	Number of subjects in additional trials	Total number of subjects
FGA vs. SGA	1	2	111	118,503	5	7	1,055	119,558
SGA vs. SGA	1	1	138	47,189	24	28	6,672	53,861
Assertive community treatment	1	1	14	2,281	1	1	118	2,399
Cognitive adaptive training	0	0	0	0	3	4	290	290
Cognitive-behavioral therapy	3	3	89	7,154	5	6	823	7,977
Cognitive remediation	2	2	57	2,885	4	5	341	3,226
Early intervention for first-episode psychosis	0	0	0	0	4	9	2,363	2,363
Family interventions	1	1	27	2,297	6	8	562	2,859
Intensive case management	1	1	10	1,652	1	1	77	1,729
Interventions for schizophrenia and co-occurring SUD	1	1	32	3,165	0	0	0	3,165
Illness self-management	1	1	13	1,404	1	1	210	1,614
Psychoeducation	1	1	10	1,125	0	0	0	1,125
Social skills training	0	0	0	0	3	4	433	433
Supported employment	1	1	14	2,265	2	3	1,477	3,742
Supportive psychotherapy	1	1	5	822	0	0	0	822

Abbreviations. FGA=first-generation antipsychotic; SGA=second-generation antipsychotic; SUD=substance use disorder.

Source. Adapted from McDonagh et al. 2017.

The APA Practice Guideline for the Treatment of Patients With Schizophrenia

TABLE B–2. **Strategy for MEDLINE (PubMed) search on treatments for neurological side effects of antipsychotic medications**

ID	Search	Hits
#1	Search "Akineton"[TIAB] OR "Amantadine"[MH] OR "Amantadine"[TIAB] OR "Artane"[TIAB] OR "Atropine"[MH] OR "Atropine"[TIAB] OR "Benadryl"[TIAB] OR "Benztropine"[MH] OR "Benztropine"[TIAB] OR "Biperiden"[MH] OR "Biperiden"[TIAB] OR "Bromocriptine"[MH] OR "bromocriptine"[TIAB] OR "Cogentin"[TIAB] OR "Cuvposa"[TIAB] OR "Dantrium"[TIAB] OR "Dantrolene"[MH] OR "Dantrolene"[TIAB] OR "Diphenhydramine"[MH] OR "Diphenhydramine"[TIAB] OR "Glycopyrrolate"[MH] OR "Glycopyrrolate"[TIAB] OR "Nitoman"[TIAB] OR "Procyclidine"[MH] OR "Procyclidine"[TIAB] OR "Robinul"[TIAB] OR "Symmetrel"[TIAB] OR "Tetrabenazine"[MH] OR "Tetrabenazine"[TIAB] OR "Trihexyphenidyl"[MH] OR "Trihexyphenidyl"[TIAB] OR "Xenazine"[TIAB] OR "beta blocker"[TIAB] OR "beta blockers"[TIAB] OR "beta adrenergic antagonist"[TIAB] OR "beta adrenergic antagonists"[TIAB] OR "beta adrenergic blocking"[TIAB] OR "beta adrenergic blocking agent"[TIAB] OR "beta adrenergic blocking agents"[TIAB] OR "adrenergic beta antagonists"[TIAB] OR "propranolol"[TIAB] OR "pindolol"[TIAB] OR "atenolol"[TIAB] OR "inderal"[TIAB] OR "muscarinic antagonists"[MeSH Terms] OR "adrenergic beta antagonists"[MeSH Terms] OR "amantadine"[MeSH Terms] OR "benztropine"[MeSH Terms] OR "diphenhydramine"[MeSH Terms] OR "trihexyphenidyl"[MeSH Terms] OR "propranolol"[MeSH Terms] OR "pindolol"[MeSH Terms] OR "atenolol"[MeSH Terms]	163,354
#2	Search "9-hydroxy-risperidone"[TIAB] OR "abilify"[TIAB] OR "antipsychotic agents"[MeSH Major Topic] OR "antipsychotic agents"[MeSH Terms] OR "antipsychotic"[TIAB] OR "antipsychotics"[TIAB] OR "aripiprazole"[NM] OR "aripiprazole"[TIAB] OR "Asenapine"[NM] OR "Asenapine"[TIAB] OR "Chlorpromazine"[MH] OR "Chlorpromazine"[NM] OR "Chlorpromazine"[TIAB] OR "Chlorprothixene"[MH] OR "Chlorprothixene"[NM] OR "Chlorprothixene"[TIAB] OR "Clopixol"[TIAB] OR "Clozapine"[MH] OR "clozapine"[NM] OR "clozapine"[TIAB] OR "clozaril"[TIAB] OR "Consta"[TIAB] OR "Droperidol"[MH] OR "droperidol"[NM] OR "droperidol"[TIAB] OR "Fanapt"[TIAB] OR "Fazaclo"[TIAB] OR "Fluanxol"[TIAB] OR "flupenthixol"[NM] OR "flupenthixol"[TIAB] OR "flupenthixol"[TIAB] OR "fluphenazine depot"[NM] OR "fluphenazine depot"[TIAB] OR "fluphenazine enanthate"[NM] OR "fluphenazine enanthate"[TIAB] OR "Fluphenazine"[MH] OR "Fluphenazine"[TIAB] OR "Geodon"[TIAB] OR "Haldol"[TIAB] OR "haloperidol decanoate"[NM] OR "haloperidol decanoate"[TIAB] OR "Haloperidol"[MH] OR "haloperidol"[NM] OR "haloperidol"[TIAB] OR "Iloperidone"[TIAB] OR "Inapsine"[TIAB] OR "Invega"[TIAB] OR "Largactil"[TIAB] OR "Loxapac"[TIAB] OR "Loxapine"[MH] OR "Loxapine"[NM] OR "Loxapine"[TIAB] OR "Loxitane"[TIAB] OR "Lurasidone"[TIAB] OR "Mellaril"[TIAB] OR "Mesoridazine"[MH] OR "Mesoridazine"[NM] OR "Mesoridazine"[TIAB] OR "Moban"[TIAB] OR "Modecate"[TIAB] OR "Molindone"[MH] OR "Molindone"[NM] OR "Molindone"[TIAB] OR "Navane"[TIAB] OR "olanzapine"[NM] OR "olanzapine"[TIAB] OR "Orap"[TIAB] OR "paliperidone palmitate"[NM] OR "Perphenazine"[MH] OR "Paliperidone"[TIAB] OR "Perphenazine"[NM] OR "Perphenazine"[TIAB] OR "Pimozide"[MH] OR "Pimozide"[NM] OR "Pimozide"[TIAB] OR "Prolixin"[TIAB] OR "quetiapine"[TIAB] OR "Relprevv"[TIAB] OR "Risperdal"[TIAB] OR "Risperidone"[MH] OR "Risperidone"[NM] OR "Risperidone"[TIAB] OR "Saphris"[TIAB] OR "Serentil"[TIAB] OR "Seroquel"[TIAB] OR "Stelazine"[TIAB] OR "Sustenna"[TIAB] OR "Symbyax"[TIAB] OR "Taractan"[TIAB] OR "Thioridazine"[MH] OR "Thioridazine"[NM] OR "Thioridazine"[TIAB] OR "Thiothixene"[MH] OR "Thiothixene"[NM] OR "Thiothixene"[TIAB] OR "Thorazine"[TIAB] OR "Trifluoperazine"[MH] OR "Trifluoperazine"[NM] OR "Trifluoperazine"[TIAB] OR "Trilafon"[TIAB] OR "Zeldox"[TIAB] OR "ziprasidone"[NM] OR "ziprasidone"[TIAB] OR "zuclopenthixol"[TIAB] OR "Zydis"[TIAB] OR "Zyprexa"[TIAB]	113,808
#3	Search "akathisia"[TIAB] OR "Akathisia, Drug-Induced"[MH] OR "drug induced parkinsonism"[TIAB] OR "Dyskinesia, Drug-Induced"[MH] OR "dystonic reaction"[TIAB] OR "dystonic reactions"[TIAB] OR "extrapyramidal reactions"[TIAB] OR "extrapyramidal side effect"[TIAB] OR "extrapyramidal side effects"[TIAB] OR "extrapyramidal signs"[TIAB] OR "extrapyramidal syndrome"[TIAB] OR "extrapyramidal syndromes"[TIAB] OR "Neuroleptic Malignant Syndrome"[MH] OR "neuroleptic malignant"[TIAB] OR "tardive dyskinesia"[TIAB] OR "tardive dystonia"[TIAB] OR "neuroleptic induced parkinsonism"[TIAB] OR "medication induced parkinsonism"[TIAB] OR "tardive akathisia"[TIAB]	16,341

ID	Search	Hits
#4	Search (("animals"[MeSH Major Topic] OR "animals"[MeSH Terms] OR "animal"[TIAB] OR "animals"[TIAB] OR "rat"[TIAB] OR "mouse"[TIAB] OR "mice"[TIAB] OR "rodent"[TIAB] OR "rodents"[TIAB] OR "rats"[TIAB]) NOT ("humans"[MAJR] OR "humans"[MH] OR "human"[TIAB] OR "humans"[TIAB]))	4,437,558
#5	Search "meta analysis"[TIAB] OR "meta analyses"[TIAB] OR "meta analytic"[TIAB] OR "metaanalysis"[TIAB] OR "metaanalysis"[TIAB] OR "systematic review"[TIAB] OR "systematic reviews"[TIAB] OR "meta analysis"[Publication Type] OR "randomized controlled trial"[PT] OR "randomised"[TIAB] OR "randomized"[TIAB] OR "randomisation"[TIAB] OR "randomization"[TIAB] OR "randomly"[TIAB] OR "placebo"[TIAB] OR "sham"[TIAB] OR "trial"[TIAB] OR "groups"[TIAB]	2,841,422
#6	Search "controlled clinical trial"[PT] OR "blinded"[TIAB] OR "case control"[TIAB] OR "clinical trial"[TIAB] OR "clinical trials"[TIAB] OR "Cohort Analysis"[TIAB] OR "cohort research"[TIAB] OR "cohort study"[TIAB] OR "cohort trial"[TIAB] OR "comparator group"[TIAB] OR "controlled studies"[TIAB] OR "controlled study"[TIAB] OR "controlled trial"[TIAB] OR "controlled trials"[TIAB] OR "double blind"[TIAB] OR "followup study"[TIAB] OR "longitudinal research"[TIAB] OR "longitudinal study"[TIAB] OR "longitudinal trial"[TIAB] OR "multicenter trial"[TIAB] OR "multicenter trials"[TIAB] OR "naturalistic research"[TIAB] OR "naturalistic study"[TIAB] OR "naturalistic trial"[TIAB] OR "prospective cohort"[TIAB] OR "prospective research"[TIAB] OR "prospective study"[TIAB] OR "prospective trial"[TIAB] OR "retrospective cohort"[TIAB] OR "retrospective research"[TIAB] OR "retrospective study"[TIAB] OR "retrospective trial"[TIAB] OR "single blind"[TIAB]	1,513,299
#7	Search (#1 AND #2) OR (#1 AND #3) OR (#2 AND #3)	15,146
#8	Search #7 NOT #4	11,508
#9	Search #8 AND (#5 OR #6)	3,156
#10	Search "english"[Language] AND #9	2,980

TABLE B–3. Strategy for Cochrane Library search on treatments for neurological side effects of antipsychotic medications

ID	Search	Hits
#1	"Akineton" OR "Amantadine" OR "Artane" OR "Atropine" OR "Benadryl" OR "Benztropine" OR "Biperiden" OR "bromocriptine" OR "Cogentin" OR "Dantrium" OR "Dantrolene" OR "Diphenhydramine" OR "Glycopyrrolate" OR "Procyclidine" OR "Robinul" OR "Symmetrel" OR "Tetrabenazine" OR "Trihexyphenidyl" OR "Xenazine" OR "beta blocker" OR "beta blockers" OR "beta adrenergic antagonist" OR "beta adrenergic antagonists" OR "beta adrenergic blocking" OR "beta adrenergic blocking agent" OR "beta adrenergic blocking agents" OR "adrenergic beta antagonists" OR "propranolol" OR "pindolol" OR "atenolol" OR "inderal":ti,ab,kw (Word variations have been searched)	21,056
#2	"9-hydroxy-risperidone" OR "abilify" OR "antipsychotic" OR "antipsychotics" OR "aripiprazole" OR "Asenapine" OR "Chlorpromazine" OR "Chlorprothixene" OR "Clopixol" OR "clozapine" OR "clozaril" OR "Consta" OR "droperidol" OR "Fanapt" OR "Fazaclo" OR "Fluanxol" OR "flupenthixol" OR "flupenthixol" OR "fluphenazine depot" OR "fluphenazine enanthate" OR "Fluphenazine" OR "Geodon" OR "Haldol" OR "haloperidol decanoate" OR "haloperidol" OR "Iloperidone" OR "Inapsine" OR "Invega" OR "Largactil" OR "Loxapac" OR "Loxapine" OR "Loxitane" OR "Lurasidone" OR "Mellaril" OR "Mesoridazine" OR "Moban" OR "Modecate" OR "Molindone" OR "Navane" OR "olanzapine" OR "Orap" OR "Paliperidone" OR "Perphenazine" OR "Pimozide" OR "Prolixin" OR "quetiapine" OR "Relprevv" OR "Risperdal" OR "Risperidone" OR "Saphris" OR "Serentil" OR "Seroquel" OR "Stelazine" OR "Sustenna" OR "Symbyax" OR "Taractan" OR "Thioridazine" OR "Thiothixene" OR "Thorazine" OR "Trifluoperazine" OR "Trilafon" OR "Zeldox" OR "ziprasidone" OR "zuclopenthixol" OR "Zydis" OR "Zyprexa"	16,885
#3	"akathisia" OR "drug induced parkinsonism" OR "dystonic reaction" OR "dystonic reactions" OR "extrapyramidal reactions" OR "extrapyramidal side effect" OR "extrapyramidal side effects" OR "extrapyramidal signs" OR "extrapyramidal syndrome" OR "extrapyramidal syndromes" OR "neuroleptic malignant" OR "tardive dyskinesia" OR "tardive dystonia" OR "neuroleptic induced parkinsonism" OR "medication induced parkinsonism" OR "tardive akathisia"	2,505
#4	(#1 and #2) OR (#1 and #3) OR (#2 and #3)	2,473
	Limited to Cochrane Reviews, Other Reviews and Trials	2,450

Full-text documents were then reviewed by one individual (L.J.F.) to determine whether they met eligibility criteria. For tardive dyskinesia, 12 systematic reviews were available, with 2 reviews of multiple treatment approaches and 1 review each related to anticholinergic medication, cholinergic medication, benzodiazepines, vitamin B_6, vitamin E, calcium channel blockers, γ-aminobutyric acid agonists, non-antipsychotic catecholaminergic drugs, miscellaneous treatments, and antipsychotic reduction or cessation. For akathisia, 3 recent systematic reviews were available, with 1 review each related to β-adrenergic blocking agents, anticholinergic agents, and mirtazapine. No additional RCTs or observational studies met inclusion criteria for other treatments of akathisia (e.g., benzodiazepines). For medication-induced parkinsonism, 1 systematic review was available, but evidence was insufficient to draw any definitive conclusions. For acute dystonia, 1 systematic review, 1 RCT, and 1 nonrandomized prospective study examined effects of anticholinergic medications in reducing the likelihood of acute dystonia; however, no studies meeting inclusion criteria examined use of anticholinergic agents as a treatment of acute dystonia. In addition, no studies meeting inclusion criteria were found that addressed treatment of neuroleptic malignant syndrome.

Appendix C.
Review of Research Evidence Supporting Guideline Statements

Assessment and Determination of Treatment Plan

STATEMENT 1: Assessment of Possible Schizophrenia

APA *recommends* **(1C)** that the initial assessment of a patient with a possible psychotic disorder include the reason the individual is presenting for evaluation; the patient's goals and preferences for treatment; a review of psychiatric symptoms and trauma history; an assessment of tobacco use and other substance use; a psychiatric treatment history; an assessment of physical health; an assessment of psychosocial and cultural factors; a mental status examination, including cognitive assessment; and an assessment of risk of suicide and aggressive behaviors, as outlined in APA's *Practice Guidelines for the Psychiatric Evaluation of Adults* (3rd edition).

Evidence for this statement comes from general principles of assessment and clinical care in psychiatric practice. Expert opinion suggests that conducting such assessments as part of the initial psychiatric evaluation improves diagnostic accuracy, appropriateness of treatment selection, and treatment safety. For additional details, see Guideline I, "Review of Psychiatric Symptoms, Trauma History, and Psychiatric Treatment History," Guideline II, "Substance Use Assessment," Guideline III, "Assessment of Suicide Risk," Guideline IV, "Assessment of Risk for Aggressive Behaviors," Guideline V, "Assessment of Cultural Factors," and Guideline VI, "Assessment of Medical Health," in the APA *Practice Guidelines for the Psychiatric Evaluation of Adults*, 3rd Edition (American Psychiatric Association 2016a). A detailed systematic review to support this statement is outside the scope of this guideline; however, less comprehensive searches of the literature did not yield any studies related to this recommendation in the context of schizophrenia treatment. Consequently, the strength of research evidence is rated as low.

Grading of the Overall Supporting Body of Research Evidence for Assessment of Possible Schizophrenia

On the basis of the limitations of the evidence for assessment of possible schizophrenia, no grading of the body of research evidence is possible.

STATEMENT 2: Use of Quantitative Measures

APA *recommends* **(1C)** that the initial psychiatric evaluation of a patient with a possible psychotic disorder include a quantitative measure to identify and determine the severity of symptoms and impairments of functioning that may be a focus of treatment.

Evidence for this statement comes from general principles of assessment and clinical care in psychiatric practice. Consequently, the strength of research evidence is rated as low. Expert opinion suggests that conducting such assessments as part of the initial psychiatric evaluation improves diagnostic accuracy, appropriateness of treatment selection, and longitudinal assessment of patient symptoms and treatment effects. This recommendation is also consistent with Guideline VII, "Quantitative Assessment," as part of the APA *Practice Guidelines for the Psychiatric Evaluation of Adults*, 3rd Edition (American Psychiatric Association 2016a).

Grading of the Overall Supporting Body of Research Evidence for Use of Quantitative Measures

On the basis of the limitations of the evidence for use of quantitative measures, no grading of the body of research evidence is possible.

STATEMENT 3: Evidence-Based Treatment Planning

APA *recommends* **(1C)** that patients with schizophrenia have a documented, comprehensive, and person-centered treatment plan that includes evidence-based nonpharmacological and pharmacological treatments.

Evidence for this statement comes from general principles of assessment and clinical care in psychiatric practice. A detailed systematic review to support this statement was outside the scope of this guideline; however, less comprehensive searches of the literature did not yield any studies that directly related to this recommendation in the context of schizophrenia treatment. Consequently, the strength of research evidence is rated as low. Nevertheless, in the bulk of the literature reviewed in the Agency for Healthcare Research and Quality (AHRQ) report (McDonagh et al. 2017), pharmacotherapy was included in all treatment arms in the studies of psychosocial interventions. Invariably, in studies of pharmacotherapies, some additional form of clinical intervention is incorporated into treatment and can include elements of patient education, supportive psychotherapy, and other brief interventions.

Grading of the Overall Supporting Body of Research Evidence for Evidence-Based Treatment Planning

On the basis of the limitations of the evidence for evidence-based treatment planning, no grading of the body of research evidence is possible.

Pharmacotherapy

STATEMENT 4: Antipsychotic Medications

APA *recommends* **(1A)** that patients with schizophrenia be treated with an antipsychotic medication and monitored for effectiveness and side effects.*

Evidence for this statement comes from the AHRQ review (McDonagh et al. 2017) as well as from other high-quality meta-analyses that examined findings from randomized controlled trials (RCTs) of antipsychotic medications in schizophrenia (Huhn et al. 2019; Leucht et al. 2017). The data from

---

*This guideline statement should be implemented in the context of a person-centered treatment plan that includes evidence-based nonpharmacological and pharmacological treatments for schizophrenia.

placebo-controlled trials are essential in making an initial determination of whether the benefits of antipsychotic medications outweigh the harms of antipsychotic medications. Placebo-controlled trial data as well as findings from head-to-head comparison studies and network analyses provide additional information on whether the benefits and harms of specific antipsychotic medications suggest preferential use (or nonuse) as compared with other antipsychotic medications. The strength of the research evidence is rated as high in demonstrating that the benefits of treatment with an antipsychotic medication outweigh the harms, although harms are clearly present and must be taken into consideration.

Primary evidence for placebo-controlled antipsychotic trial data came from the systematic review, Bayesian meta-analysis, and meta-regression conducted by Leucht et al. (2017), which included 167 studies (total $N = 28,102$) published from 1955 to 2016 that were randomized and double-blinded with placebo control groups. The authors excluded studies of acute treatment with short-acting intramuscular antipsychotic medications and relapse prevention (including studies of long-acting injectable [LAI] antipsychotic agents). Studies of clozapine were excluded because of possible superior efficacy, and studies conducted in China were excluded because of concerns about study quality. Studies were also excluded if subjects had primarily negative symptoms or significant comorbidity in either psychiatric or physical health conditions. The median study duration was 6 weeks, with almost all studies lasting 12 weeks or less in terms of primary study outcomes. None of the studies was focused on first-episode or treatment-resistant samples of subjects, and the mean illness duration was 13.4 years (standard deviation [SD] 4.7), with a mean subject age of 38.7 (SD 5.5). The number of studies available on each drug was highly variable, with chlorpromazine, haloperidol, olanzapine, and risperidone being most often studied, and limited information was available on some antipsychotic medications. Results are provided in Table C–1.

The authors found a moderate benefit of antipsychotic medications, with positive symptoms improving the most but improvements in negative symptoms, depression, quality of life, and social functioning also noted with treatment (Leucht et al. 2017). Side effects were also present but differed substantially among medications. The authors also found, however, that effect sizes for antipsychotic medications have decreased with time over the past 60 years. This seems to result from increasing placebo response rates rather than decreasing medication response, although the benefit of haloperidol as compared with placebo has decreased with time. Not surprisingly, these trends are likely to confound comparisons of newer versus older medications. Although industry sponsorship was associated with a lower effect size as compared with studies funded by other mechanisms, publication bias was observed because of the tendency to avoid publishing studies with no effect of treatment.

In the AHRQ review (McDonagh et al. 2017), few head-to-head comparison studies were available for most of the antipsychotic medications. In terms of functioning, the strength of evidence (SOE) was low. Older second-generation antipsychotics (SGAs; risperidone, olanzapine, quetiapine, ziprasidone) and paliperidone did not differ in terms of global functioning or employment rates, although social functioning with risperidone in an LAI formulation was better than with quetiapine in a single study (Rouillon et al. 2013). Measures of quality of life also showed no difference among older SGAs or between older SGAs and FGAs (specifically, haloperidol and perphenazine) on the basis of a low to moderate SOE.

In terms of response rates (McDonagh et al. 2017), there was no difference between haloperidol and risperidone (16 RCTs, $N=3,452$; relative risk [RR] 0.94, 95% confidence interval [CI] 0.87–1.02; moderate SOE), aripiprazole (5 RCTs, $N=2,185$; RR 1.01, 95% CI 0.76–1.34; low SOE), quetiapine (6 RCTs, $N=1,421$; RR 0.99, 95% CI 0.76–1.30; low SOE), and ziprasidone (6 RCTs, $N=1,283$; RR 0.98, 95% CI 0.74–1.30; low SOE). However, response with olanzapine was significantly better than with haloperidol (14 RCTs, $N=4,099$; RR 0.86, 95% CI 0.78–0.96; low SOE). In addition, a network meta-analysis of 46 head-to-head RCTs showed a significantly greater likelihood of response with olanzapine (odds ratio [OR] 1.71, 95% CI 1.11–2.68) and risperidone (OR 1.41, 95% CI 1.01–2.00) than quetiapine (low SOE). Olanzapine was also associated with higher remission rates as compared with haloper-

TABLE C–1. Results of meta-analysis on placebo-controlled trials of antipsychotic treatment

	Number of studies	Number of subjects	Measure	95% CI	I²	Comments
All studies	167	28,102				
Drug effect size	105	22,741	Mean effect size=0.47	0.42, 0.51	52%	
Any response with drug vs. placebo	97	20,690	Response ratio=1.93	1.72, 2.19		NNT=6
Good response	30	8,408	Response ratio=1.96	1.65, 2.44		NNT=8; 23% good response with antipsychotic vs. 14% with placebo
At least minimal response	46	8,918	Response ratio=1.75	1.59, 1.07		NNT=5; 51% minimal response with antipsychotic vs. 30% with placebo
Discontinuation for any reason	105	22,851	Risk ratio=1.25	1.20, 1.31		NNT=11; 38% discontinuation with antipsychotic vs. 56% with placebo
Discontinuation for inefficacy	94	23,017	Risk ratio=2.09	1.90, 2.32		NNT=7; 13% discontinuation with antipsychotic vs. 26% with placebo
Positive symptoms	64	18,174	SMD=0.45	0.40, 0.50	56%	
Negative symptoms	69	18,632	SMD=0.35	0.31, 0.40	42%	
Depression	33	9,658	SMD=0.27	0.20, 0.34	50%	
Quality of life	6	1,900	SMD=0.35	0.16, 0.51	43%	
Social functioning	10	3,077	SMD=0.34	0.21, 0.47	46%	
Use of antiparkinsonian medications	63	14,942	Risk ratio=1.93	1.65, 2.29		NNH=12; 19% with antipsychotic vs. 10% with placebo
Sedation	86	18,574	Risk ratio=2.80	2.30, 3.55	54%	14% with antipsychotic vs. 6% with placebo
Weight gain	59	15,219	SMD=−0.43	−0.55, −0.30	73%	
Prolactin increase	51	15,219	SMD=−0.43	−0.55, −0.30	91%	
QTc prolongation	29	9,833	SMD=−0.19	−0.29, −0.08	80%	

Abbreviations. CI=confidence interval; NNH=number needed to harm; NNT=number needed to treat; SMD=standardized mean difference.

Source. Data from Leucht et al. 2017.

idol (3 RCTs; pooled RR 0.65, 95% CI 0.45–0.94; I^2=54%; low SOE), but there was no difference in remission rates between haloperidol and ziprasidone (3 RCTs; RR 0.89, 95% CI 0.71–1.12; low SOE).

In terms of core illness symptoms (e.g., delusions, hallucinations, disorganized thinking), all SGAs that were studied were superior to placebo (standardized mean difference [SMD] –0.33 to –0.88; low SOE; McDonagh et al. 2017). Risperidone (21 RCTs, N=4,020; mean difference [MD] 3.24, 95% CI 1.62–4.86) and olanzapine (15 RCTs, N=4,209; MD 2.31, 95% CI 0.44–4.18) were associated with greater improvements in total Positive and Negative Syndrome Scale (PANSS) score as compared with haloperidol (moderate SOE), but no differences were noted in other comparisons of FGAs and SGAs (low SOE). With comparisons among SGAs, clozapine improved core illness symptoms more than other SGAs except for olanzapine (network meta-analysis of 212 RCTs; SMDs on PANSS or Brief Psychiatric Rating Scale [BPRS] –0.32 to –0.55; low SOE); olanzapine and risperidone improved core illness symptoms more than the other SGAs except for each other and paliperidone (SMDs –0.13 to –0.26; low SOE); and paliperidone improved core illness symptoms more than lurasidone and iloperidone (SMDs –0.17; low SOE).

For negative symptoms (McDonagh et al. 2017), haloperidol was less effective than olanzapine (5 RCTs, N=535; MD based on the Scale for the Assessment of Negative Symptoms scores 2.56, 95% CI 0.94–4.18; moderate SOE), aripiprazole (3 RCTs, N=1,701; MD 0.80, 95% CI 0.14–1.46), olanzapine (14 RCTs, N=3,742; MD 1.06, 95% CI 0.46–1.67), and risperidone (22 RCTs, N=4,142; MD 0.80, 95% CI 0.14–1.46), with the latter findings based on negative symptom scores of the PANSS and having a low SOE. Other comparisons of FGAs versus SGAs showed no effects on negative symptoms (low SOE).

In an additional network meta-analysis of 32 antipsychotic medications, Huhn et al. (2019) included 402 placebo-controlled and head-to-head randomized controlled trials that included a total of 53,463 adult participants with acute symptoms and a diagnosis of schizophrenia or a related disorder. Not included were studies that focused on individuals with a first episode of psychosis or treatment resistance and studies in which individuals had concomitant medical illnesses or a predominance of negative or depressive symptoms. For the majority of antipsychotic medications, treatment was associated with a statistically significant reduction in overall symptoms as compared with placebo, and there were few significant differences between individual drugs. With antipsychotic medications that did not differ significantly from placebo, there were numerical differences favoring the antipsychotic medication, and the number of subjects in the network meta-analysis was small, yielding a wide credible interval (CrI). Only clozapine, amisulpride, zotepine, olanzapine, and risperidone exhibited greater efficacy than many other antipsychotic medications for overall symptoms, with the greatest benefit noted with clozapine (SMD –0.89, 95% CrI –1.08 to –0.71). Discontinuation rates for inefficacy paralleled the findings for treatment efficacy (Huhn et al. 2019). In terms of positive symptoms, negative symptoms, and depressive symptoms, the majority of the medications showed a statistically significant difference from placebo, with the exception of several antipsychotic agents for which sample sizes were small and CrIs were wide. Few studies had assessed effects of antipsychotic medications on social functioning. As in the Leucht et al. (2017) meta-analysis, side-effect profiles differed considerably among the antipsychotic medications.

Few studies assessed effects of antipsychotic medications on self-harm, but among patients at high risk, the International Suicide Prevention Trial (InterSePT; Meltzer et al. 2003) found that clozapine was superior to olanzapine in preventing significant suicide attempts or hospitalization to prevent suicide (hazard ratio [HR] 0.76, 95% CI 0.58–0.97; low SOE).

In terms of dose-response effects on antipsychotic medication effectiveness, standard doses of antipsychotic medications are superior to low or very low dose treatment in reducing the risk of relapse (Uchida et al. 2011a). In addition, there is evidence of a dose-response relationship for many antipsychotic medications in short-term trials of acute efficacy (Davis and Chen 2004).

Overall discontinuation rates and time to discontinuation reflect whether a treatment is effective but also whether it is tolerable. In this regard, a network meta-analysis of 111 studies (McDonagh et al. 2017) found that rates of discontinuation were lower with the following medications:

- Olanzapine and clozapine as compared with asenapine, cariprazine, iloperidone, lurasidone, olanzapine LAI, quetiapine, risperidone, and ziprasidone (ORs range from 0.42 for clozapine vs. iloperidone to 0.69 for clozapine vs. risperidone)
- Clozapine as compared with monthly paliperidone palmitate LAI (OR 0.56, 95% CI 0.33–0.96)
- Olanzapine as compared with paliperidone (OR 0.67, 95% CI 0.50–0.89)
- Quetiapine extended release (XR) as compared with iloperidone, olanzapine LAI, or quetiapine (ORs 0.26–0.35)
- Risperidone and aripiprazole as compared with iloperidone or quetiapine (ORs 0.61–0.77).
- Risperidone and monthly aripiprazole LAI as compared with iloperidone (ORs 0.52 and 0.62, respectively)

Findings on time to discontinuation are more limited and need replication (low SOE), but they suggest that olanzapine may have a longer time to discontinuation than quetiapine, risperidone, and ziprasidone (4 months on the basis of trial data; 1.5–2.2 months shorter on the basis of observational data); clozapine may have a longer time to discontinuation than olanzapine, risperidone, or quetiapine (7.2–7.8 months in Phase 2E of the Clinical Antipsychotic Trials of Intervention Effectiveness [CATIE] study); and risperidone LAI may have a longer time to discontinuation than aripiprazole, clozapine, olanzapine, quetiapine, or ziprasidone (2.6–4 months).

A network meta-analysis (McDonagh et al. 2017), which used data from 90 head-to-head trials of greater than 6 weeks' duration, found the risk of withdrawals due to adverse events was less with the following medications:

- Risperidone LAI as compared with clozapine (OR 0.27, 95% CI 0.10–0.71), lurasidone (OR 0.39, 95% CI 0.18–0.84), quetiapine XR (OR 0.43, 95% CI 0.22–0.81), risperidone (OR 0.50, 95% CI 0.25–0.99), and ziprasidone (OR 0.40, 95% CI 0.20–0.82)
- Olanzapine as compared with clozapine (OR 0.39, 95% CI 0.19–0.79), lurasidone (OR 0.57, 95% CI 0.34–0.94), quetiapine (OR 0.62, 95% CI 0.44–0.87), risperidone (OR 0.72, 95% CI 0.55–0.96), and ziprasidone (OR 0.58, 95% CI 0.41–0.82)
- Aripiprazole as compared with clozapine (OR 0.43, 95% CI 0.21–0.88) and ziprasidone (OR 0.64, 95% CI 0.44–0.94)
- Cariprazine as compared with clozapine (OR 0.40, 95% CI 0.17–0.95)
- Iloperidone as compared with clozapine (OR 0.34, 95% CI 0.13–0.91)

These findings had a low SOE, and head-to-head comparison data were not available for all available antipsychotic medications. For haloperidol, withdrawals due to adverse events were significantly higher than with SGAs (moderate SOE), specifically, aripiprazole (8 RCTs, $N=3,232$; RR 1.25, 95% CI 1.07–1.47; $I^2=0\%$), olanzapine (24 RCTs, $N=5,708$; RR 1.89, 95% CI 1.57–2.27; $I^2=0\%$), risperidone (25 RCTs, $N=4,581$; RR 1.32, 95% CI 1.09–1.60; $I^2=0\%$), and ziprasidone (7 RCTs, $N=1,597$; RR 1.68, 95% CI 1.26–2.23; $I^2=0\%$).

Overall adverse event rates also favored SGAs as compared with haloperidol (moderate SOE), specifically aripiprazole (3 RCTs, $N=1,713$; RR 1.11, 95% CI 1.06–1.17; $I^2=0\%$), risperidone (8 RCTs, $N=1,313$; RR 1.20, 95% CI 1.01–1.42; $I^2=84\%$), and ziprasidone (6 RCTs, $N=1,448$; RR 1.13, 95% CI 1.03–1.23; $I^2=31\%$). Among comparisons between SGAs, no differences in overall adverse events were noted (low to moderate SOE).

In terms of mortality, comparisons were difficult because of the short duration of most studies and the small number of reported events in these clinical trials (incidence rates 0%–1.17%). Nevertheless, there were no significant mortality differences found between asenapine versus olanzapine (2 RCTs; RR 2.49, 95% CI 0.54–11.5; low SOE), quetiapine versus risperidone (2 RCTs; RR 3.24, 95% CI 0.72–14.6; low SOE), and paliperidone palmitate LAI (monthly) versus risperidone LAI (2 RCTs; RR 1.26, 95% CI 0.21–7.49; low SOE). Additional findings from retrospective cohort studies found no significant difference in the risk of all-cause (1 study, $N=48,595$) or cardiovascular (2 studies, $N=55,582$) mortality between risperidone, olanzapine, and quetiapine (low SOE).

For the additional harms data described in the AHRQ report (McDonagh et al. 2017), evidence was relatively limited and did not adjust for known factors that confound risk. Data on cardiac disease are mixed. A large, good-quality retrospective cohort study found no significant differences in the risk of cardiovascular death, acute coronary syndrome, or ischemic stroke between risperidone and olanzapine or quetiapine in patients ages 18–64 years within the first year of starting the drug. However, a large adverse event database study found that clozapine was significantly associated with myocarditis or cardiomyopathy, whereas olanzapine, quetiapine, and risperidone were not. In contrast, other limited evidence suggested an increased risk of cardiac arrest and arrhythmia with risperidone compared with clozapine, and data from CATIE suggested a higher estimated 10-year risk of coronary heart disease with olanzapine compared with risperidone. As compared with FGAs, the SGA aripiprazole showed a lower likelihood of cardiomyopathy or coronary heart disease.

Findings on neurological side effects such as akathisia and parkinsonism also showed significant variability among the head-to-head comparison studies, which makes it difficult to draw overall conclusions about side-effect rates or risk. For new-onset tardive dyskinesia, overall rates were low (3% of subjects treated with risperidone as compared with 1%–2% for other medications). Nevertheless, findings from observational trials suggested a significant increase in risk with risperidone as compared with olanzapine (OR 1.70, 95% CI 1.35–2.14).

Metabolic effects varied with study duration, but clinically important weight gain (defined as a 7% or more increase from baseline) was greater with olanzapine than with aripiprazole (RR 2.31), asenapine (RR 2.59), clozapine (RR 1.71), quetiapine (RR 1.82), risperidone (RR 1.81), and ziprasidone (RR 5.76) across 3.7–24 months. Olanzapine had a significantly greater risk of metabolic syndrome than risperidone (pooled OR 1.60, 95% CI 1.10–2.21; $I^2=0\%$; follow-up of 6 weeks to 3 months) or aripiprazole (pooled OR 2.50, 95% CI 1.32–4.76; $I^2=0\%$; follow-up of 3.5–12 months). In adults, observational evidence indicated an increased risk of new-onset diabetes with olanzapine compared with risperidone (OR 1.16, 95% CI 1.03–1.31). A single study found diabetic ketoacidosis to be increased with olanzapine compared with risperidone (OR 3.5, 95% CI 1.7–7.9), but a second study found no difference in diabetic ketoacidosis, hyperglycemia, or hyperglycemic hyperosmolar state between risperidone and olanzapine, regardless of age group, but a significantly lower risk with quetiapine compared with risperidone in older patients (adjusted HR 0.69, 95% CI 0.53–0.90).

Taken together, the findings of the AHRQ review (McDonagh et al. 2017) complement the meta-analyses of Leucht et al. (2017) and Huhn et al. (2019) in showing efficacy of antipsychotic medications, particularly for core illness symptoms but also for other outcomes. Furthermore, research evidence demonstrates no clear and consistent superiority of one antipsychotic medication as compared with other antipsychotic medications, with the exception of clozapine. In addition, the systematic reviews suggest considerable variability in side-effect profiles among antipsychotic medications, without a clear continuum of risk for individual medications when all side effects are considered.

Grading of the Overall Supporting Body of Research Evidence for Efficacy of Antipsychotic Medications

- **Magnitude of effect:** *Moderate.* The magnitude of effect varies among individual antipsychotic medications but is moderate overall on the basis of findings from meta-analyses of placebo-controlled trials.
- **Risk of bias:** *Medium.* Studies are RCTs that are summarized in multiple good-quality meta-analyses. Although the risk of bias of individual RCTs varies, most have some limitations, and, in older trials, reporting of study design features is often incomplete. Among head-to-head comparison trials, some studies are observational trials and are associated with a higher risk of bias.

- **Applicability:** The included trials all involve individuals with schizophrenia. Some studies also include individuals with other diagnoses such as schizoaffective disorder. The studies include subjects from countries around the world, with the exception of China. The doses of medication used are representative of usual clinical practice.
- **Directness:** *Direct.* Studies measure functioning, quality of life, core illness symptoms, negative symptoms, and response to treatment.
- **Consistency:** *Consistent.* When multiple studies that included a given comparison are available, results are generally consistent. In addition, the overall direction of effects is generally consistent among antipsychotic medications in placebo-controlled trials.
- **Precision:** *Variable.* For many comparisons, particularly when multiple RCTs are available, findings are precise. However, for other comparisons, imprecision is present because of wide confidence intervals that often cross the threshold for clinically significant benefit of the intervention.
- **Dose-response relationship:** *Present.* There is evidence of a dose-response relationship in acute treatment trials as well as in studies of antipsychotic medications for relapse prevention.
- **Confounding factors:** *Present.* In placebo-controlled trials, effect sizes have decreased over the past 60 years, apparently due to increases in placebo response rates; these trends are likely to confound comparisons of older and newer medications.
- **Publication bias:** *Suspected.* Among placebo-controlled trials, studies with no effect of treatment appear to have had lower rates of publication.
- **Overall strength of research evidence:** *High.* There are a large number of randomized, double-blind, placebo-controlled trials of antipsychotic medication as well as a smaller number of head-to-head comparison RCTs. Although many studies have a medium risk of bias and publication bias appears to be present, there is also consistency in overall study findings and a dose-response relationship is present, strengthening confidence in the conclusions.

Grading of the Overall Supporting Body of Research Evidence for Harms of Antipsychotic Medications

- **Magnitude of effect:** *Small to moderate.* The magnitude of effect for harms of antipsychotic medication differs by drug and by side effect but is small to moderate overall.
- **Risk of bias:** *Medium to high.* Studies are RCTs that are summarized in multiple good-quality meta-analyses. Particularly in older clinical trials, side effects tend not to be assessed or reported as systematically as efficacy and effectiveness-related outcomes.
- **Applicability:** The included trials all involve individuals with schizophrenia. Some studies also include individuals with other diagnoses such as schizoaffective disorder. The studies include subjects from around the world, with the exception of China. The doses of medication used are representative of usual clinical practice.
- **Directness:** *Variable.* Most studies measure overall adverse events, and some measure specific adverse effects, each of which is a direct measure. Other studies measure study withdrawal rates due to adverse effects, which is an indirect measure.
- **Consistency:** *Consistent.* In studies that compare the same medication with placebo, side effect–related outcomes are generally consistent in their direction and relative degree. Head-to-head comparison data are less consistent.
- **Precision:** *Precise.* Confidence intervals are narrow for comparisons in which multiple studies with good sample sizes are available. For comparisons with a small number of studies or small samples, imprecision is present because of wide confidence intervals. Head-to-head comparisons also have imprecision due to outcomes that cross the threshold for clinically significant harms of the intervention.
- **Dose-response relationship:** *Suspected.* There is less systematic information available on dose-response relationships for side effects of antipsychotic medication; however, the available evidence suggests that greater doses are associated with a greater degree of medication-related side effects.

- **Confounding factors:** *Present.* Cohort effects that are present in efficacy and effectiveness studies of antipsychotic medication are also likely to be relevant when assessing harms of antipsychotic medication.
- **Publication bias:** *Suspected.* Among placebo-controlled trials, studies with no effect of treatment appear to have had lower rates of publication.
- **Overall strength of research evidence:** *Moderate.* Available studies are RCTs that are generally of moderate quality and have good sample sizes. Findings are consistent, with narrow confidence intervals for many comparisons, and are likely to exhibit a dose-response relationship.

Antipsychotic Medications in First-Episode Schizophrenia

In subgroup analyses, the AHRQ review (McDonagh et al. 2017) found that patients experiencing a first episode of schizophrenia did not show significant differences in response or remission when treated with olanzapine, quetiapine, risperidone, ziprasidone, aripiprazole, or paliperidone. Another systematic review (Zhu et al. 2017) in individuals with a first episode of schizophrenia found that amisulpride, olanzapine, ziprasidone, and risperidone reduced overall symptoms more than haloperidol, but the evidence was noted as being of very low to moderate quality, and only 13 studies were available to address this clinical question.

Treatment Approaches to Partial Response or Nonresponse

High Doses of Antipsychotic Medication

A limited amount of evidence suggests no benefit from high doses of an antipsychotic medication in individuals who have not responded to typical doses of the medication. A systematic review and meta-analysis by Dold et al. (2015) found 5 trials, which included a total of 348 patients and studied this question with FGAs or SGAs. Dose escalation was not found to confer any benefits in terms of study attrition, response rates, or symptoms (as measured by PANSS or BPRS). A subsequent systematic review and meta-analysis by Samara et al. (2018) found 10 relevant RCTs, which included a total of 675 participants. Although no clear differences in response were noted between subjects who received the same dose of medication as compared with those who received a higher dose, many of the studies had a medium to high risk of bias. There were also no differences in other outcomes, including the proportion of individuals who left the study early because of adverse effects or for any reason.

Augmentation Pharmacotherapy

A number of pharmacotherapies have been studied as augmentation strategies in individuals with treatment-resistant schizophrenia. Evidence has been primarily from small short-term, open-label studies that have yielded mixed findings. Correll et al. (2017b) conducted a systematic search for meta-analyses that addressed the effects of combining an antipsychotic medication with another pharmacotherapy in individuals with schizophrenia. They found 29 meta-analyses that together encompassed 19,833 subjects in 381 trials and that evaluated 42 augmentation strategies. Although 14 of these augmentation therapies showed better outcomes than comparison treatment, the meta-analyses with the highest effect sizes had the lowest quality of included studies, undermining confidence in the benefits of augmentation.

In terms of augmentation of clozapine, Siskind et al. (2018) conducted a systematic review and meta-analysis of augmentation strategies for individuals with clozapine-refractory schizophrenia and found 46 studies of 25 interventions. They noted possible benefits of memantine for negative symptoms and aripiprazole, fluoxetine, and sodium valproate for overall psychotic symptoms but found that many of the studies had a poor study quality and short periods of follow-up, which limited the ability to draw conclusions. Wagner et al. (2019a) conducted a systematic meta-review of 21 meta-analyses that examined strategies for augmenting treatment with clozapine. Although the best evidence was available for combination treatment of clozapine with FGAs or SGAs for psychotic symptoms and with antidepressants for persistent negative symptoms, these authors also concluded that additional high-quality clinical trials are essential before making definitive statements about clozapine augmentation. Furthermore, their findings are consistent with those of Correll et al. (2017b), who did not identify any combination medication strategies with clozapine that led to better outcomes than comparator treatments and found that available studies were of low quality.

Other meta-analyses have also examined the effects of using more than one antipsychotic medication as compared with antipsychotic monotherapy. Galling et al. (2017) found a possible benefit of aripiprazole augmentation in terms of greater improvement in negative symptoms and reductions in prolactin levels and body weight. However, they noted that the apparent benefits of antipsychotic augmentation in reducing total symptoms were no longer seen when the analysis was restricted to double-blind trials of higher quality. A Cochrane review of antipsychotic combination treatments for schizophrenia (Ortiz-Orendain et al. 2017) also found that evidence on combinations of antipsychotic medications was of very low quality. Nevertheless, data from a large nationwide cohort study in Finland suggested that use of two different antipsychotic medications may have some benefits as compared with monotherapy. Tiihonen et al. (2019) studied 62,250 patients with a diagnosis of schizophrenia and compared hospitalization rates within the same individual during periods of antipsychotic monotherapy and periods with use of more than one antipsychotic medication. They found that rehospitalization rates with clozapine were lower than with other monotherapies and that individuals receiving more than one antipsychotic medication had a 7%–13% lower risk of psychiatric rehospitalization than individuals treated with monotherapy ($P<0.001$). Use of multiple antipsychotic medications was also associated with a reduction in secondary outcomes (e.g., all-cause hospitalization, nonpsychiatric hospitalization, mortality). Thus, there is weak and inconsistent evidence suggesting possible benefits of combined treatment with more than one antipsychotic medication, but more research is needed.

On the other hand, augmentation of antipsychotic therapy with an antidepressant medication may be helpful, particularly for patients with negative symptoms or depression. Stroup et al. (2019) used U.S. Medicaid data on 81,921 adult outpatients ages 18–64 years who had a diagnosis of schizophrenia. The authors employed propensity score matching and weighted Cox proportional hazards regression models to examine the effect of adding an antidepressant, a benzodiazepine, a mood stabilizer, or another antipsychotic medication to existing treatment with an antipsychotic medication. These authors found that the addition of an antidepressant medication was associated with a reduced risk for psychiatric hospitalization or emergency visits. In addition, Helfer et al. (2016) conducted a systematic review and meta-analysis of the addition of antidepressant medication to antipsychotic treatment. Data from 82 RCTs that included 3,608 subjects indicated that antidepressant augmentation was associated with improvements in quality of life (SMD –0.32, 95% CI –0.57 to –0.06) and rates of response (risk ratio 1.52, 95% CI 1.29–1.78; NNT=5, 95% CI 4–7) as well as greater reductions in depressive symptoms (SMD –0.25, 95% CI –0.38 to –0.12), positive symptoms (SMD –0.17, 95% CI –0.33 to –0.01), negative symptoms (SMD –0.30, 95% CI –0.44 to –0.16), and overall symptoms (SMD –0.24, 95% CI –0.39 to –0.09).

STATEMENT 5: Continuing Medications

APA *recommends* (1A) that patients with schizophrenia whose symptoms have improved with an antipsychotic medication continue to be treated with an antipsychotic medication.*

Evidence in support of this statement is based primarily on the evidence for antipsychotic efficacy in improving symptoms and quality of life as well as promoting functioning (see Statement 4 earlier in the appendix). Thus, the strength of research evidence is rated as high.

---

*This guideline statement should be implemented in the context of a person-centered treatment plan that includes evidence-based nonpharmacological and pharmacological treatments for schizophrenia.

Additional evidence supporting this statement comes from registry database studies and from discontinuation studies. For example, in a nationwide prospective registry study ($N=6{,}987$) with a 5-year follow-up of individuals with first-onset schizophrenia (Kiviniemi et al. 2013), there was a significant decrease in all-cause mortality in individuals taking SGAs as compared with individuals who were not taking antipsychotic medication (OR 0.69; $P=0.005$).

Another nationwide study ($N=8{,}719$) using prospectively collected registry data found that the lowest rates of rehospitalization or death occurred in individuals who received continuing treatment with an antipsychotic medication for up to 16.4 years (Tiihonen et al. 2018). Individuals who discontinued antipsychotic medication had a risk of death that was 174% higher than that in continuous users of antipsychotic medications (HR 2.74, 95% CI 1.09–6.89), whereas the risk of death was 214% higher (HR 3.14, 95% CI 1.29–7.68) in nonusers of antipsychotic medications as compared with continuous users. Rates of treatment failure, which included rehospitalization as well as death, were also lower in individuals who received continuous treatment with an antipsychotic medication. More specifically, 38% of those who discontinued treatment experienced treatment failure as compared with a matched group of continuous users of an antipsychotic medication, in which the rate of treatment failure was 29.3%. For nonusers of antipsychotic medication, treatment failure occurred in 56.5% as compared with 34.3% of a matched group of continuous antipsychotic medication users.

Several meta-analyses have examined mortality-related data with antipsychotic treatment. A meta-analysis of studies with follow-up periods of at least 1 year found that mortality was increased in individuals who did not receive antipsychotic medication as compared with those who were treated with an antipsychotic medication (pooled risk ratio 0.57, 95% CI 0.46–0.76; $P<0.001$ based on 22,141 deaths in 715,904 patient years in 4 cohort studies) (Vermeulen et al. 2017). With continuous treatment with clozapine, mortality was found to be lower in long-term follow-up (median 5.4 years) as compared with treatment with other antipsychotic medications (mortality rate ratio 0.56, 95% CI 0.36–0.85, $P=0.007$ based on 1,327 deaths in 217,691 patient years in 24 studies) (Vermeulen et al. 2019).

On the basis of 10 RCTs (total $N=776$) with mean study duration of 18.6 ± 5.97 months, a meta-analysis of discontinuation studies (Kishi et al. 2019) concluded that relapse rates were lower in individuals with schizophrenia who continued treatment with an antipsychotic medication as compared with those who discontinued treatment (RR 0.47, 95% CI 0.35–0.62; $P<0.00001$; $I^2=31\%$; NNT=3). An additional meta-analysis (Thompson et al. 2018), using somewhat different inclusion and exclusion criteria for studies, also found that relapse rates were lower in individuals who received maintenance treatment ($N=230$; 19%; 95% CI 0.05%–37%) as compared with those who stopped the antipsychotic medication ($N=290$; 53%; 95% CI 39%–68%). Although caution may be needed in interpreting these results because of methodological considerations (Moncrieff and Steingard 2019), the findings align with expert opinion on the benefits of maintenance treatment with an antipsychotic medication (Goff et al. 2017).

Grading of the Overall Supporting Body of Research Evidence for the Efficacy of Continuing Treatment With an Antipsychotic Medication

- **Magnitude of effect:** *Large.* The magnitude of effect is large in terms of lower relapse rates and lower mortality for individuals who received maintenance treatment with antipsychotic medications as compared with discontinuation of antipsychotic medication.
- **Risk of bias:** *Medium.* Studies include RCTs of antipsychotic discontinuation and observational studies using registry data. Although the registry studies have a greater risk of bias than RCTs, they use prospectively collected data and have good observational study designs.
- **Applicability:** The included trials all involve individuals with schizophrenia. Some studies also include individuals with other diagnoses such as schizoaffective disorder. The doses of medica-

tion used are representative of usual clinical practice. The observational studies include data from a nationwide registry and have broad generalizability, in contrast to RCTs with more restrictive inclusion and exclusion criteria. However, the applicability of registry data from Nordic countries may be reduced by differences in the health care delivery system as compared with that of the United States.

- **Directness:** *Direct*. Studies measured relapse rates and mortality.
- **Consistency:** *Consistent*. Findings showing benefits of maintenance antipsychotic treatment are consistent among the different studies and study designs.
- **Precision:** *Variable*. Most meta-analyses have narrow confidence intervals that do not cross the threshold for clinically significant benefit of treatment; however, some studies have wider confidence intervals.
- **Dose-response relationship:** *Not assessed*.
- **Confounding factors:** *Unclear*. It is possible that missing data or cohort-related effects may influence the results from multiyear registry databases. For long-term follow-up studies, which are needed to assess long-term effects of antipsychotic medication, loss of individuals to follow-up and changes in treatment over time may also confound data interpretation.
- **Publication bias:** *Not assessed*.
- **Overall strength of research evidence:** *High*. Available studies include RCTs with a medium risk of bias. These RCTs are complemented by prospective registry studies with very large sample sizes. Confidence intervals for most outcomes are relatively narrow, and findings are consistent in showing substantial benefit for continued antipsychotic medication treatment.

Grading of the Overall Supporting Body of Research Evidence for the Harms of Continuing Treatment With an Antipsychotic Medication

See Statement 4, subsection "Grading of the Overall Supporting Body of Research Evidence for Harms of Antipsychotic Medications," earlier in the appendix.

STATEMENT 6: Continuing the Same Medications

APA *suggests* **(2B)** that patients with schizophrenia whose symptoms have improved with an antipsychotic medication continue to be treated with the same antipsychotic medication.*

Evidence in support of this statement includes the evidence described for antipsychotic efficacy (see Statement 4 earlier in the appendix) and the evidence for continuing with antipsychotic treatment (see Statement 5 earlier in the appendix). Additional evidence that specifically addresses this guideline statement comes from randomized trials of a change in antipsychotic medication. On the basis of these studies, the strength of research evidence is rated as moderate.

The CATIE study provided important findings on medication changes (Essock et al. 2006). At the time of randomization, some individuals happened to be randomly assigned to a medication that they were already taking, whereas other individuals were assigned to a different antipsychotic medication. Individuals who were assigned to change to a different antipsychotic medication ($N=269$) had an earlier time to all-cause treatment discontinuation than those assigned to continue taking the same antipsychotic medication ($N=129$; Cox proportional HR 0.69; $P=0.007$). Although a change from olanzapine to a different antipsychotic medication was beneficial in terms of weight gain, there were no other differences in outcome measures for individuals who switched medications as compared with those who continued with the same treatment (Rosenheck et al. 2009).

---

*This guideline statement should be implemented in the context of a person-centered treatment plan that includes evidence-based nonpharmacological and pharmacological treatments for schizophrenia.

Additional evidence comes from an RCT aimed at reducing the metabolic risk of antipsychotic treatment by changing medication from olanzapine, quetiapine, or risperidone to aripiprazole (Stroup et al. 2011). Individuals were followed for 24 weeks after being assigned to continue taking their current medication (N=106) or to switch to aripiprazole (N=109). Although the two groups did not differ in the proportion of individuals with medication efficacy (as measured by the PANSS total score or change in Clinical Global Impression [CGI] severity score), individuals who switched medication were more likely to stop medication (43.9% vs. 24.5%; P=0.0019), and treatment discontinuation occurred earlier in those who switched medication as compared with those who did not (HR 0.456, 95% CI 0.285–0.728; P=0.0010). However, modest but statistically significant changes did occur in weight, serum non-high-density lipoprotein cholesterol, and serum triglycerides in individuals who switched to aripiprazole as compared with those who continued with olanzapine, quetiapine, or risperidone.

Together, these findings suggest that changes in antipsychotic medications may be appropriate for addressing significant side effects such as weight or metabolic considerations, but switching medications may also confer an increased risk of medication discontinuation, with associated risks of increased relapse and increased mortality.

Grading of the Overall Supporting Body of Research Evidence for the Efficacy of Continuing the Same Antipsychotic Medication

- **Magnitude of effect:** *Moderate.* Evidence from two RCTs suggests that a change in medication is associated with a moderate risk of earlier treatment discontinuation compared with continuing the same medication.
- **Risk of bias:** *Medium.* Studies are RCTs with a medium risk of bias based on their descriptions of randomization, blinding procedures, and study dropouts.
- **Applicability:** The included trials all involve individuals with schizophrenia. Some studies also include individuals with other diagnoses such as schizoaffective disorder. The studies were conducted in the United States. Doses of medication used are representative of usual clinical practice. The available RCTs examine changes in medication aimed at reducing metabolic effects of treatment, and a change from a high metabolic risk medication to a low metabolic risk medication may not be representative of other medication changes.
- **Directness:** *Indirect.* Studies measure all-cause treatment discontinuation, which combines effects due to inefficacy and lack of tolerability.
- **Consistency:** *Consistent.* The two studies are consistent in showing benefits of continuing with the same antipsychotic medication.
- **Precision:** *Precise.* Confidence intervals are narrow and do not cross the threshold for clinically significant benefit of the intervention.
- **Dose-response relationship:** *Not assessed.*
- **Confounding factors:** *Absent.*
- **Publication bias:** *Unable to be assessed.*
- **Overall strength of research evidence:** *Moderate.* The two RCTs that assess changing from one antipsychotic to another have good sample sizes and a medium risk of bias. Their findings are consistent with each other and with the results of studies discussed for Statements 4 and 5 on the benefits of antipsychotic medication treatment.

Grading of the Overall Supporting Body of Research Evidence for the Harms of Continuing the Same Antipsychotic Medication

See Statement 4, subsection "Grading of the Overall Supporting Body of Research Evidence for Harms of Antipsychotic Medications," earlier in the appendix.

Statement 7: Clozapine in Treatment-Resistant Schizophrenia

APA *recommends* **(1B)** that patients with treatment-resistant schizophrenia be treated with clozapine.*

Evidence on clozapine comes from multiple RCTs, observational studies (including clinical trials and studies using administrative databases), and meta-analyses. In some instances, the studies were limited to individuals with treatment-resistant schizophrenia, whereas in other studies a formal determination of treatment resistance was not reported or possible. Nevertheless, most information about clozapine will be of relevance to patients with treatment-resistant schizophrenia because, in current practice, most individuals receive clozapine only after a lack of response to other treatments.

In comparisons of SGAs, the AHRQ report (McDonagh et al. 2017) found that, independent of prior treatment history, clozapine improved core illness symptoms more than other SGAs (except for olanzapine) and was associated with a lower risk of suicide or suicide attempts than olanzapine, quetiapine, and ziprasidone (low SOE). In addition, in treatment-resistant patients, clozapine treatment was associated with a lower rate of treatment discontinuation due to lack of efficacy than the other SGAs that were studied. It is not clear whether rates of overall treatment discontinuation with clozapine may be influenced by the increased frequency of clinical interactions related to the more intensive monitoring with clozapine as compared with other antipsychotic medications.

The AHRQ review drew on several meta-analyses related to treatment-resistant schizophrenia (Ranasinghe and Sin 2014; Samara et al. 2016; Souza et al. 2013); however, some additional studies are also relevant to this guideline statement. A meta-analysis by Siskind et al. (2016b) had considerable overlap with the meta-analysis of Samara et al. (2016) in terms of the included studies. Despite this, the findings of the two meta-analyses were somewhat different, likely due to differences in the inclusion criteria and analytic approach (Samara and Leucht 2017). Samara et al. (2016) found few significant differences in outcomes and did not find clozapine to be significantly better than most other drugs in treatment-resistant schizophrenia. Siskind et al. (2016b) found no difference for clozapine compared with other antipsychotic medications in long-term studies but did find clozapine to be superior to other medications in short-term studies and across all studies in reducing total psychotic symptoms (24 studies, $N=1,858$; $P<0.005$). Similarly, in terms of response to treatment (as reflected by a 20%–30% reduction in symptoms), clozapine showed higher rates of response than comparators in short-term studies of treatment-resistant schizophrenia (8 studies, total $N=598$ for clozapine, 620 for comparators; RR 1.17, 95% CI 1.07–2.7; $P=0.03$; absolute risk reduction 12.48%, 95% CI 7.52–17.43; NNT=9). Again, however, studies that assessed long-term response showed no difference between clozapine and comparators. A greater benefit of clozapine than comparators was also seen when the analysis was limited to non-industry-funded trials (6 studies, $N=208$; RR 1.68, 95% CI 1.20–2.35; $P=0.002$). In a subsequent meta-analysis using data from the same studies, Siskind et al. (2017b) found that 40.1% of treatment-resistant individuals who received clozapine had a response, with a reduction of PANSS scores of 25.8% (22 points on the PANSS) from baseline.

In an additional network meta-analysis of 32 antipsychotic medications, Huhn et al. (2019) analyzed 402 placebo-controlled and head-to-head RCTs that included a total of 53,463 adult participants with acute symptoms and a diagnosis of schizophrenia or a related disorder. Studies that focused on individuals with a first episode of psychosis or treatment resistance were excluded, as were studies in which individuals had concomitant medical illnesses or a predominance of negative or depressive symptoms. Only clozapine, amisulpride, zotepine, olanzapine, and risperidone exhibited greater efficacy than many other antipsychotic medications for overall symptoms, with the greatest benefit

---

*This guideline statement should be implemented in the context of a person-centered treatment plan that includes evidence-based nonpharmacological and pharmacological treatments for schizophrenia.

noted with clozapine (SMD –0.89, 95% CrI –1.08 to –0.71). Clozapine also was statistically better than placebo and the majority of the other antipsychotic medications in terms of all-cause discontinuation (SMD 0.76, 95% CrI 0.59–0.92) and its effects on positive symptoms (SMD –0.64, 95% CrI –1.09 to –0.19), negative symptoms (SMD 0.62, 95% CrI –0.84 to –0.39), and depressive symptoms (SMD –0.52, 95% CrI –0.82 to –0.23).

Findings from studies using administrative databases also suggest benefits of treatment with clozapine. For example, a prospective nationwide study conducted over a 7.5-year period in Sweden (Tiihonen et al. 2017) found significantly reduced rates of rehospitalization with the use of clozapine as compared with no antipsychotic treatment (HR 0.53, 95% CI 0.48–0.58). In addition, the reduction in rehospitalization with clozapine was comparable to reductions in rehospitalization with LAI antipsychotic medications, whereas other oral formulations of antipsychotic medications had higher risks of rehospitalization. In comparison with oral olanzapine, clozapine had a lower rate of treatment failure (HR 0.58, 95% CI 0.53–0.63) that was comparable to the rate of treatment failure with LAI antipsychotic medications (range of HRs 0.65–0.80).

Similar benefits of clozapine were found in analysis of prospective registry data from Finland obtained for all persons with schizophrenia who received inpatient care from 1972 to 2014 (Taipale et al. 2018a). Of the 62,250 individuals in the prevalent cohort, 59% were readmitted during follow-up time of up to 20 years (median follow-up duration 14.1 years). Among oral antipsychotic medications, clozapine was associated with the lowest risk for psychiatric readmission compared with no antipsychotic use (HR 0.51, 95% CI 0.49–0.53) and for all-cause readmission (HR 0.60, 95% CI 0.58–0.61). For the 8,719 individuals with a first episode of schizophrenia, risks of psychiatric readmission and all-cause readmission were also reduced (HR 0.45, 95% CI 0.40–0.50 and HR 0.51, 95% CI 0.47–0.56, respectively).

A meta-analysis that examined effects of clozapine on hospital use also found benefits for clozapine (Land et al. 2017). Although the vast majority of studies in the meta-analysis were observational studies, use of clozapine as compared with other antipsychotic medications was associated with a significant decrease in the proportion of individuals who were hospitalized (22 studies, N=44,718; RR 0.74, 95% CI 0.69–0.80; P<0.001), although the time to rehospitalization did not differ.

In terms of suicide risk, subjects in the InterSePT study (Meltzer et al. 2003) who met criteria for treatment-resistant schizophrenia showed benefits of clozapine that were comparable to the benefits seen in the overall sample. For the sample as a whole, clozapine was superior to olanzapine in preventing significant suicide attempts or hospitalization to prevent suicide in high-risk patients (HR 0.76, 95% CI 0.58–0.97). Fewer clozapine-treated patients in the InterSePT study attempted suicide (P=0.03); required hospitalizations (P=0.05) or rescue interventions (P=0.01) to prevent suicide; or required concomitant treatment with antidepressants (P=0.01) or with anxiolytics or soporifics (P=0.03). Subjects treated with clozapine were also less likely to have CGI severity of suicidality scale ratings of "much worse" or "very much worse" (HR 0.78, 95% CI 0.61–0.99) than subjects treated with olanzapine.

In terms of mortality risk, a population-based cohort study of 2,370 patients with treatment-resistant schizophrenia found a higher rate of self-harm in individuals treated with non-clozapine antipsychotic medications than in those treated with clozapine (HR 1.36, 95% CI 1.04–1.78) (Wimberley et al. 2017). There was also a higher rate of all-cause mortality in patients not receiving clozapine than in those treated with clozapine (HR 1.88, 95% CI 1.16–3.05); however, the comparator group included individuals who were not taking any antipsychotic medication. When the study subjects were limited to those who were adhering to treatment, the higher mortality during treatment with other antipsychotic medications did not reach statistical significance. In the year after clozapine discontinuation, an increase in mortality was observed (HR 2.65, 95% CI 1.47–4.78), consistent with benefits of clozapine treatment in reducing overall mortality. Another cohort study also found significant benefits of clozapine on all-cause mortality in individuals with treatment-resistant schizophrenia (adjusted HR 0.61, 95% CI 0.38–0.97; P=0.04) (Cho et al. 2019). These findings are also consistent with results of a meta-analysis that showed significantly lower rates of long-term crude mortality in patients who received continuous treatment with clozapine as compared with patients treated with other antipsychotic medications (mortality rate ratio 0.56, 95% CI 0.36–0.85; $P=0.007$) (Vermeulen et al. 2019).

In terms of side effects with clozapine, a network meta-analysis conducted as part of the AHRQ report (McDonagh et al. 2017) showed that clozapine had a higher risk of study withdrawal due to adverse events than some other SGAs (low SOE) but did not show differences in overall rates of adverse events as compared with risperidone (low SOE). In the meta-analysis by Siskind et al. (2016b), individuals treated with clozapine had a higher likelihood of experiencing sialorrhea ($P<0.001$; number needed to harm [NNH]=4), seizures ($P<0.05$; NNH=17), tachycardia ($P<0.01$; NNH=7), fever ($P<0.01$; NNH=19), dizziness ($P<0.01$; NNH=11), sedation ($P<0.001$; NNH=7), constipation ($P<0.05$; NNH=12), and nausea or vomiting ($P<0.05$; NNH=19) than individuals treated with comparator antipsychotic medications. In the meta-analysis by Leucht et al. (2013), all-cause treatment discontinuation was less likely with clozapine than placebo (OR 0.46, 95% CI 0.32–0.65), as were extrapyramidal side effects (OR 0.3, 95% CI 0.17–0.62). In contrast, weight gain (SMD 0.65, 95% CI 0.31–0.99) and sedation (OR 8.82, 95% CI 4.72–15.06) were more likely with clozapine than placebo.

In an Australian national survey of 1,049 people with a diagnosis of schizophrenia or schizoaffective disorder who reported taking any antipsychotic medication (Siskind et al. 2017a), the proportion of individuals with diabetes, obesity, and metabolic syndrome was higher in individuals taking clozapine as compared with other antipsychotic medications (adjusted ORs 1.744, 1.899, and 2.300, respectively; $P<0.001$). In addition, clozapine was associated with a greater proportion of individuals with dry or watery mouth (adjusted OR 2.721; $P<0.001$), difficulty swallowing (adjusted OR 1.754; $P<0.01$), constipation (adjusted OR 1.996; $P<0.001$), dizziness/vertigo (adjusted OR 1.571; $P<0.01$), and palpitations (adjusted OR 1.543; $P<0.05$). The proportion of individuals who reported trembling or shaking was significantly less in those treated with clozapine as compared with other antipsychotic agents (adjusted OR 0.581; $P<0.01$).

In the network meta-analysis by Huhn et al. (2019), individuals treated with clozapine were less likely to require use of an antiparkinsonian medication (SMD 0.46, 95% CrI 0.19–0.88) than those treated with other antipsychotic agents or placebo. However, clozapine was associated with a greater degree of weight gain (SMD 2.37, 95% CrI 1.43–3.32), sedation (SMD 3.02, 95% CrI 2.52–3.37), and experiencing at least one anticholinergic side effect (SMD 2.21, 95% CrI 1.26–3.47) than placebo.

Grading of the Overall Supporting Body of Research Evidence for Efficacy of Clozapine in Treatment-Resistant Schizophrenia

- **Magnitude of effect:** *Moderate*. The magnitude of clozapine's effect varies with the study design and inclusion criteria. Some meta-analyses of RCTs show no difference for clozapine, but most studies show significant benefit, at least in the short term. Observational studies also show a magnitude of effect that is at least moderate.
- **Risk of bias:** *Medium*. Studies include RCTs and observational studies, primarily registry studies. Most studies have some limitations based on their descriptions of randomization, blinding procedures, and study dropouts.
- **Applicability:** The included trials all involve individuals with schizophrenia. Some studies also include individuals with other diagnoses such as schizoaffective disorder. Most individuals who receive treatment with clozapine have had at least one trial of another antipsychotic medication, and most would meet usual clinical criteria for treatment-resistant schizophrenia, even when this is not well specified in the study description. The doses of medication used are representative of usual clinical practice.
- **Directness:** *Variable*. Studies measure psychotic symptoms, response to treatment, all-cause treatment discontinuation, psychiatric hospitalization, all-cause hospitalization, depression,

and mortality. Some of these outcomes are directly related to the review questions, and some are indirectly related.

- **Consistency:** *Inconsistent.* Although most meta-analyses and observational studies show benefits for clozapine, not all meta-analyses show superiority of clozapine to other antipsychotic medications in individuals with treatment-resistant schizophrenia.
- **Precision:** *Variable.* Some confidence intervals are narrow without overlapping the threshold for clinically significant benefits, whereas other confidence intervals are wide or overlapping.
- **Dose-response relationship:** *Present.* Increases in dose and corresponding increases in blood levels of clozapine appear to be related to improved clinical efficacy in nontoxic ranges of dosing.
- **Confounding factors:** *Present.* Confounding factors may increase the observed effect. Additional monitoring and an increased frequency of clinical contacts with clozapine may enhance the effects of the medication relative to other antipsychotic medications, at least in observational studies.
- **Publication bias:** *Unclear.* Although publication bias for clozapine-specific studies was not tested, publication bias is relatively common in studies of psychopharmacology because of nonpublication of negative studies.
- **Overall strength of research evidence:** *Moderate.* The available studies include RCTs of moderate quality and good sample sizes. The effect sizes for clozapine vary among meta-analyses and outcomes. However, most studies, including RCTs and prospective observational studies, show benefits of clozapine as compared with other antipsychotic medications.

Grading of the Overall Supporting Body of Research Evidence for Harms of Clozapine

- **Magnitude of effect:** *Moderate.* The magnitude of effect is moderate overall but varies with the specific side effect. As compared with other antipsychotic medications, clozapine is associated with a greater risk of weight gain, sialorrhea, sedation, metabolic effects, seizures, constipation, anticholinergic side effects, tachycardia, and dizziness but a lower risk of all-cause treatment discontinuation, extrapyramidal side effects, or need for anticholinergic medication.
- **Risk of bias:** *Medium.* Studies include RCTs and a large observational study of patient-reported side effects. RCTs are of low to medium risk of bias based on their descriptions of randomization, blinding procedures, and study dropouts, whereas the observational study has a high risk of bias.
- **Applicability:** The included trials all involve individuals with schizophrenia. Some studies also include individuals with other diagnoses such as schizoaffective disorder. The doses of medication used are representative of usual clinical practice.
- **Directness:** *Variable.* Studies measure observed and reported side effects of clozapine, as well as treatment discontinuation (all cause and due to adverse effects).
- **Consistency:** *Consistent.* Study findings are consistent in the relative magnitude and direction of effects for specific side effects and for treatment discontinuation.
- **Precision:** *Precise.* Confidence intervals are narrow and do not cross the threshold for clinically significant benefit of the intervention.
- **Dose-response relationship:** *Not assessed.* However, clinical observations suggest that many side effects do increase in occurrence or severity with the dose of clozapine.
- **Confounding factors:** *Unclear.* Not all studies assess side effects in a systematic fashion, and patients may be less likely to report some side effects if they are not directly assessed.
- **Publication bias:** *Not assessed.* Nevertheless, publication bias is relatively common in studies of psychopharmacology because of nonpublication of negative studies.
- **Overall strength of research evidence:** *Low to moderate.* Available studies include RCTs and an observational study. Data from several meta-analyses suggest a moderate strength of research evi-

dence for outcomes related to clozapine harms, but the AHRQ review found a low strength of research evidence in a network meta-analysis, and the observational study also has a high risk of bias.

Other Interventions for Treatment-Resistant Schizophrenia

Use of Antipsychotic Medications Other Than Clozapine

The network analysis conducted as part of the AHRQ review (McDonagh et al. 2017) found that treatment-resistant patients had a small benefit with olanzapine over other older SGAs in core illness symptom improvement and negative symptoms, whereas response rates and all-cause treatment discontinuations were not different. Negative symptoms were also significantly reduced with olanzapine as compared with haloperidol ($N=2,207$; MD 1.28, 95% CI 0.11–2.44), and patients treated with ziprasidone showed better response than those treated with haloperidol ($N=120$; RR 1.54, 95% CI 1.19–2.00).

Electroconvulsive Therapy

Some studies have shown evidence for benefits of electroconvulsive therapy (ECT) in combination with antipsychotic medications. Pompili et al. (2013) conducted a systematic review that included RCTs and observational studies, including case-control studies, and concluded that ECT in combination with antipsychotic medications may be helpful for a subgroup of individuals who have treatment resistance, catatonia, aggression, or suicidal behavior, particularly when rapid improvement is needed.

Zheng et al. (2016) conducted a systematic review and meta-analysis of RCTs comparing antipsychotic medications other than clozapine with antipsychotic medication in combination with ECT in patients with treatment-resistant schizophrenia. In the 11 studies, which included 818 patients, the addition of ECT was associated with greater improvements in symptoms (SMD –0.67; $P<0.00001$) and greater rates of study-defined response (RR 1.48; $P<0.0001$; NNT=6) and remission (RR 2.18; $P=0.0002$; NNT=8) as well as greater rates of headache ($P=0.02$; NNH=6) and memory impairment ($P=0.001$; NNH=3).

In terms of ECT augmentation of clozapine in treatment-resistant schizophrenia, Petrides et al. (2015) conducted a randomized, single-blind, 8-week trial in which patients who had not responded to clozapine alone received a constant dose of clozapine or clozapine plus bilateral ECT (three times per week for 4 weeks and then twice weekly for 4 weeks for 20 total treatments). Fifty percent of the 20 patients treated with ECT plus clozapine experienced a reduction in psychotic symptoms of at least 40% and also achieved a CGI improvement rating of "much improved" and a CGI severity rating of "borderline mentally ill" or "not at all ill." This contrasts with 19 patients who received clozapine but not ECT in the randomized phase of the trial, none of whom showed response by these criteria. When the latter group of patients received ECT in the unblinded crossover phase of the trial, the rate of response was 47%. Global cognitive outcomes did not differ for the two randomized groups. In contrast, in another randomized trial of 23 patients who received 12 sessions of ECT as compared with sham ECT, no differences were found in PANSS score reductions, although both groups showed improvement during the study (Melzer-Ribeiro et al. 2017).

Lally et al. (2016b) conducted a systematic review and found 5 trials (4 open-label studies plus the study by Petrides and colleagues, with a total of 71 subjects) in which the pooled response rate to clozapine plus ECT was 54%. When cohort studies, nonblinded randomized trials, case series, and case reports were considered, the overall response rate for clozapine plus ECT was 76% (83 of 126 patients), even though clozapine doses and serum levels were relatively high (mean serum clozapine level of 772.6 ng/mL at a mean daily dose of 506.9 mg for the 52 patients with an available clozapine level; mean daily dose 412.3 mg for the sample as a whole).

G. Wang et al. (2018) conducted a systematic review and meta-analysis of RCTs of ECT augmentation of clozapine for clozapine-resistant schizophrenia that included Chinese and non-Chinese studies. Findings from 18 RCTs that included 1,769 subjects showed benefits of adjunctive ECT compared with clozapine alone for symptomatic improvement at post-ECT and endpoint assessments (SMD –0.88, $P=0.0001$ and SMD –1.44, $P<0.00001$, respectively). Significant benefits of adjunctive ECT were also seen in study-defined response rates and in remission rates at both assessments ($P<0.00001$, NNT=3 and NNT=4, respectively, for response and $P\leq0.0001$, NNT=13 and NNT=14, respectively, for remission); however, subjective memory issues and headache were more frequent in the group that received adjunctive ECT ($P<0.0001$, NNH=4 and $P=0.005$, NNH=8, respectively).

These studies and meta-analyses suggest a beneficial effect of ECT in combination with antipsychotic medication in individuals with treatment-resistant schizophrenia and clozapine-resistant schizophrenia despite the small number of studies and low quality of observational trials. The increases in reported rates of headache and memory impairment, however, suggest a need to weigh the potential benefits and risks of ECT for the individual patient as compared with the risks of treatment-resistant schizophrenia.

Transcranial Magnetic Stimulation in Treatment-Resistant Schizophrenia

Studies have also been done with transcranial magnetic stimulation (TMS) for treatment of hallucinations and for treatment of negative symptoms in individuals with schizophrenia. He et al. (2017) conducted a meta-analysis of studies published in English or Chinese that studied low (1 Hz) or high (10 Hz) frequency TMS in individuals with schizophrenia. In 13 studies of 1 Hz TMS, auditory hallucinations showed greater improvement with active TMS as compared with sham treatment, but publication bias was noted, and sensitivity analysis also indicated that the meta-analytic finding was unstable and likely to change with additional research. In 7 studies of 10 Hz TMS, there was no effect of active treatment on negative symptoms as compared with sham TMS.

Aleman et al. (2018) conducted a meta-analysis of studies of TMS applied to the dorsolateral prefrontal cortex as compared with sham TMS for treatment of negative symptoms and found a mean weighted effect size of 0.64 (0.32–0.96, total $N=827$); however, sham TMS showed a significant improvement of negative symptoms from baseline to posttreatment, with a mean weighted effect size of 0.31 (0.09–0.52, total $N=333$). Interpretation of the findings was also complicated by the use of several different coil placements (i.e., right, left, bilateral) and variability in other stimulation parameters (e.g., frequency, intensity, number of stimuli per session, duration of treatment). A meta-analysis by Dollfus et al. (2016) of 13 parallel design trials of TMS for treatment of auditory hallucinations in schizophrenia also showed a significant placebo effect, which was greatest with the 45° position coil and was viewed as introducing substantial bias in determining TMS efficacy.

In terms of addition of TMS to clozapine, Wagner et al. (2019b) used data from the TMS for the Treatment of Negative Symptoms in Schizophrenia (RESIS) trial and examined a subgroup of patients who received treatment with clozapine with the addition of active ($N=12$) or sham ($N=14$) TMS applied to the left dorsolateral prefrontal cortex for 3 weeks, with five treatment sessions per week. There was no effect of active TMS on negative symptoms, although there was significant benefit of TMS on secondary outcomes (i.e., PANSS positive symptom and general subscales; total PANSS).

These findings on benefits of TMS may change with further research using larger samples and rigorous study designs; however, at present, there is limited evidence for benefits of TMS in reducing either auditory hallucinations or negative symptoms, and findings are confounded by significant placebo effects and publication biases.

STATEMENT 8: Clozapine in Suicide Risk

APA *recommends* **(1B)** that patients with schizophrenia be treated with clozapine if the risk for suicide attempts or suicide remains substantial despite other treatments.*

---

*This guideline statement should be implemented in the context of a person-centered treatment plan that includes evidence-based nonpharmacological and pharmacological treatments for schizophrenia.

For individuals with schizophrenia who are at substantial risk for suicide, evidence on the use of clozapine comes from retrospective cohort studies and a large pragmatic, open-label RCT (N=980). Consequently, the strength of research evidence is rated as moderate.

On the basis of findings from the InterSePT study (Meltzer et al. 2003), the AHRQ report (McDonagh et al. 2017) concluded that clozapine was superior to olanzapine in preventing significant suicide attempts or hospitalization to prevent suicide in high-risk patients (HR 0.76, 95% CI 0.58–0.97; moderate SOE). Fewer clozapine-treated patients in the InterSePT study attempted suicide (P=0.03); required hospitalizations (P=0.05) or rescue interventions (P=0.01) to prevent suicide; or required concomitant treatment with antidepressants (P=0.01) or with anxiolytics or soporifics (P=0.03). Although there was not a significant difference in suicide deaths (5 for clozapine and 3 for olanzapine), Kaplan-Meier life table estimates indicated a significant reduction in the 2-year event rate in the clozapine group (P=0.02), with an NNT of 12. Data from other RCTs, in which suicide-related outcomes were reported as adverse events, showed very low event rates and no differences among antipsychotic medications.

One large retrospective study (Kiviniemi et al. 2013) used a nationwide registry to follow up with patients presenting with a first episode of schizophrenia (N=6,987). At 5 years, the risk of suicide in patients treated with clozapine was significantly reduced (OR 0.29, 95% CI 0.14–0.63), whereas suicide risk in those treated with risperidone, olanzapine, or quetiapine was comparable to the risk with no antipsychotic treatment. Another large nationwide study (N=9,567) of patients newly starting treatment with SGAs found lower rates of suicide attempts in those beginning with clozapine as compared with other drugs studied (Bitter et al. 2013). Suicide attempt rates were 1.1% at 1 year in those treated with clozapine in contrast to suicide attempt rates that ranged from 2.1% to 3.7% for other SGAs at 1 year. The suicide attempt rate with clozapine treatment was also reduced as compared with the 6 months prior to clozapine initiation (2.2% prior to clozapine as compared with 1.1% after clozapine initiation).

For a discussion of the evidence related to the side effects of clozapine, see Statement 7 earlier in the appendix.

Grading of the Overall Supporting Body of Research Evidence for Efficacy of Clozapine in Individuals With Substantial Risk Factors for Suicide Attempts or Suicide

- **Magnitude of effect:** *Moderate to large.* In the randomized controlled InterSePT study, moderate effects are present for clozapine as compared with olanzapine in reducing suicide attempts and hospitalizations to prevent suicide. As compared with other antipsychotic medications, larger effects of clozapine on suicide attempts and suicide are found in observational registry studies with longer periods of follow-up and larger sample sizes.
- **Risk of bias:** *Medium.* Studies include an RCT and observational studies. There is low risk of bias in the RCT on most outcomes but a medium to high risk of bias for the observational studies because of their lack of randomization, lack of blinding, and retrospective study design.
- **Applicability:** The included trials all involve individuals with schizophrenia. Some studies also include individuals with other diagnoses such as schizoaffective disorder. Doses of clozapine used in the RCT are representative of usual clinical practice. In addition, the RCT includes individuals with an increased risk of suicide, whereas the observational studies assessed suicide-related outcomes without preselecting for high-risk individuals. Nevertheless, rates of suicide are increased among individuals with schizophrenia, making the observational study findings of relevance to routine clinical practice.
- **Directness:** *Variable.* In the RCT, studies measured suicide attempts and deaths due to suicide, but mortality was infrequent, making statistical comparisons invalid. For the observational studies, suicide attempts and deaths from suicide were also studied. Nevertheless, observational study findings are indirect because of the lack of selection of patients at high risk of suicide.

- **Consistency:** *Consistent.* Reductions in suicide attempts are consistent in the RCT and in observational studies. The reduction in suicide deaths in larger samples with longer follow-up periods is consistent with the reduction in suicide attempts.
- **Precision:** *Precise.* Confidence intervals are narrow and do not cross the threshold for clinically significant benefit of the intervention.
- **Dose-response relationship:** *Not assessed.*
- **Confounding factors:** *Present.* In the RCT, effects on suicide deaths may be reduced by the need to intervene with increased monitoring, hospitalization, or study withdrawal if suicidal risk is significant. Additional monitoring and an increased frequency of clinical contacts with clozapine may enhance the effects of the medication relative to other antipsychotic medications, at least in observational studies.
- **Publication bias:** *Unable to be assessed.* The small number of relevant studies makes assessment of publication bias impossible.
- **Overall strength of research evidence:** *Moderate.* In terms of clozapine effects on suicidal behaviors and suicide, available studies include an RCT and several observational studies with large samples and long periods of follow-up. Confidence intervals are relatively narrow, and the findings are consistent.

Grading of the Overall Supporting Body of Research Evidence for Harms of Clozapine in Individuals With Substantial Risk Factors for Suicide Attempts or Suicide

See Statement 7, subsection "Grading of the Overall Supporting Body of Research Evidence for Harms of Clozapine," earlier in the appendix.

STATEMENT 9: Clozapine in Aggressive Behavior

APA *suggests* **(2C)** that patients with schizophrenia be treated with clozapine if the risk for aggressive behavior remains substantial despite other treatments.*

Evidence for the use of clozapine for individuals with substantial aggressive behavior is limited, and the strength of research evidence is rated as low. A systematic review on pharmacological management of persistent hostility and aggression in persons with schizophrenia spectrum disorders found 92 articles with sufficient methodological information to evaluate, although none were at low risk of bias (Victoroff et al. 2014). The authors found two studies (1 RCT, *N*=157; 1 open-label, *N*=44) showing that in inpatients with schizophrenia spectrum disorders, clozapine was superior to haloperidol in reducing scores on the Overt Aggression Scale (Conley et al. 2003; Ratey et al. 1993). Another RCT conducted in physically assaultive inpatients (*N*=100) also found clozapine to be superior to haloperidol or olanzapine in reducing scores on the Overt Aggression Scale (Krakowski et al. 2006, 2008). In reducing hostility (as measured by PANSS or BPRS hostility items), 4 RCTs (3 in inpatients, 1 in outpatients) reported superiority of clozapine as compared with FGAs. Two of these studies (*N*=48 and *N*=151) compared clozapine with chlorpromazine (Claghorn et al. 1987; Niskanen et al. 1974), and the other 2 studies (*N*=167 and *N*=71) compared clozapine with haloperidol (Citrome et al. 2001; Kane et al. 2001).

These findings support the opinions of many experts in viewing clozapine as beneficial in patients at substantial risk of aggressive behaviors. Nevertheless, additional evidence from well-designed clinical trials is needed. For a discussion of the evidence related to the side effects of clozapine, see Statement 7 earlier in the appendix.

---

*This guideline statement should be implemented in the context of a person-centered treatment plan that includes evidence-based nonpharmacological and pharmacological treatments for schizophrenia.

Grading of the Overall Supporting Body of Research Evidence for Efficacy of Clozapine in Individuals With Substantial Risk Factors for Aggressive Behaviors

- **Magnitude of effect:** *Unclear.* Available studies report statistical superiority, but there are no good estimates of the magnitude effect either within or among studies.
- **Risk of bias:** *High.* Most of the available studies, including RCTs and open-label studies, have a significant risk of bias and a lack of reported details about randomization, blinding, and other features of study design.
- **Applicability:** The included trials all involve individuals with schizophrenia. Some studies also include individuals with other diagnoses such as schizoaffective disorder. Most studies are focused on inpatients, including forensic psychiatry populations, who exhibit physically assaultive behavior. The doses of medication used are within normal to high dose ranges for usual clinical practice.
- **Directness:** *Variable.* Studies measure multiple different outcomes, including hostility items on PANSS or BPRS, time in restraint, episodes of restraint, and episodes of assaultive behavior.
- **Consistency:** *Consistent.* Studies generally report reductions in hostility or aggressive behavior.
- **Precision:** *Unknown.* Confidence intervals are not reported in all studies or in the available meta-analysis. Nevertheless, a lack of precision is likely due to the small samples in most studies.
- **Dose-response relationship:** *Not assessed.*
- **Confounding factors:** *Present.* In observational outpatient studies, additional monitoring and an increased frequency of clinical contacts with clozapine may enhance medication effects relative to other antipsychotic medications. The high risk of bias in many of these studies suggests that confounding factors may be present but unrecognized.
- **Publication bias:** *Unable to be assessed.* The relatively small number of studies and the heterogeneity of study designs make it difficult to assess publication bias. However, publication bias seems possible because of the tendency for negative clinical trial results to go unpublished.
- **Overall strength of research evidence:** *Low.* The available studies include RCTs and open-label studies with a high risk of bias. Although the findings are consistent, the applicability to typical clinical practice is limited. Other sources of possible bias were unable to be assessed but are likely to be present.

Grading of the Overall Supporting Body of Research Evidence for Harms of Clozapine in Individuals With Substantial Risk Factors for Aggressive Behaviors

See Statement 7, subsection "Grading of the Overall Supporting Body of Research Evidence for Harms of Clozapine," earlier in the appendix.

STATEMENT 10: Long-Acting Injectable Antipsychotic Medications

APA *suggests* **(2B)** that patients receive treatment with a long-acting injectable antipsychotic medication if they prefer such treatment or if they have a history of poor or uncertain adherence.*

---

*This guideline statement should be implemented in the context of a person-centered treatment plan that includes evidence-based nonpharmacological and pharmacological treatments for schizophrenia.

Evidence for this guideline statement comes from the AHRQ review (McDonagh et al. 2017) as well as from other RCTs, registry database studies, cohort studies, "mirror image" studies, and meta-analyses of such trials. The findings from these studies are mixed because RCTs show few differences in outcomes between LAI antipsychotic medications and oral antipsychotic agents, whereas observational trials show consistent benefits of LAI formulations. There are a number of possible explanations for these apparent disparities related to the design of the studies and differences in study populations (Correll et al. 2016; Fagiolini et al. 2017). Individuals who are agreeable to participating in a randomized clinical trial are more likely to be adherent to treatment than a broader population of individuals with a particular diagnosis. A greater focus on adherence-related questions and a greater frequency of visits may occur in an RCT as compared with treatment as usual, which may also influence adherence or outcomes. Consequently, the possible advantages of LAIs over oral formulations in promoting or assuring adherence may be less salient in RCTs as compared with observational trials. Although each type of study has advantages and disadvantages, observational trials that use registry databases are also able to examine outcomes among large numbers of individuals over many years of follow-up in contrast to the smaller numbers and shorter follow-up periods of RCTs.

In the AHRQ review (McDonagh et al. 2017), the ability to draw conclusions about the comparative effectiveness of LAI antipsychotic medications is limited by the relatively small number of head-to-head comparison studies among LAI antipsychotic medications or for LAI formulations as compared with oral agents. Few studies assessed differences in symptoms with treatment, but clozapine was noted to be superior to aripiprazole LAI (monthly or every 6 weeks), olanzapine LAI, paliperidone LAI (monthly and every 3 months), and risperidone LAI, whereas paliperidone LAI every 3 months was superior to oral lurasidone (low SOE). For the few comparisons where data on response were available, no differences were found (low SOE). Risperidone LAI was significantly better than quetiapine in social function over 24 months but did not differ from quetiapine on measures of quality of life (low SOE). No difference in social function was found between monthly paliperidone palmitate LAI and biweekly risperidone LAI (low SOE). In terms of quality of life, oral aripiprazole and monthly aripiprazole LAI did not differ from one another with up to 2 years of follow-up (low SOE).

In terms of findings on harms, a network meta-analysis of 90 head-to-head RCTs showed that risperidone LAI had a significantly lower risk of withdrawal due to adverse events than clozapine (OR 0.27, 95% CI 0.10–0.71), lurasidone (OR 0.39, 95% CI 0.18–0.84), quetiapine XR (OR 0.43, 95% CI 0.22–0.81), risperidone (OR 0.50, 95% CI 0.25–0.99), or ziprasidone (OR 0.40, 95% CI 0.20–0.82). No differences in overall adverse events were found between aripiprazole as compared with monthly aripiprazole LAI or between paliperidone or monthly paliperidone palmitate LAI as compared with risperidone LAI (low SOE). In addition, no differences in extrapyramidal side effects were seen in a 28-week trial of aripiprazole and monthly paliperidone LAI or a network meta-analysis comparing monthly and 4- to 6-week aripiprazole LAI. However, monthly aripiprazole LAI had a greater incidence of extrapyramidal side effects (RR 1.88) and worse akathisia than oral aripiprazole in the short term but not at 1 year. For mortality, no significant difference was found between monthly paliperidone palmitate LAI versus risperidone LAI (RR 1.26, 95% CI 0.21–7.49) on the basis of 2 RCTs of 4–24 months' duration (low SOE).

A number of other meta-analyses of RCTs are also available and provide complementary information to the findings in the AHRQ review. Ostuzzi et al. (2017) conducted a systematic review and meta-analysis of RCTs that compared the oral and LAI formulations of the same antipsychotic medication and included risperidone (6 studies), olanzapine (2 studies), aripiprazole (3 studies), zuclopenthixol (1 study), fluphenazine (7 studies), and haloperidol (2 studies). There was a small benefit for aripiprazole LAI (2 studies, $N=986$; RR 0.78, 95% CI 0.64–0.95; high SOE) as compared with oral aripiprazole for all-cause discontinuation, a small benefit for oral olanzapine as compared with olanzapine LAI for discontinuation due to inefficacy (2 studies, $N=1,445$; RR 1.52, 95% CI 1.12–2.07; low SOE), and a small benefit for risperidone LAI as compared with oral risperidone for hyperprolactinemia (5 studies, $N=891$; RR 0.81, 95% CI 0.68–0.98; moderate SOE). The other comparisons showed no differences for these outcomes, and there were also no differences noted for nonresponse rate, relapse rate, dropouts for adverse events, extrapyramidal symptoms, or weight gain.

Kishimoto et al. (2014) examined the relative efficacy of LAI antipsychotic medications as compared with oral antipsychotic medications in relapse prevention and found that LAIs were similar to oral agents in outpatient studies lasting ≥1 year (12 studies; RR 0.93, 95% CI 0.71–1.07; $P=0.31$) and at the longest study time point across all settings (21 studies, $N=4,950$; RR 0.93, 95% CI 0.80–1.08; $P=0.35$). When analyzed by drug, fluphenazine LAI showed greater benefit than oral antipsychotic agents in preventing relapse (RR 0.79, 95% CI 0.65–0.96; $P=0.02$); however, the authors note that this may be mediated by a cohort effect rather than a drug-specific effect because all of the fluphenazine studies predated 1992. For drug inefficacy, calculated as the sum of relapses plus discontinuations due to inefficacy, fluphenazine LAI was again superior to oral antipsychotic agents (8 studies, $N=826$; RR 0.78, 95% CI 0.66–0.91; $P=0.002$), whereas olanzapine LAI was inferior to oral antipsychotic agents ($N=1,445$; RR 1.52, 95% CI 1.12–2.07; $P=0.007$). In preventing hospitalization, fluphenazine LAI was also superior to oral antipsychotic agents (4 studies, $N=197$; RR 0.82, 95% CI 0.67–0.99, $P=0.04$); however, pooled data for LAIs as compared with oral antipsychotic agents showed no statistically significant effects (10 studies, $N=2,296$; RR 0.88, 95% CI 0.75–1.03; $P=0.09$). No differences in all-cause discontinuation were noted in pooled analyses or for individual LAIs (fluphenazine, haloperidol, zuclopenthixol, risperidone, olanzapine).

A separate meta-analysis (Kishi et al. 2016b) examined the efficacy of paliperidone LAI or risperidone LAI as compared with oral antipsychotic agents in patients with a recent-onset psychotic disorder. Although there was significant heterogeneity in the study findings, LAIs and oral agents were comparable overall in relapse prevention (3 studies; $N=875$). The LAIs did have fewer study discontinuations because of inefficacy (RR 0.34, NNT=−50) or nonadherence (RR 0.30, NNT=−33), but LAIs also had a higher incidence of tremor (RR 2.38) or at least one adverse effect (RR 1.13). In terms of mortality with LAIs as compared with oral antipsychotic agents, another meta-analysis of 52 RCTs (Kishi et al. 2016a) found no difference between LAIs and placebo or oral antipsychotics in all-cause death or death due to suicide (total $N=17,416$; LAI antipsychotics=11,360, oral antipsychotics=3,910, and placebo=2,146; LAI antipsychotics vs. placebo=28.9, LAI antipsychotics vs. oral antipsychotics=64.5).

Another RCT, the Preventing Relapse Oral Antipsychotics Compared to Injectables Evaluating Efficacy (PROACTIVE) study (P. F. Buckley et al. 2015), was a multisite trial conducted at 8 academic centers in the United States. The researchers randomly assigned patients with schizophrenia or schizoaffective disorder to risperidone LAI or the physician's choice of an oral SGA for up to 30 months. Subjects were outpatients who were neither resistant to treatment nor experiencing a first episode of psychosis. Approximately half of the subjects (161 of 305) discontinued treatment before the end of the trial. There was no significant difference noted in the proportion with a relapse (42% for risperidone LAI vs. 32% for oral SGA; $P=0.08$), time to first relapse ($P=0.13$), or time to first hospitalization ($P=0.30$). In addition, no significant differences between risperidone LAI and oral SGAs were noted for the bulk of symptom ratings (anxiety-depression, negative symptoms, excitement, affective flattening, avolition, asociality-anhedonia, CGI severity and CGI improvement). However, changes in symptom scores did differ between the treatment arms, with lower Scale for the Assessment of Negative Symptoms (SANS) alogia scores with oral SGAs and greater improvement in psychotic symptoms and BRPS total scores with risperidone LAI. In patients followed after an initial relapse, 32 (11%) had two relapses, and 13 (4%) had three relapses, with no significant differences in the rate or time to successive relapse between those treated with risperidone LAI and those treated with oral SGAs (Buckley et al. 2016).

In contrast to the findings from RCTs, observational studies often find benefits of LAI antipsychotic formulations as compared with oral antipsychotic formulations. Tiihonen et al. (2017) used a prospective national database in Sweden (with individuals as their own controls) to examine the risk of treatment failure, which was defined as psychiatric rehospitalization, admissions due to a suicide attempt, discontinuation of antipsychotic medication or switch to another antipsychotic medication, or death. Of the 29,823 patients, 43.7% were rehospitalized, and 71.7% met criteria for treatment failure. The LAI formulations of antipsychotic medications were associated with a 20%–30% lower risk of rehospitalization as compared with oral formulations of an antipsychotic (HR 0.78, 95% CI 0.72–0.84 for the total cohort; HR 0.68, 95% CI 0.53–0.86 for the incident cohort). For specific LAI antipsychotic medications as compared with no use of antipsychotic medication, rehospitalization risk was lowest with once-monthly paliperidone LAI (HR 0.51, 95% CI 0.41–0.64), zuclopenthixol LAI (HR 0.53, 95% CI 0.48–0.57), perphenazine LAI (HR 0.58, 95% CI 0.52–0.65), and olanzapine LAI (HR 0.58, 95% CI 0.44–0.77). Of the oral medications, rehospitalization rates were lowest with clozapine (HR 0.53, 95% CI 0.48–0.58). Rates of treatment failure were also lowest with clozapine (HR 0.58, 95% CI 0.53–0.63) and with LAI antipsychotic formulations as compared with other oral formulations (HR values for LAI formulations: perphenazine LAI 0.65, haloperidol LAI 0.67, zuclopenthixol LAI 0.69, paliperidone LAI 0.72, flupentixol LAI 0.75, olanzapine LAI 0.77, and risperidone LAI 0.80).

Tiihonen et al. (2011) also compared LAI antipsychotics with their equivalent oral formulation in a nationwide cohort of 2,588 consecutive patients in Finland who had an initial admission with a diagnosis of schizophrenia. Of those individuals, only 58.2% used an antipsychotic medication after discharge, and 45.7% of the cohort continued to take an antipsychotic for at least 30 days. For rehospitalization as well as for all-cause discontinuation, LAI antipsychotic had a lower adjusted hazard ratio (aHR) than the equivalent oral formulation (aHR 0.36, 95% CI 0.17–0.75; $P=0.007$ and aHR 0.41, 95% CI 0.27–0.61; $P=<0.0001$, respectively). For each LAI antipsychotic as compared with its oral equivalent, rehospitalization was lower with haloperidol LAI (aHR 0.12, 95% CI 0.01–1.13; $P=0.06$) but not perphenazine LAI (aHR 0.53, 95% CI 0.22–1.28; $P=0.16$) or risperidone LAI (aHR 0.57, 95% CI 0.30–1.08; $P=0.09$). Use of an LAI antipsychotic was also associated with lower rates of all-cause discontinuation for haloperidol LAI, perphenazine LAI, and risperidone LAI as compared with their oral equivalents (aHR 0.27, 95% CI 0.08–0.88; $P=0.03$; aHR 0.32, 95% CI 0.19–0.53; $P=<0.0001$; and aHR 0.44, 95% CI 0.31–0.62; $P=<0.0001$, respectively). Zuclopenthixol LAI showed no difference from its equivalent oral formulation in either rehospitalization or all-cause discontinuation.

Taipale et al. (2018a) used the same nationwide Finnish health care registry to assess the long-term effectiveness of antipsychotic medications on the risk of psychiatry rehospitalization over follow-up periods of up to 20 years (median of 14.1 years). The sample included a prevalence cohort of 62,250 individuals as well as 8,719 individuals who were followed prospectively after a first episode of psychosis. The risk of psychiatric rehospitalization was lower with LAI antipsychotic medications than with oral antipsychotic formulations (LAI FGAs HR 0.46, 95% CI 0.40–0.54; LAI SGAs HR 0.45, 95% CI 0.39–0.52; oral FGAs HR 0.67, 95% CI 0.60–0.74; oral SGAs HR 0.57, 95% CI 0.53–0.61) in first-episode patients, as was the risk of all-cause hospitalization (LAI FGAs HR 0.58, 95% CI 0.51–0.66; LAI SGAs HR 0.56, 95% CI 0.50–0.63; oral FGAs HR 0.80, 95% CI 0.74–0.87; oral SGAs HR 0.69, 95% CI 0.66–0.73), with similar patterns noted in the prevalence cohort.

A nationwide registry was also used by Taipale et al. (2018b) to examine all-cause mortality and its relationship to medication treatment among patients with schizophrenia in Sweden. Information was available on 29,823 individuals between 2006 and 2013, of which 4,603 patients were in the incident cohort. For LAI SGAs, the cumulative mortality rate was about one-third lower than the mortality rate for equivalent oral antipsychotics in pairwise analyses (aHRs 0.67, 95% CI 0.56–0.80). Those taking an LAI formulation of an SGA had the lowest cumulative mortality (7.5%), with median follow-up of 6.9 years. Corresponding rates of cumulative mortality were 8.5% for oral SGAs, 12.2% for oral FGAs, 12.3% for LAI FGAs, and 15.2% in those who were not taking an antipsychotic medication. As compared with LAI SGAs, corresponding aHRs were 1.52 (95% CI 1.13–2.05) for oral SGAs, 1.37 (95% CI 1.01–1.86) for LAI FGAs, 1.83 (95% CI 1.33–2.50) for oral FGAs, and 3.39 (95% CI 2.53–4.56) in those who were not taking an antipsychotic medication.

MacEwan et al. (2016b) used a multistate database of U.S. Medicaid patients to examine the probability of rehospitalization after an index admission with LAI antipsychotic treatment as compared with oral antipsychotic treatment. Using multivariate logistic regression with propensity score matching for 1,450 patients with a diagnosis of schizophrenia, an LAI antipsychotic medication was associated with a lower probability of readmission at 60 days postdischarge (adjusted OR 0.60, 95% CI 0.41–0.90) but not at 30 days postdischarge.

Kishimoto and colleagues conducted meta-analyses of cohort studies and mirror image studies to compare the effectiveness of LAIs versus oral antipsychotic agents in terms of hospitalization and treatment discontinuation (Kishimoto et al. 2013, 2018). On the basis of 42 prospective and retrospective cohort studies (total $N=101,624$; mean follow-up 18.6 ± 10.0 months), LAIs were found to be superior to oral antipsychotics in terms of all-cause discontinuations (10 studies, $N=37,293$; risk ratio 0.78, 95% CI 0.67–0.91; $P=0.001$) and hospitalization rates (15 studies, 68,009 person-years; rate ratio 0.85, 95% CI 0.78–0.93; $P<0.001$) but not hospitalization risk or days of hospitalization (Kishimoto et al. 2018). However, the patients treated with an LAI antipsychotic medication had longer illness durations than those treated with oral formulations of antipsychotic medication, which may have influenced the findings. In 25 mirror image studies that followed patients for at least 6 months before and after a transition between medication formulations, LAI antipsychotic medications were superior to oral antipsychotic medications in preventing hospitalization (16 studies, $N=4,066$; risk ratio 0.43, 95% CI 0.35–0.53; $P<0.001$) and in decreasing the number of hospitalizations (15 studies, 6,342 person-years; rate ratio 0.38, 95% CI 0.28–0.51; $P<0.001$) (Kishimoto et al. 2013).

Grading of the Overall Supporting Body of Research Evidence for the Efficacy of LAI Antipsychotic Medications

- **Magnitude of effect:** *Variable*. In RCTs, there are few differences in outcomes between LAI and oral formulations of antipsychotic medications. However, significant benefits with a moderate magnitude of effect are noted in observational studies, including prospective registry database studies and mirror image studies.
- **Risk of bias:** *Medium*. Studies include RCTs that have some limitations in study design or reporting of features such as randomization or blinding. Observational studies based on prospective registry data are well designed but have at least a medium risk of bias because of a lack of randomization or blinding.
- **Applicability:** The included trials all involve individuals with schizophrenia. Some studies also include individuals with schizoaffective disorder. The doses of medication used are not always stated but appear to be representative of usual clinical practice. The observational studies include data from a nationwide registry and have broad generalizability, in contrast to RCTs with more restrictive inclusion and exclusion criteria. However, the applicability of registry data from Nordic countries may be reduced by differences in the health care delivery system as compared with that of the United States.
- **Directness:** *Variable*. Most studies measure direct outcomes, including differences in symptoms, quality of life, functioning, relapse prevention, and rehospitalization. However, some studies assess indirect outcomes, including all-cause treatment discontinuation.
- **Consistency:** *Inconsistent*. RCTs generally show little or no benefit of LAI as compared with oral formulations of antipsychotic medications, whereas observational studies show moderate benefits. However, findings are consistent for different types of observational studies, including prospective registry database studies and mirror image analyses.
- **Precision:** *Imprecise*. For RCTs, confidence intervals cross the threshold for clinically significant benefit of the intervention.
- **Dose-response relationship:** *Not assessed*.
- **Confounding factors:** *Unclear*. Confounding factors may be present for the observational studies because of the lack of randomization. Individuals with poor adherence or more severe symptoms may be more likely to receive an LAI, which would give LAI-treated patients a greater risk of relapse or rehospitalization.

- **Publication bias:** *Not suspected.* Publication bias was not detected in the meta-analyses that specifically examined this question.
- **Overall strength of research evidence:** *Moderate.* Available evidence includes data from several types of observational studies, each of which shows consistent benefits for LAI as compared with oral formulations of antipsychotic medication. The potential benefit of LAI formulations in assuring adherence may not be observable in RCTs in which patients are already selected for high adherence. Although trials are of varying quality, most have good sample sizes. When beneficial effects are noted, most confidence intervals are narrow. There is some variation from drug to drug, but registry data show better outcomes with LAI formulations as a group as compared with oral formulations of antipsychotic medication as a group.

Grading of the Overall Supporting Body of Research Evidence for the Harms of LAI Antipsychotic Medications

- **Magnitude of effect:** *Variable.* In general, there appear to be few differences between harms of LAI antipsychotic medications and oral formulations of antipsychotic medications, particularly when LAI and oral formulations of the same drug are compared. When differences are noted in rates of specific side effects, the magnitude of those effects is small.
- **Risk of bias:** *Medium.* In RCTs, some limitations in study design are present. In other studies, harms of treatment were not systematically assessed.
- **Applicability:** The included trials all involve individuals with schizophrenia. Some studies also include individuals with other diagnoses such as schizoaffective disorder. The doses of medication used are not always stated but appear to be representative of usual clinical practice. The observational studies include data from a nationwide registry and have broad generalizability, in contrast to RCTs with more restrictive inclusion and exclusion criteria. However, the applicability of registry data from Nordic countries may be reduced by differences in the health care delivery system as compared with that of the United States.
- **Directness:** *Variable.* When assessments of adverse effects are conducted, studies measure specific side effects. However, other studies measure study withdrawals due to adverse effects.
- **Consistency:** *Inconsistent.* Some comparisons show differences between LAI and oral formulations on specific side effects, but these are not consistent among medications or meta-analyses.
- **Precision:** *Imprecise.* Confidence intervals cross the threshold for clinically significant benefit of the intervention.
- **Dose-response relationship:** *Not assessed.* Data from studies of oral medications suggest that increases in dose are likely to be associated with increases in medication side effects.
- **Confounding factors:** *Unclear.* Adverse effects are not always assessed in a systematic fashion, and reporting biases may be present.
- **Publication bias:** *Not suspected.* Publication bias was not detected in the meta-analyses that specifically examined this question.
- **Overall strength of research evidence:** *Low.* Available studies include RCTs that assess side effects of LAI and oral formulations of antipsychotic medications. Meta-analyses and network meta-analyses are also available that include head-to-head comparison trials. In terms of ascertainment and reporting of information on side effects, studies have at least a medium risk of bias, and there is significant inconsistency in the findings among the available studies, making it difficult to draw conclusions with any degree of confidence.

STATEMENT 11: Anticholinergic Medications for Acute Dystonia

APA *recommends* **(1C)** that patients who have acute dystonia associated with antipsychotic therapy be treated with an anticholinergic medication.

This recommendation is based on expert opinion and is supported by studies of the prophylactic use of anticholinergic medications to reduce the risk of acute dystonia in the initial phases of antipsychotic therapy. The strength of research evidence for this guideline statement is rated as low. No studies were found that specifically examined the treatment of acute dystonia with anticholinergic medications in a randomized or controlled manner, although intramuscular administration of an anticholinergic agent is widely viewed as the treatment of choice for acute dystonia associated with antipsychotic therapy (Stanilla and Simpson 2017).

Information on the use of anticholinergic medications to prevent acute dystonia associated with antipsychotic therapy comes from a review of 9 studies (Arana et al. 1988), of which 4 were randomized, blinded trials (total $N=232$); 2 were open trials (total $N=856$); and 3 were retrospective studies (total $N=278$). On the basis of data from all of these studies, prophylactic use of an anticholinergic medication was associated with 1.9-fold reduction in risk of acute dystonia (14.8% without prophylaxis vs. 7.7% with prophylaxis). In patients who received a high-potency antipsychotic agent (e.g., haloperidol), the benefits of prophylactic anticholinergic medication were even more pronounced (5.4-fold reduction in risk; 46.8% without prophylaxis vs. 8.7% with prophylaxis).

A subsequent study of consecutive psychiatric admissions ($N=646$) showed a lower rate of acute dystonia in patients who received anticholinergic prophylaxis (8.5% without anticholinergic prophylaxis vs. 2.8% with anticholinergic prophylaxis), and rates of acute dystonia were greater in individuals treated with a high-potency antipsychotic agent (Spina et al. 1993). A small double-blind RCT ($N=29$) showed a decrease in acute dystonia associated with antipsychotic therapy in patients who received benztropine as compared with placebo, but the results did not reach statistical significance (Goff et al. 1991). These studies suggest therapeutic effects of anticholinergic medications in acute dystonia associated with antipsychotic therapy, and although the studies were conducted in patients who received FGAs, they likely would also apply to acute dystonia when it occurs with use of SGAs.

Grading of the Overall Supporting Body of Research Evidence for Anticholinergic Medications for Acute Dystonia

On the basis of the limitations of the evidence for anticholinergic medications for acute dystonia, no grading of the body of research evidence is possible.

STATEMENT 12: Treatments for Parkinsonism

APA *suggests* **(2C)** the following options for patients who have parkinsonism associated with antipsychotic therapy: lowering the dosage of the antipsychotic medication, switching to another antipsychotic medication, or treating with an anticholinergic medication.

This statement is based on expert opinion, and, consequently, the strength of research evidence is rated as low. Knowledge of pharmacology and pharmacokinetics suggests that side effects such as parkinsonism may be diminished by reducing the dose of a medication or changing to a medication with a different side-effect profile and a lesser propensity for treatment-related parkinsonism. Clinical experience also suggests that an anticholinergic medication can be used to treat antipsychotic-associated parkinsonism (Stanilla and Simpson 2017). A good-quality systematic review assessed the use of anticholinergic medication compared with placebo for parkinsonism associated with antipsychotic therapy (Dickenson et al. 2017). Although many studies of anticholinergic treatment for parkinsonism were conducted decades ago and suggested benefits of anticholinergics, few of these studies met the systematic review's inclusion criteria. In addition, sample sizes in the two included studies were small, and no definitive conclusions could be drawn from the systematic review.

Grading of the Overall Supporting Body of Research Evidence for Treatments for Parkinsonism

On the basis of the limitations of the evidence for treatments for parkinsonism, no grading of the body of research evidence is possible.

STATEMENT 13: Treatments for Akathisia

APA *suggests* (2C) the following options for patients who have akathisia associated with antipsychotic therapy: lowering the dosage of the antipsychotic medication, switching to another antipsychotic medication, adding a benzodiazepine medication, or adding a beta-adrenergic blocking agent.

This statement is based on expert opinion, and, consequently, the strength of research evidence is rated as low. Knowledge of pharmacology and pharmacokinetics suggests that side effects such as akathisia may be diminished by reducing the dose of a medication or changing to a medication with a different side-effect profile and a lesser propensity for treatment-related akathisia. A good-quality systematic review identified some benefits of benzodiazepines for akathisia associated with antipsychotic therapy (Lima et al. 2002), but only 2 studies (total $N=27$) met the inclusion criteria. Another good-quality systematic review assessed the use of β-adrenergic blocking agents in akathisia and also found insufficient evidence to draw conclusions about therapeutic benefits (3 RCTs, total $N=51$; Lima et al. 2004). In addition, no reliable evidence was found to support or refute the use of anticholinergic agents as compared with placebo for akathisia associated with antipsychotic therapy (Rathbone and Soares-Weiser 2006). The literature search did not identify well-designed trials published after these systematic reviews that shed additional light on any of these treatment approaches.

Grading of the Overall Supporting Body of Research Evidence for Treatments for Akathisia

On the basis of the limitations of the evidence for treatments for akathisia, no grading of the body of research evidence is possible.

STATEMENT 14: VMAT2 Medications for Tardive Dyskinesia

APA *recommends* (1B) that patients who have moderate to severe or disabling tardive dyskinesia associated with antipsychotic therapy be treated with a reversible inhibitor of the vesicular monoamine transporter 2 (VMAT2).

This statement is based on information from a good-quality systematic review (Solmi et al. 2018b) on deutetrabenazine and valbenazine treatment; information on tetrabenazine comes from less robust clinical trials. The strength of research evidence for this guideline statement is rated as moderate.

For deutetrabenazine, data were available from 2 double-blind, placebo-controlled RCTs (Anderson et al. 2017; Fernandez et al. 2017) that enrolled subjects with moderate to severe tardive dyskinesia. Each trial lasted 12 weeks, and the dosage of deutetrabenazine was 12–48 mg/day. Treatment with deutetrabenazine was associated with a significant decrease in total Abnormal Involuntary Movement Scale (AIMS) scores ($N=413$; SMD –0.40, 95% CI –0.19 to –0.62, $P<0.001$; weighted mean difference [WMD] –1.44, 95% CI –0.67 to –2.19, $P<0.001$) and significantly greater rates of response (defined as an AIMS score reduction of at least 50%; RR 2.13, 95% CI 1.10–4.12, $P=0.024$; NNT=7, 95% CI 3–333, $P=0.046$) (Solmi et al. 2018b). The rate of treatment response increased with treatment duration during the open-label extension phase of the study (Hauser et al. 2019). Deutetrabenazine was well tolerated, with trial completion rates and rates of adverse effects similar to rates with placebo (Solmi et al. 2018b).

For valbenazine, data were available from 4 double-blind, placebo-controlled trials (total $N=488$) of 4–6 weeks each using a valbenazine dosage of 12.5–100 mg/day in individuals with moderate to severe tardive dyskinesia (Citrome 2017b; Correll et al. 2017a; Factor et al. 2017; Hauser et al. 2017; Josiassen et al. 2017; Kane et al. 2017; O'Brien et al. 2015). Treatment with valbenazine was associated with a significant decrease in total AIMS scores ($N=421$; SMD –0.58, 95% CI –0.26 to –0.91, $P<0.001$; WMD –2.07, 95% CI –1.08 to –3.05, $P<0.001$) and significantly greater rates of response (RR 3.05, 95% CI 1.81–5.11, $P<0.001$; NNT=4, 95% CI 3–6, $P<0.001$; Solmi et al. 2018b). With valbenazine, as with deutetrabenazine, the rate of treatment response increased with treatment duration during the open-label extension phase of the study (Factor et al. 2017). Furthermore, in the randomized KINECT 3 study, a dose-response relationship was observed, with greater benefit at dosages of 80 mg/day as compared with 40 mg/day (Hauser et al. 2017). Valbenazine was well tolerated, with trial completion rates and rates of adverse effects that were similar to rates with placebo (Solmi et al. 2018b).

For tetrabenazine, prospective placebo-controlled data are more limited and include a single-blind trial of 20 subjects (Ondo et al. 1999), a double-blind crossover trial of 6 subjects (Godwin-Austen and Clark 1971), and another double-blind crossover trial of 24 subjects (Kazamatsuri et al. 1972). Although benefits of tetrabenazine were seen at dosages of up to 150 mg/day, the quality of evidence is not sufficient to draw robust conclusions or conduct meta-analyses (Leung and Breden 2011; Solmi et al. 2018b). Adverse effects that were more frequent with tetrabenazine than placebo included drowsiness, sedation or somnolence, parkinsonism, insomnia, anxiety, depression, and akathisia.

Although this statement specifically relates to the use of a reversible inhibitor of the vesicular monoamine transporter 2 (VMAT2) (e.g., deutetrabenazine, tetrabenazine, valbenazine), the guideline writing group also reviewed evidence for other possible treatments for tardive dyskinesia. Amantadine has been mentioned in the literature as a treatment for tardive dyskinesia, but evidence for its use is extremely limited. One randomized double-blind crossover trial (Angus et al. 1997) included only 16 patients and had significant attrition. Another randomized double-blind crossover trial (Pappa et al. 2010) also had a small sample ($N=22$), and the period of treatment was only 2 weeks. Thus, data from these trials are insufficient to support use of amantadine for treatment of tardive dyskinesia. Other studies of treatments for tardive dyskinesia have been discussed in systematic reviews, as summarized in Table C–2. On the basis of these findings, there is insufficient evidence to support a guideline statement on use of these treatments in individuals with tardive dyskinesia.

Intervention	Reference	Comments
Anticholinergic agents	Bergman and Soares-Weiser 2018	2 trials (total $N=30$) had very low-quality evidence
Benzodiazepines	Bergman et al. 2018a	4 trials (total $N=75$) of very low-quality evidence showed no clinically significant difference relative to placebo
Calcium channel blockers	Soares-Weiser and Rathbone 2011	No studies met inclusion criteria
Cessation or reduction of antipsychotic	Bergman et al. 2018b	2 trials (total $N=17$) had very low-quality evidence
Change to clozapine	Mentzel et al. 2018	In 4 trials (total $N=48$), subjects who had clinically significant tardive dyskinesia showed improvement with a change to clozapine (standardized mean change –2.56, 95% CI –4.85 to –0.28; $P=0.02$), which is consistent with observational data (Lieberman et al. 1991; Naber et al. 1989; Pinninti et al. 2015)
Cholinergic medication	Tammenmaa-Aho et al. 2018	Low-quality evidence showed no clinically important improvement in tardive dyskinesia symptoms (4 trials; $N=27$) or effect on deterioration of tardive dyskinesia symptoms (8 trials; $N=147$) when compared with placebo
Gamma-aminobutyric acid agonists	Alabed et al. 2018	Low-quality evidence showed no clinically important improvement in tardive dyskinesia symptoms (5 trials; $N=36$), and a greater rate of side effects and attrition was suggested
Ginkgo biloba extract	Soares-Weiser et al. 2018b	1 trial ($N=157$) showed benefit compared with placebo (RR 0.88, 95% CI 0.81–0.96) in a moderate-quality study, but this requires replication
Non-antipsychotic catecholaminergic drugs	El-Sayeh et al. 2018	10 trials ($N=261$) showed very low-quality evidence, and there were only 1–2 trials per therapeutic comparison
Vitamin B$_6$ (pyridoxal 5'-phosphate)	Adelufosi et al. 2015	In 3 trials (total $N=80$), inpatients followed for 9–26 weeks showed significant improvement in tardive dyskinesia symptoms when compared with placebo, but evidence was of low quality, with wide CIs
Vitamin E	Soares-Weiser et al. 2018a	13 trials (total $N=478$) of low quality showed possible blunting of additional deterioration but no clear difference when compared with placebo in terms of clinically important improvement
Miscellaneous agents, including branched-chain amino acids, buspirone, dihydrogenated ergot alkaloids, estrogen, γ-linolenic acid, insulin, isocarboxazid, lithium, melatonin, pemoline, promethazine, ritanserin, and selegiline	Soares-Weiser et al. 2018b	In 1–2 short-term trials (total $N=10–52$ for each medication), low- to very low-quality evidence was inconclusive

Abbreviations. CI=confidence interval; RR=relative risk.

Grading of the Overall Supporting Body of Research Evidence for Efficacy of VMAT2 Inhibitors

- **Magnitude of effect:** *Moderate.* Effects are at least moderate in terms of the proportion of individuals who are much improved or very much improved with valbenazine or deutetrabenazine as compared with placebo. Statistically significant differences are also found for rates of response and for decreases in total AIMS scores. Fewer data are available for tetrabenazine, and its magnitude of effect is unclear.
- **Risk of bias:** *Low to medium.* Studies are RCTs with a low to medium risk of bias based on their descriptions of randomization, blinding procedures, and study dropouts.
- **Applicability:** The included trials all involve individuals with moderate to severe tardive dyskinesia, although some studies include individuals with diagnoses other than schizophrenia. The doses of medication used are representative of usual clinical practice.
- **Directness:** *Direct.* Studies measure changes in signs of tardive dyskinesia on the AIMS and proportions of individuals who showed at least 50% response or who were much improved or very much improved on a global measure of benefit.
- **Consistency:** *Consistent.* Studies are consistent in showing benefits of valbenazine and deutetrabenazine. Studies of tetrabenazine are more limited in number, sample size, and design but also show benefit in individuals with tardive dyskinesia.
- **Precision:** *Imprecise.* Confidence intervals are wide but do not cross the threshold for clinically significant benefit of the intervention.
- **Dose-response relationship:** *Present.* Valbenazine and deutetrabenazine show an increase in clinical benefit with an increase in dose.
- **Confounding factors:** *Unclear.* No specific confounding factors are noted for valbenazine or deutetrabenazine, but confounding factors may be present for tetrabenazine because of weaknesses in study methodologies.
- **Publication bias:** *Unable to be assessed.* The small number of available studies precludes assessment of publication bias.
- **Overall strength of research evidence:** *Moderate.* The available studies of valbenazine and deutetrabenazine are of good quality with good sample sizes. However, not all confidence intervals are narrow. In addition, the duration of the randomized phase of the trials was relatively short, as little as 4–6 weeks in some studies. The long-term follow-up data are based only on open-label extension phases of these RCTs. Data on tetrabenazine have a higher risk of bias, smaller samples sizes, and inadequate blinding, yielding a low strength of research evidence.

Grading of the Overall Supporting Body of Research Evidence for Harms of VMAT2 Inhibitors

- **Magnitude of effect:** *Minimal to small.* For deutetrabenazine and valbenazine, there are no significant differences from placebo in rates of adverse effects. For tetrabenazine, some adverse effects are more frequent than with placebo, but the magnitude of the difference is still relatively small.
- **Risk of bias:** *Medium to high.* Studies of valbenazine and deutetrabenazine determine adverse events in a systematic fashion, but the duration of the randomized phase of the clinical trials is relatively short, and the open-label extension phases have a greater risk of bias. Studies of tetrabenazine have a greater number of limitations in study design, with a high risk of bias overall.
- **Applicability:** The included trials all involve individuals with moderate to severe tardive dyskinesia, although some studies include individuals with diagnoses other than schizophrenia. The doses of medication used are representative of usual clinical practice.
- **Directness:** *Direct.* Studies measure occurrence of specific side effects.

- **Consistency:** *Variable.* Studies of deutetrabenazine and valbenazine are consistent in showing negligible side effects as compared with placebo. Studies of tetrabenazine generally show greater rates of some side effects than placebo.
- **Precision:** *Imprecise.* Confidence intervals cross the threshold for clinically significant benefit of the intervention.
- **Dose-response relationship:** *Not assessed.* Although effects of dose on side effects were not evaluated, dose-response relationships are noted for efficacy of valbenazine and deutetrabenazine.
- **Confounding factors:** *Unclear.* No specific confounding factors are noted for valbenazine or deutetrabenazine, but confounding factors may be present for tetrabenazine because of weaknesses in the study methodologies.
- **Publication bias:** *Unable to be assessed.* The small number of available studies precludes assessments of publication bias.
- **Overall strength of research evidence:** *Low.* Available studies of valbenazine and deutetrabenazine include RCTs of short duration, as well as longer-term open-label follow-up phases. Findings for these medications are consistent in showing no apparent difference in side effects relative to placebo. For tetrabenazine, studies have significant limitations and a high risk of bias but show more frequent side effects than placebo. Overall, studies are generally applicable to individuals with moderate to severe tardive dyskinesia, including individuals with a diagnosis of schizophrenia.

Psychosocial Interventions

STATEMENT 15: Coordinated Specialty Care Programs

APA *recommends* **(1B)** that patients with schizophrenia who are experiencing a first episode of psychosis be treated in a coordinated specialty care program.*

This recommendation is based on evidence from four clinical trials as presented in the AHRQ review (McDonagh et al. 2017) as well as an additional study (Anderson et al. 2018) that showed reduced mortality at 2 years for those who had participated in an early intervention program. The strength of research evidence for this statement is rated as moderate on the basis of the moderate SOE found for multiple key outcomes.

Many studies of coordinated specialty care programs were not included in the AHRQ review, although there is a long history of using such programs worldwide for early identification and treatment of attenuated psychosis syndrome, related syndromes of high psychosis risk, or first-episode psychosis (J. Addington et al. 2017; Cotton et al. 2016; Malla and McGorry 2019); however, these programs were not within the scope of this guideline recommendation because they include individuals who do not have a psychiatric diagnosis or who have diagnoses other than schizophrenia at later follow-up times (Fusar-Poli et al. 2016; Iorfino et al. 2019). Only one of the studies in a meta-analysis of early intervention programs (Marshall and Rathbone 2011) was included in the AHRQ analysis; all other studies were excluded because of such factors as small sample size, enrollment of inpatients, lack of applicability to the U.S. population, and/or use of a one-off intervention.

Pooled results from studies of individuals with a first episode of psychosis (McDonagh et al. 2017) found that up to 2 years of treatment with a coordinated specialty care program was associated with higher global functioning based on Global Assessment of Functioning (GAF) and Global Assessment Scale scores (3 RCTs; WMD 3.88, 95% CI 0.91–6.85; moderate SOE), significantly more

---

*This guideline statement should be implemented in the context of a person-centered treatment plan that includes evidence-based nonpharmacological and pharmacological treatments for schizophrenia.

people working or in school (3 RCTs; RR 1.22, 95% CI 1.01–1.47; moderate SOE), significantly higher ratings of quality of life (2 RCTs; effect size 0.84, 95% CI 0.14–1.55; moderate SOE), and a greater rate of retention in treatment (RR 1.27, 95% CI 1.16–1.38; Cochran's Q=0.03, degrees of freedom=1; high SOE) as compared with usual care. Coordinated specialty care program participants were also less likely to relapse compared with those in usual care (2 RCTs; RR 0.64, 95% CI 0.52–0.79; moderate SOE). These treatment effects were not sustained and had generally dissipated by 5 years after treatment discontinuation. In addition, as compared with usual care, there were no significant effects of coordinated specialty care programs on housing status (2 RCTs; low SOE), self-harm (N=506; RR 0.93, 95% CI 0.06–14.81), or total PANSS scores (3 RCTs; WMD –2.53, 95% CI –5.45 to 0.39; low SOE).

One study (Bertelsen et al. 2007; Nordentoft et al. 2002; Secher et al. 2015) found no differences in rates of accidental death (RR 0.31, 95% CI 0.01–7.59) or unexplained death (RR 0.31, 95% CI 0.01–7.56) at 2 years and no difference in mortality at 10-year follow-up (RR 0.92, 95% CI 0.45–1.88) between individuals who received a coordinated specialty care intervention as compared with usual care. In contrast, in an early intervention program for psychosis in Ontario, Canada (Anderson et al. 2018), rates of self-harm behavior (HR 0.86, 95% CI 0.18–4.24) and suicide (HR 0.73, 95% CI 0.29–1.80) did not differ during the initial 2 years after enrollment as compared with usual care, but rates of all-cause mortality were lower in the coordinated specialty care intervention group (HR 0.24, 95% CI 0.11–0.53; absolute risk reduction 2.5%; NNT=40). As compared with those who received usual care, individuals in the coordinated specialty care program also saw a psychiatrist more rapidly (user median days=13 compared with nonuser median days=78), were more likely to have contact with a psychiatrist (HR 6.05, 95% CI 5.30–6.91), and were more likely to be hospitalized (HR 1.42, 95% CI 1.18–1.71) but were less likely to have emergency department visits (HR 0.71, 95% CI 0.60–0.83) or primary care contacts (HR 0.46, 95% CI 0.41–0.52).

Grading of the Overall Supporting Body of Research Evidence for Efficacy of Coordinated Specialty Care Programs

- **Magnitude of effect:** *Moderate.* CSC programs are associated with significant benefits in terms of retention in treatment, with smaller benefits on quality of life, functioning, and relapse reduction.
- **Risk of bias:** *Medium.* Studies are RCTs with a medium risk of bias based on their descriptions of randomization, blinding procedures, and study dropouts.
- **Applicability:** The included trials all involve individuals with schizophrenia as well as individuals with a first episode of psychosis in the context of other diagnoses. In usual practice, coordinated specialty care programs follow the same model as research programs and would be expected to be comparable.
- **Directness:** *Direct.* Studies measure core illness symptoms, functioning, quality of life, relapse, and treatment retention.
- **Consistency:** *Consistent.* Findings are generally consistent among the available RCTs.
- **Precision:** *Variable.* Confidence intervals are generally narrow and do not cross the threshold for clinically significant benefit of the intervention for the majority of outcomes. For some outcomes, however, imprecision was noted because of wide confidence intervals.
- **Dose-response relationship:** *Not assessed.* Studies do not examine effects of varying treatment duration or visit frequency.
- **Confounding factors:** *Present.* Confounding factors may increase the observed effect. Subjects and treating clinicians are aware of the treatment arm to which subjects were assigned. This may cause confounding of effects due to expectancies.
- **Publication bias:** *Unable to be assessed.* A small number of studies met inclusion criteria for the AHRQ review, which precludes assessment of publication bias.

- **Overall strength of research evidence:** *Moderate.* The strength of research evidence is moderate for most outcomes, although a high strength of evidence is noted for rates of treatment retention, and a low strength of research evidence is noted for housing status and core illness symptoms as measured by the PANSS. Neither of the latter outcomes showed an effect of coordinated specialty care programs. Trials vary in sample size, but several had large samples and findings were generally consistent among the available RCTs.

Grading of the Overall Supporting Body of Research Evidence for Harms of Coordinated Specialty Care Programs

Harms of coordinated specialty care programs were not systematically studied, and no grading of the evidence for harms is possible.

STATEMENT 16: Cognitive-Behavioral Therapy

APA *recommends* **(1B)** that patients with schizophrenia be treated with cognitive-behavioral therapy for psychosis (CBTp).*

Evidence in support of this statement comes from multiple RCTs and meta-analyses as described in the AHRQ review (McDonagh et al. 2017). The strength of the research evidence is rated as moderate on the basis of the evidence of CBTp benefits for core illness symptoms and short-term functioning.

In terms of overall symptoms, the AHRQ report relied primarily on a systematic review of 34 RCTs (Jauhar et al. 2014) that found CBTp to be more effective than usual care at improving overall symptoms based on symptom-based rating scales such as the PANSS and BPRS (SMD –0.33, 95% CI –0.47 to –0.19; I^2=68%; moderate SOE). The effect was less pronounced but remained significant (95% CI –0.27 to –0.03) when the analysis was restricted to trials with blinded outcome assessments. Because this review did not conduct stratified analysis by format, it is not possible to tell whether distinctions in outcome exist for individual as compared with group CBTp. Although the included studies ranged in duration from 8 weeks to 5 years, analysis of shorter as compared with longer durations of treatment was not conducted, limiting the ability to determine whether more prolonged treatment is able to maintain shorter-term treatment gains. For negative symptoms, there was no meaningful difference noted between CBTp and usual care based on data from two systematic reviews (Jauhar et al. 2014; Velthorst et al. 2015) (low SOE).

The AHRQ report (McDonagh et al. 2017) also found CBTp to be associated with improvements in global function in the short term (≤6 months since CBTp initiation) as measured using the GAF scale (6 trials: MD 5.35, 95% CI 1.05–9.65; I^2=77%). Removing the one study that used group CBTp from the analysis strengthened the effect and eliminated statistical heterogeneity. In one study that focused on global function (van der Gaag et al. 2011), a higher proportion of CBTp patients had normal functioning after 6 months of treatment as compared with patients who received usual care (28% vs. 14%; RR 2.21, 95% CI 1.25–3.93). Another study (Zimmer et al. 2007) found short-term benefits of an integrated cognitive-behavioral intervention on social and/or occupational function (as measured by the Social and Occupational Functioning Assessment Scale and overall functioning (GAF mean difference 5.69, 95% CI 2.05–10.97; p=0.000). Benefits of CBTp on global, social, and occupational function were not maintained for more than 6 months after treatment cessation (low SOE). CBTp also improved quality of life more than usual care in the short term but not with longer periods of follow-up (low SOE).

---

*This guideline statement should be implemented in the context of a person-centered treatment plan that includes evidence-based nonpharmacological and pharmacological treatments for schizophrenia.

Grading of the Overall Supporting Body of Research Evidence for Efficacy of Cognitive-Behavioral Therapy for Psychosis

- **Magnitude of effect:** *Moderate*. With outcomes for which an effect is observed (such as core illness symptoms and short-term functioning improvements), there is a moderate magnitude of benefit. For other outcomes, either no benefit is seen or evidence is inconclusive.
- **Risk of bias:** *Medium*. Studies in meta-analyses and other RCTs have a moderate degree of study limitations based on their descriptions of randomization, blinding procedures, and study dropouts.
- **Applicability:** The included trials all involve individuals with schizophrenia. Some studies also include individuals with other diagnoses such as schizoaffective disorder. When delivered in clinical practice, CBTp may be conducted with a lesser degree of fidelity than when delivered in research contexts.
- **Directness:** *Direct*. Studies measure core illness symptoms; negative symptoms; and social, occupational, and global function.
- **Consistency:** *Variable*. For outcomes with an observed effect, study findings are consistent. For outcomes with no observed effect, study findings are less consistent.
- **Precision:** *Precise*. Confidence intervals are narrow and do not cross the threshold for clinically significant benefit of the intervention for outcomes with an observed effect. For outcomes with no observed effect, findings are imprecise for most outcomes.
- **Dose-response relationship:** *Not assessed*. The impact of differences in the numbers or frequency of treatment sessions is unclear.
- **Confounding factors:** *Present*. Confounding factors may increase the observed effect. Subjects and treating clinicians are aware of the treatment arm to which subjects were assigned. This may cause confounding of effects due to expectancies.
- **Publication bias:** *Unclear*. At least one meta-analysis of CBTp suggests that publication bias may be present, but analysis for possible publication bias based on all of the included studies was not available.
- **Overall strength of research evidence:** *Moderate*. For outcomes that show an effect of CBTp, there is a moderate strength of research evidence. For other outcomes that did not show an effect, the strength of research evidence is low or insufficient.

Grading of the Overall Supporting Body of Research Evidence for Harms of Cognitive-Behavioral Therapy for Psychosis

Harms of the treatment were rarely reported in studies of CBTp and were not systematically studied. Information was available from only a single RCT, and the AHRQ report notes that the evidence is insufficient to draw any conclusions (McDonagh et al. 2017). Thus, no grading of the evidence for harms is possible.

STATEMENT 17: Psychoeducation

APA *recommends* **(1B)** that patients with schizophrenia receive psychoeducation.*

Evidence in support of this statement comes from a good-quality systematic review as described in the AHRQ report (McDonagh et al. 2017). The strength of the research evidence is rated as moderate on the basis of the evidence of psychoeducation benefits on relapse rates.

---

*This guideline statement should be implemented in the context of a person-centered treatment plan that includes evidence-based nonpharmacological and pharmacological treatments for schizophrenia.

The 10 RCTs (total $N=1{,}125$) of psychoeducation included in the systematic review (Pekkala and Merinder 2002) varied in length (with duration of follow-up as long as 5 years), included diverse interventions, and used individual and group techniques. Although most of the studies included stabilized outpatients and were conducted in North America and northern Europe, many studies contained some individuals with a diagnosis other than schizophrenia. On the basis of the data from 6 trials, psychoeducation had a greater effect than usual care on relapse rates (with or without readmission) at 9–18 months of follow-up (RR 0.80, 95% CI 0.70–0.92; moderate SOE). Psychoeducation was also superior to usual care in terms of global functional outcomes at 1 year of follow-up (3 RCTs; MD –5.23, 95% CI –8.76 to –1.71; low SOE).

In terms of potential harms, few studies reported adverse outcomes. Nevertheless, for psychoeducation as compared with usual care, no differences were observed in the number of deaths, which were small in both groups, and rates of all-cause study dropout were also comparable between study groups (McDonagh et al. 2017).

Grading of the Overall Supporting Body of Research Evidence for Efficacy of Psychoeducation

- **Magnitude of effect:** *Small.* A modest benefit is seen for psychoeducation in terms of relapse rates and global functional outcomes. Effects on other outcomes are less robust or are inconclusive.
- **Risk of bias:** *Medium.* Studies are RCTs, including RCTs as part of a meta-analysis, and have a medium risk of bias based on their descriptions of randomization, blinding procedures, and study dropouts.
- **Applicability:** The included trials all involve individuals with schizophrenia. However, many of the trials also include individuals with other diagnoses. There is considerable variability in the content and format of interventions; however, variability is also present in the delivery of psychoeducation in usual clinical practice.
- **Directness:** *Direct.* Studies measure relapse rates, symptoms, functioning, and quality of life.
- **Consistency:** *Consistent.* When outcome data are available from multiple studies, findings are consistent.
- **Precision:** *Variable.* The confidence interval is narrow for relapse at 9–18 months, but other outcomes have wide confidence intervals.
- **Dose-response relationship:** *Not assessed.*
- **Confounding factors:** *Present.* Confounding factors may increase the observed effect. Subjects and treating clinicians are aware of the treatment arm to which subjects were assigned. This may cause confounding of effects due to expectancies.
- **Publication bias:** *Unclear.* The most recent meta-analysis of psychoeducation in schizophrenia did not assess whether publication bias was present.
- **Overall strength of research evidence:** *Moderate.* Available RCTs on effects of psychoeducation have reasonable sample sizes and precise, consistent findings on relapse. For functioning, the overall strength of research evidence is low.

Grading of the Overall Supporting Body of Research Evidence for Harms of Psychoeducation

Harms of psychoeducation were reported in only a few studies but appeared comparable to usual care; no grading of the evidence for harms is possible because of the small amount of available evidence.

STATEMENT 18: Supported Employment Services

APA *recommends* **(1B)** that patients with schizophrenia receive supported employment services.*

Evidence in support of this statement comes from one study comparing supported employment with usual care and an RCT and meta-analysis comparing supported employment with other vocational interventions as described in the AHRQ report (McDonagh et al. 2017). The strength of the research evidence is rated as moderate on the basis of the evidence of benefits for supported employment on obtaining competitive work.

The AHRQ review (McDonagh et al. 2017) found that supported employment, using the individual placement and support (IPS) model, results in better employment outcomes than usual care with 2 years of follow-up. Patients receiving IPS in one fair-quality trial ($N=204$) were significantly more likely to obtain competitive work than those receiving usual care (75% vs. 27.5%, $P=0.001$; Mueser et al. 2004). They were also more likely to obtain any form of paid work than those receiving usual care (73.9% vs. 53.6%). A large RCT ($N=1,273$), with both usual care and vocational training comparisons, showed similar benefits of IPS (55% vs. 34%, $P<0.001$ overall and 22% vs. 12%, $P<0.001$ in the subgroup of study subjects with schizophrenia) (Cook et al. 2005). These findings are consistent with findings of a good-quality systematic review of 14 RCTs ($N=2,265$) in which other vocational training interventions were used as controls (Kinoshita et al. 2013). Together, these studies provide a moderate SOE for benefits of supported employment using IPS. Although associated with a lower SOE, supported employment also showed benefits in terms of working more than 20 hours per week (13% vs. 34%, $P=0.00$), having more weeks of employment overall (24 more weeks competitive and 11 more weeks any employment, $P<0.001$), and longer tenure per individual job (4 weeks, $P=0.048$) than those in either usual care, other vocational interventions, or both. Patients receiving IPS also reported earning more money than those in usual care ($2,078/month vs. $617.59/month, $P<0.001$).

Several other meta-analyses of supported employment using somewhat different analytic methods and different inclusion and exclusion criteria than the AHRQ review found similar benefits of supported employment using the IPS approach (Frederick and VanderWeele 2019; Suijkerbuijk et al. 2017). In terms of outcomes unrelated to work, findings are less consistent but suggest potential advantages to supported employment in reducing symptoms and hospitalization risk (Burns et al. 2007; Hoffmann et al. 2014; Luciano et al. 2014).

Grading of the Overall Supporting Body of Research Evidence for Efficacy of Supported Employment Services

- **Magnitude of effect:** *Moderate.* Moderate effects are present for the proportion of individuals attaining competitive employment or any form of paid employment as compared with usual care or vocational training comparisons.
- **Risk of bias:** *Medium.* Studies are RCTs (including meta-analyses of RCTs) and have a medium risk of bias based on descriptions of randomization, blinding procedures, and study dropouts.
- **Applicability:** The included trials all involve individuals with schizophrenia. However, many of the trials also include individuals with other diagnoses. Supported employment interventions, particularly those using the IPS model, appear to be representative of usual clinical practice.
- **Directness:** *Direct.* Studies measure the duration of competitive employment and the proportion of individuals attaining paid or competitive employment, as well as less direct outcomes such as wages earned.

---

*This guideline statement should be implemented in the context of a person-centered treatment plan that includes evidence-based nonpharmacological and pharmacological treatments for schizophrenia.

- **Consistency:** *Consistent.* When outcome data are available from more than one study, findings are consistent. In addition, several meta-analyses using somewhat different inclusion and exclusion criteria reached similar findings.
- **Precision:** *Precise.* Narrow confidence intervals are present for the proportion of individuals in competitive employment or working at least 20 hours per week, as well as for mean weeks worked and mean wages earned.
- **Dose-response relationship:** *Not assessed.*
- **Confounding factors:** *Present.* Confounding factors may increase the observed effect. Subjects and treating clinicians are aware of the treatment arm to which subjects were assigned. This may cause confounding of effects due to expectancies.
- **Publication bias:** *Suspected.* There appears to be a lack of reporting of smaller trials with negative results based on network meta-analysis and associated funnel plots to identify publication bias (Suijkerbuijk et al. 2017).
- **Overall strength of research evidence:** *Moderate.* There is a moderate overall strength of research evidence for the proportion of individuals attaining competitive employment, any form of paid employment, mean weeks worked, or monthly wages earned as compared with usual care or vocational training comparisons. Trials are of varying quality, but many have a good sample size; large numbers of study subjects are included in meta-analyses.

Grading of the Overall Supporting Body of Research Evidence for Harms of Supported Employment Services

Harms of supported employment services were not systematically studied, and no grading of the evidence for harms is possible.

Statement 19: Assertive Community Treatment

APA *recommends* **(1B)** that patients with schizophrenia receive assertive community treatment if there is a history of poor engagement with services leading to frequent relapse or social disruption (e.g., homelessness; legal difficulties, including imprisonment).*

This recommendation is based on information from the AHRQ review (McDonagh et al. 2017), which used a good-quality systematic review (14 RCTs; N=2,281) as a primary source (Marshall and Lockwood 2000) and also considered one additional RCT (N=118; Sytema et al. 2007). The strength of research evidence for this guideline statement is rated as moderate on the basis of the moderate SOE found for multiple key outcomes.

The AHRQ review (McDonagh et al. 2017) focused on assertive community treatment (ACT) alone as compared with usual care and did not include a recent review in which evidence for ACT was combined with evidence for intensive case management. Significant variability was noted in study populations, with a range of ages, demographic characteristics, diagnoses, and eligibility criteria (e.g., frequent or recent hospitalization, other risk factors for reduced continuity of care). In addition, the degree of fidelity to ACT principles was often unclear, which may influence effectiveness.

Individuals who received ACT were less likely to discontinue treatment and be lost to follow-up than individuals who received usual care (12 trials; OR 0.51, 95% CI 0.41–0.63; moderate SOE). They were also less likely to be admitted to a hospital compared with individuals who received usual care (6 RCTs; OR 0.59, 95% CI 0.41–0.85; I^2=73%), and many of the reported studies also showed a decrease in the number of days in the hospital. Furthermore, individuals who received ACT were

---

*This guideline statement should be implemented in the context of a person-centered treatment plan that includes evidence-based nonpharmacological and pharmacological treatments for schizophrenia.

less likely to be unemployed (3 trials; OR 0.46, 95% CI 0.21–0.99; I^2=34%), homeless (4 trials; OR 0.20, 95% CI 0.09–0.47; I^2=52%), or living nonindependently (4 trials; OR 0.52, 95% CI 0.35–0.79; I^2=0%) compared with usual care (moderate SOE). Core illness symptoms also improved with ACT, but the degree of improvement was comparable to that in the usual care group (3 trials, N=255; MD –0.14, 95% CI –0.36 to 0.08; moderate SOE). As compared with usual care, there was no significant difference in social function (pooled analysis of 3 studies; MD 0.03, 95% CI –0.28 to 0.34; low SOE) and no significant differences in arrests (2 trials, total N=604; OR 1.17, 95% CI 0.60–2.29; I^2=0%), imprisonment (4 trials, total N=471; OR 1.19, 95% CI 0.70–2.01; I^2=27%), or police contacts (2 trials, total N=149; OR 0.76, 95% CI 0.32–1.79; I^2=84%) with ACT (low SOE). Findings from the additional RCT were generally consistent with the meta-analytic results. Only 2 trials reported information on quality of life, with one finding a small but statistically significant difference and the other showing no difference.

In individuals with co-occurring schizophrenia and a substance use disorder, one good-quality systematic review of 32 trials (N=3,165) examined differences between integrated ACT and usual care (Hunt et al. 2013). For most outcomes of interest, only one or two of the studies from the systematic review contributed relevant data; however, these limited data showed no differences between integrated ACT and usual care for substance use, treatment discontinuation, function, or mortality through follow-up durations of up to 36 months.

Grading of the Overall Supporting Body of Research Evidence for Efficacy of Assertive Community Treatment

- **Magnitude of effect:** *Moderate.* On several important outcomes, there is at least a moderate effect. These outcomes include treatment discontinuation and likelihood of hospitalization, unemployment, or homelessness. On other outcomes, however, there is no difference between ACT and treatment as usual.
- **Risk of bias:** *Medium.* Evidence comes from an RCT and a meta-analysis of RCTs, but individual studies have a medium risk of bias based on their descriptions of randomization, blinding procedures, and study dropouts.
- **Applicability:** The included trials all involve individuals with schizophrenia. However, many of the trials also include individuals with other diagnoses. The delivery of ACT in the trials is likely to be representative of usual clinical practice, although program fidelity may be diminished in usual practice.
- **Directness:** *Direct.* Studies measured core illness symptoms, functioning, quality of life, employment, housing status, and interactions with the criminal justice system.
- **Consistency:** *Variable.* Findings of benefits for having housing or employment are consistent, whereas other outcomes show inconsistencies among individual studies within the meta-analysis.
- **Precision:** *Imprecise.* Confidence intervals for most outcomes are wide, and many cross the threshold for clinically significant benefit of the intervention.
- **Dose-response relationship:** *Not applicable.*
- **Confounding factors:** *Present.* Confounding factors may increase the observed effect. Subjects and treating clinicians are aware of the treatment arm to which subjects were assigned. This may cause confounding of effects due to expectancies.
- **Publication bias:** *Not assessed.*
- **Overall strength of research evidence:** *Moderate.* A significant number of RCTs of ACT are available and, compared with usual care, show that ACT is associated with a lower likelihood of being unemployed and a lower likelihood of not living independently or being homeless. Many trials are moderate in quality, although there is some variability.

Grading of the Overall Supporting Body of Research Evidence for Harms of Assertive Community Treatment

Harms of assertive community treatment were not systematically studied, and no grading of the evidence for harms is possible.

STATEMENT 20: Family Interventions

APA *suggests* **(2B)** that patients with schizophrenia who have ongoing contact with family receive family interventions.*

This guideline statement is based on 1 fair-quality systematic review (27 non-Chinese studies, total $N=2,297$; Pharoah et al. 2010) and 6 additional studies (total $N=562$; Barrowclough et al. 1999; Dyck et al. 2000; Garety et al. 2008; Kopelowicz et al. 2012; Mayoral et al. 2015; Sellwood et al. 2001, 2007; Valencia et al. 2007) as described in the AHRQ review (McDonagh et al. 2017). Because most family interventions are aimed at reducing relapse, the strength of research evidence for this statement is rated as moderate on the basis of the moderate SOE found for relapse in the AHRQ review with medium-term follow-up, although other outcomes had a low SOE.

The studies of family intervention described in the AHRQ review (McDonagh et al. 2017) had significant variation in content and methods of the delivered intervention (e.g., psychoeducation, motivational interviewing, behavioral family therapy, support groups, 24-hour support, communication training, stress management, role-play, homework, goal setting, development of social networks), measured outcomes, study design (e.g., setting, treatment duration, treatment frequency, follow-up duration, single-family versus multiple-family format, family members only vs. family members plus patient), and demographics of the study population (e.g., age, illness duration, symptom severity at baseline). Most studies had small sample sizes, and most had some risk of bias due to lack of reporting of randomization procedures or outcome assessment blinding. Studies conducted in China were excluded because of concerns about their applicability to Canadian and U.S. populations.

In the AHRQ review (McDonagh et al. 2017), family interventions resulted in significantly lower relapse rates than usual care when measured at 0–6 months (3 RCTs; $N=244$; 23% vs. 37%; RR 0.62, 95% CI 0.41–0.92; low SOE), 7–12 months (19 RCTs; $N=1,118$; 30% vs. 44%; RR 0.67, 95% CI 0.54–0.83; moderate SOE), 13–24 months (9 RCTs; $N=517$; 49% vs. 61%; RR 0.75, 95% CI 0.58–0.99; low SOE), and 5 years posttreatment (2 RCTs; $N=140$; 78% vs. 94%; RR 0.82, 95% CI 0.72–0.94; low SOE) but not at 25–36 months. The strongest evidence for effects of family interventions on relapse occurred in studies that included at least 10 treatment sessions over 7–12 months.

Improvements in core illness symptoms (4 RCTs; $N=223$; SMD –0.46, 95% CI –0.73 to –0.20; low SOE) and negative symptoms (3 trials; $N=163$; SMD –0.38, 95% CI –0.69 to –0.07; low SOE) were also found with family intervention compared with usual care. Unemployment (4 trials; $N=230$; 75% vs. 66% after 6–12 months of follow-up; RR 1.09, 95% CI 0.91–1.29; $I^2=0\%$; low SOE), independent living (3 RCTs; $N=164$; 57% vs. 63% at 1 year; RR 0.83, 95% CI 0.66–1.03; low SOE), and reduction in self-harm (6 trials; $N=314$; 4% vs. 6%; RR 0.85, 95% CI 0.24–3.02; $I^2=23\%$; low SOE) were not found to be different between family intervention and usual care groups (low SOE). For social functioning, quality of life, family burden, and nonsuicide mortality, there was insufficient evidence to draw any conclusions from the available studies. Rates of treatment discontinuation varied with time in the study, but family interventions either did not differ from usual care or had fewer treatment dropouts than usual care (McDonagh et al. 2017; low SOE).

---

*This guideline statement should be implemented in the context of a person-centered treatment plan that includes evidence-based nonpharmacological and pharmacological treatments for schizophrenia.

Grading of the Overall Supporting Body of Research Evidence for Efficacy of Family Interventions

- **Magnitude of effect:** *Moderate*. For outcomes that show an effect of family interventions, such as effects on relapse rate and illness symptoms, the magnitude of the effect is generally moderate.
- **Risk of bias:** *Medium*. Evidence comes from RCTs, including RCTs in a fair-quality systematic review. These studies have a medium risk of bias based on their descriptions of randomization, blinding procedures, and study dropouts.
- **Applicability:** The included trials all involve individuals with schizophrenia. However, many of the trials also include individuals with other diagnoses. Studies from China are excluded from the analysis because of concerns about their applicability to Canadian and U.S. populations. There is considerable variability in the content and methods of the family interventions that are studied; however, there is also considerable variability in interventions that are delivered in clinical practice.
- **Directness:** *Direct*. Studies measure relapse, core illness symptoms, and outcomes related to functioning.
- **Consistency:** *Consistent*. For outcomes with data from more than one study, findings among the studies are consistent.
- **Precision:** *Imprecise*. Confidence intervals for all outcomes are wide or cross the threshold for clinically significant benefit of the intervention.
- **Dose-response relationship:** *Present*. The strongest evidence for effects of family interventions on relapse occurs in studies that include at least 10 treatment sessions over 7–12 months.
- **Confounding factors:** *Present*. Confounding factors may increase the observed effect. Subjects and treating clinicians are aware of the treatment arm to which subjects were assigned. This may cause confounding of effects due to expectancies.
- **Publication bias:** *Not assessed*. The most recent meta-analysis of family interventions did not assess whether publication bias was present.
- **Overall strength of research evidence:** *Moderate*. For relapse at 7–12 months, there is a moderate strength of research evidence, but for most other outcomes, the strength of research evidence is low. The strength of research evidence is influenced by a lack of precision, as well as by the small sample sizes for some of the outcomes.

Grading of the Overall Supporting Body of Research Evidence for Harms of Family Interventions

Harms of family interventions were not systematically studied, and no grading of the evidence for harms is possible.

STATEMENT 21: Self-Management Skills and Recovery-Focused Interventions

APA *suggests* **(2C)** that patients with schizophrenia receive interventions aimed at developing self-management skills and enhancing person-oriented recovery.*

This guideline statement is based on evidence provided by a fair-quality systematic review (13 studies; total *N*=1,404; Zou et al. 2013) and 1 additional fair-quality study (*N*=210; Hasson-Ohayon et al.

---

*This guideline statement should be implemented in the context of a person-centered treatment plan that includes evidence-based nonpharmacological and pharmacological treatments for schizophrenia.

2007) as described in the AHRQ review (McDonagh et al. 2017), as well as a meta-analysis of person-oriented recovery approaches (7 RCTs, $N=1,739$; Thomas et al. 2018). The strength of research evidence for this statement is rated as low on the basis of the low SOE found for the majority of outcomes in the AHRQ review and a significant risk of bias (consistent with a low SOE) for most of the studies in the meta-analysis of person-oriented recovery approaches.

For illness self-management training and for recovery-focused interventions, interpretation of the evidence can be challenging because of the degree of heterogeneity in the content and format of the interventions. For example, illness self-management training programs are designed to improve knowledge, management of symptoms, and social and occupational functioning, with a primary goal of reducing the risk of relapse by focusing on medication management, recognizing signs of relapse, and developing a relapse prevention plan and coping skills for persistent symptoms (McDonagh et al. 2017; Substance Abuse and Mental Health Services Administration 2010a). Recovery-focused interventions can include similar approaches but are focused primarily on supporting a recovery-oriented vision that strives for community integration in the context of individual goals, needs, and strengths (Le Boutillier et al. 2011; Thomas et al. 2018). Activities of recovery-focused interventions incorporate opportunities for participants to share experiences and receive support as well as practicing strategies for success in illness self-management. With illness self-management, the interventions were typically administered in a group format, whereas recovery-focused interventions included a mix of group and individual formats as well as a mix of peer- and professional-led activities. Both illness self-management and recovery-focused interventions had significant variations in session content, duration, and number.

In terms of outcomes with illness self-management, the AHRQ review (McDonagh et al. 2017) noted a reduction in core illness symptom severity based on the BPRS (5 RCTs; pooled WMD –4.19, 95% CI –5.84 to –2.54; moderate SOE) and a reduced likelihood of relapse with completion of 10 or more self-management sessions (OR 0.41, 95% CI 0.21–0.79; low SOE). Effects of intervention were reduced if low-fidelity treatment was given or if fewer self-management sessions were completed. No significant effect of illness self-management was noted for negative symptoms (low SOE).

With recovery-focused interventions (Thomas et al. 2018), individuals in the intervention group showed a modest improvement in person-oriented recovery, empowerment, and hope immediately after the intervention (effect size 0.24, 95% CI 0.04–0.44) and at follow-up (effect size 0.21, 95% CI 0.06–0.35). Moderator analysis suggested that the greatest improvement was seen when mental health professionals and peer providers collaborated in treatment delivery.

Grading of the Overall Supporting Body of Research Evidence for Efficacy of Self-Management Skills and Recovery-Focused Interventions

- **Magnitude of effect:** *Small.* Modest changes were noted in core illness symptom severity, likelihood of relapse, measures of person-oriented recovery, empowerment, and hope.
- **Risk of bias:** *Medium.* Studies are RCTs, including RCTs as part of a meta-analysis, and have a medium risk of bias based on their descriptions of randomization, blinding procedures, and study dropouts.
- **Applicability:** The included trials all involve individuals with schizophrenia. However, many of the trials also include individuals with other diagnoses. There is considerable variability in the content and format of delivered interventions; however, there is also wide variation in illness self-management and recovery-focused interventions in clinical practice.
- **Directness:** *Direct.* Studies measure functioning, symptoms, and relapse.
- **Consistency:** *Variable.* Consistent for symptoms and relapse but inconsistent for functioning.
- **Precision:** *Variable.* Precise for symptoms as measured by the BPRS but imprecise for other outcomes because of wide confidence intervals.
- **Dose-response relationship:** *Present.* Effects of illness self-management were less prominent if fewer self-management sessions were completed.

- **Confounding factors:** *Present.* Confounding factors may increase the observed effect. Subjects and treating clinicians are aware of the treatment arm to which subjects were assigned. This may cause confounding of effects due to expectancies.
- **Publication bias:** *Not assessed.*
- **Overall strength of research evidence:** *Low.* Studies are RCTs, including a meta-analysis of RCTs, and have a medium risk of bias. The strength of research evidence is moderate for effects on symptoms; it is low or insufficient for other outcomes. Although a dose-response effect seems to be present, increasing confidence in the findings, this is offset by the lack of precision for most outcomes.

Grading of the Overall Supporting Body of Research Evidence for Harms of Self-Management Skills and Recovery-Focused Interventions

Harms of self-management skills and recovery-focused interventions were not systematically studied, and no grading of the evidence for harms is possible.

STATEMENT 22: Cognitive Remediation

APA *suggests* **(2C)** that patients with schizophrenia receive cognitive remediation.*

This guideline statement is based on evidence provided by 2 good-quality systematic reviews (57 studies, total $N=2,885$; Cella et al. 2017; Wykes et al. 2011), 1 good-quality trial ($N=90$; Deste et al. 2015; Vita et al. 2011), and 3 fair-quality trials ($N=56–156$; Farreny et al. 2012; Mueller et al. 2015; Twamley et al. 2012). The strength of research evidence for this statement is rated as low on the basis of the low SOE found for the majority of outcomes.

Studies included in the AHRQ review (McDonagh et al. 2017) used standard cognitive remediation principles (Saperstein and Medalia 2012) and usual care control comparisons, but other population and study characteristics varied (e.g., population demographics, treatment setting, individual vs. group format, drill and practice vs. drill plus strategy methodology, sessions per week, treatment duration, follow-up duration, extent of treatment fidelity, baseline symptom severity, computerized vs. noncomputerized content delivery, presence of active comparator condition).

Overall, as compared with usual care, use of cognitive remediation for 15–16 weeks of treatment was associated with small positive effects on core illness symptoms (2 trials, $N=153$; SMD –0.62, 95% CI –1.01 to –0.24; low SOE), but effects were inconsistent among the studies, and symptom improvement was not sustained following treatment removal (8 RCTs; effect size 0.17, 95% CI –0.03 to 0.48). Cognitive remediation as compared with usual care was also associated with improvements in negative symptoms (1 systematic review of 18 RCTs; effect size –0.36, 95% CI –0.52 to –0.20; moderate SOE) as well as small positive effects on social, occupational, and global function (6 RCTs; effect sizes of 0.16–0.40; low SOE). Effects of intervention on cognitive functioning were outside the scope of the AHRQ review, but some evidence suggests that improved cognitive function can result from treatment with cognitive remediation, with indirect benefits for global function (Harvey et al. 2018). Only 1 study reported on health-related quality of life, and study limitations preclude drawing conclusions on this outcome. Treatment with cognitive remediation did not differ from usual care in terms of rates of treatment discontinuation (McDonagh et al. 2017). Cognitive remediation also seems to be acceptable to individuals who receive treatment in clinical settings as compared with research settings (Medalia et al. 2019).

Although the AHRQ review did not specifically assess cognitive outcomes with cognitive remediation, this has been a major focus of study and the primary target of cognitive remediation as an in-

---

This guideline statement should be implemented in the context of a person-centered treatment plan that includes evidence-based nonpharmacological and pharmacological treatments for schizophrenia.

tervention. Results from meta-analyses (Revell et al. 2015; Wykes et al. 2011) and more recent randomized trials (D'Amato et al. 2011; Donohoe et al. 2018; Gomar et al. 2015; Keefe et al. 2012; McGurk et al. 2016; Mueller et al. 2015; Reeder et al. 2017) have been mixed, with significant heterogeneity in the degree of cognitive improvement (if any), the domains of cognitive improvement, and the persistence and generalizability of improvements. This may not be surprising given the wide variety of cognitive remediation approaches and formats that have been used in an effort to enhance cognitive processes such as attention, memory, executive function, social cognition, or meta-cognition (Delahunty and Morice 1996; Medalia et al. 2018; Pentaraki et al. 2017; Reeder et al. 2016; Wykes et al. 2011). There are also no clear-cut factors that are predictive of whether cognitive improvement will occur (Reser et al. 2019), which makes it difficult to determine how to target the intervention to individuals who are most likely to respond. Nevertheless, cognitive remediation does seem to result in improvements in cognition in individuals with schizophrenia, at least on a short-term basis (Harvey et al. 2018; Revell et al. 2015).

Grading of the Overall Supporting Body of Research Evidence for Efficacy of Cognitive Remediation

- **Magnitude of effect:** *Small.* Small but significant effects are seen for core illness symptoms and negative symptoms as well as for cognitive processes in some domains. However, significant heterogeneity is present in the degree of benefit as well as the persistence and generalizability of benefits.
- **Risk of bias:** *Medium.* RCTs, including those in systematic reviews, have a medium risk of bias based on their descriptions of randomization, blinding procedures, and study dropouts.
- **Applicability:** The included trials all involve individuals with schizophrenia. Multiple different approaches to delivering cognitive remediation are used in the clinical trials. In addition, the use of cognitive remediation remains limited outside research settings, which makes it difficult to compare the study methods with current practice.
- **Directness:** *Direct.* Studies measure core illness symptoms, functioning, quality of life, and treatment discontinuation as well as cognitive effects.
- **Consistency:** *Consistent.* Within each outcome, study findings were consistent.
- **Precision:** *Imprecise.* Confidence intervals are relatively wide for many outcomes.
- **Dose-response relationship:** *Not assessed.* It is not clear whether using a different frequency or duration of cognitive remediation sessions will affect outcomes.
- **Confounding factors:** *Present.* Confounding factors may increase the observed effect. Subjects and treating clinicians are aware of the treatment arm to which subjects were assigned. This may cause confounding of effects due to expectancies.
- **Publication bias:** *Not suspected.* On the basis of analyses conducted as part of meta-analyses on cognitive remediation, there is no evidence of publication bias.
- **Overall strength of research evidence:** *Low.* Ratings of the strength of evidence are low for global, social, and occupational function and for core illness symptoms and moderate for negative symptoms. There is significant variability in the findings, perhaps related to the many differences in the study populations and treatment-related characteristics. Nevertheless, this reduces confidence in conclusions related to cognitive remediation.

Grading of the Overall Supporting Body of Research Evidence for Harms of Cognitive Remediation

Harms of cognitive remediation were not systematically studied, and no grading of the evidence for harms is possible.

STATEMENT 23: Social Skills Training

APA *suggests* **(2C)** that patients with schizophrenia who have a therapeutic goal of enhanced social functioning receive social skills training.*

This guideline statement is based on 3 fair-quality RCTs (total $N=384$; Bartels et al. 2014; Mueser et al. 2010; Valencia et al. 2007, 2013) as described in the AHRQ review (McDonagh et al. 2017). The strength of research evidence for this statement is rated as low on the basis of the low SOE found for outcomes in the AHRQ review with social skills training.

In the trials of social skills training that were included in the AHRQ review (McDonagh et al. 2017), sessions were held weekly for 24–52 weeks and included specific, progressive intervention modules on such topics as management of symptoms and medication, improving social and family relationships, and increasing functional skills such as money management. Goals of social skills training included enhanced psychosocial function and reductions in relapse and need for hospitalization. Demographic parameters, diagnoses of participants, and outcome measures varied among the trials.

Social function was noted to be significantly improved with social skills training as compared with usual care (SMD on GAF at 6 months 1.60, 95% CI 1.19–2.02; SMD on GAF at 1 year 2.02, 95% CI 1.53–2.52; SMD on Multnomah Community Ability Scale at 2 years 0.65, 95% CI 0.36–0.95; low SOE), but it was not clear whether gains were maintained after treatment discontinuation. Core illness symptoms, as measured by the PANSS, also showed more improvement with social skills training as compared with usual care (SMD at 6 months –1.50, 95% CI –1.92 to –1.09; SMD at 2 years –0.81, 95% CI –1.22 to –0.40; low SOE). Negative symptoms also improved with social skills training as compared with usual care (SMD at 6 months –1.30, 95% CI –1.70 to –0.90; SMD at 1 year –0.82, 95% CI –1.23 to –1.40; SMD at 2 years –0.45, 95% CI –0.74 to –0.15; low SOE), and in one study gains were maintained 1 year after treatment had ended. It was unclear whether relapse rates were affected by social skills training because of a small number of studies, small sample sizes, and small numbers of individuals who experienced relapse. In terms of treatment discontinuation, individuals who received social skills training did not differ from those in the usual care group (RR 1.10 at 1 year, 95% CI 0.92–1.31; RR 1.01 at 2 years, 95% CI 0.88–1.16; low SOE), with high rates of treatment retention in both groups.

Grading of the Overall Supporting Body of Research Evidence for Efficacy of Social Skills Training

- **Magnitude of effect:** *Small.* A modest effect of social skills training was noted on social function, core illness symptoms, and negative symptoms.
- **Risk of bias:** *Medium.* Studies are RCTs with a medium risk of bias based on their descriptions of randomization, blinding procedures, and study dropouts.
- **Applicability:** The included trials all involve individuals with schizophrenia. However, many of the trials also include individuals with other diagnoses. Typically, individuals also had decreases in social functioning.
- **Directness:** *Direct.* Studies measure social functioning, core illness symptoms, negative symptoms, relapse, and ability to maintain treatment.
- **Consistency:** *Variable.* Findings in the 3 included studies are consistent for negative symptom improvements but inconsistent for improvements in functioning and core illness symptoms.
- **Precision:** *Imprecise.* Confidence intervals for some outcomes cross the threshold for clinically significant benefit of the intervention in some studies.

---

*This guideline statement should be implemented in the context of a person-centered treatment plan that includes evidence-based nonpharmacological and pharmacological treatments for schizophrenia.

- **Dose-response relationship:** *Not assessed*.
- **Confounding factors:** *Present*. Confounding factors may increase the observed effect. Subjects and treating clinicians are aware of the treatment arm to which subjects were assigned. This may cause confounding of effects due to expectancies.
- **Publication bias:** *Not suspected*. A meta-analysis conducted subsequent to the AHRQ review showed no significant publication bias for studies of social skills training (Turner et al. 2018).
- **Overall strength of research evidence:** *Low*. Available RCTs have medium risk of bias, have variable consistency, and lack precision, reducing the strength of the evidence.

Grading of the Overall Supporting Body of Research Evidence for Harms of Social Skills Training

Harms of social skills training were not systematically studied, and no grading of the evidence for harms is possible.

STATEMENT 24: Supportive Psychotherapy

APA *suggests* **(2C)** that patients with schizophrenia be treated with supportive psychotherapy.*

This guideline statement is based on studies that compared supportive psychotherapy with usual care (total $N=822$) in 1 good-quality systematic review (L. A. Buckley et al. 2015) as described in the AHRQ review (McDonagh et al. 2017). The strength of research evidence for this statement is rated as low on the basis of the low SOE found for study outcomes in the AHRQ review.

The studies in the systematic review (L. A. Buckley et al. 2015) were aimed primarily at helping patients with coping abilities and maintaining levels of functioning. In other respects, there was significant variation in measured outcomes, study design (e.g., setting, treatment duration, treatment frequency, follow-up duration), and demographics of the study population (e.g., age, illness duration, symptom severity at baseline). In addition, most of the included studies had some risk of bias.

The AHRQ review (McDonagh et al. 2017) found no difference in global or social function on the basis of 2 studies, but study results were not able to be pooled for analysis. Four RCTs reported information on study attrition, and no significant difference was noted between supportive psychotherapy and usual care ($N=354$; RR 0.86, 95% CI 0.53–1.40; low SOE). For other outcomes, evidence was available from only a single study and sample sizes were small, making it difficult to draw reliable conclusions.

Grading of the Overall Supporting Body of Research Evidence for Efficacy of Supportive Psychotherapy

- **Magnitude of effect:** *Not present*. On the basis of a small number of studies, there is no difference from usual care in global functioning or treatment discontinuation.
- **Risk of bias:** *Medium*. Studies are RCTs that have a medium risk of bias based on their descriptions of randomization, blinding procedures, and study dropouts.
- **Applicability:** The included trials all involve individuals with schizophrenia. However, some trials also include individuals with other diagnoses. There is significant variation in the duration and frequency of treatment; however, variability in the delivery of supportive psychotherapy is also common in usual clinical practice.

---

*This guideline statement should be implemented in the context of a person-centered treatment plan that includes evidence-based nonpharmacological and pharmacological treatments for schizophrenia.

- **Directness:** *Direct.* Studies measure functioning, core symptoms, negative symptoms, relapse, quality of life, and treatment discontinuation.
- **Consistency:** *Consistent.* For outcomes that are studied in more than one trial, findings are generally consistent.
- **Precision:** *Imprecise.* Confidence intervals are wide and cross the threshold for clinically significant benefit of the intervention for many outcomes.
- **Dose-response relationship:** *Not assessed.*
- **Confounding factors:** *Unclear.* Supportive therapy is similar to the type of therapy that is commonly delivered in usual care, so expectancy effects of receiving a novel intervention are likely to be minimal.
- **Publication bias:** *Unable to be assessed.* The number of studies on supportive therapy is too small to be able to assess for the presence or absence of publication bias.
- **Overall strength of research evidence:** *Low.* The overall strength of evidence is low for global functioning and study discontinuation. There is insufficient evidence to draw conclusions about other outcomes. The available trials vary in their sample sizes. Study designs also differ, which makes comparison of findings difficult.

Grading of the Overall Supporting Body of Research Evidence for Harms of Supportive Psychotherapy

Harms of supportive psychotherapy were not systematically studied, and no grading of the evidence for harms is possible.

Appendix D.
Strength of Evidence

The strength of evidence tables in this appendix are adapted from the Agency for Healthcare Research and Quality (AHRQ) review (McDonagh et al. 2017), in which key outcomes are prioritized in terms of clinical and patient-centered outcomes. The prioritized outcomes are listed below, per intervention area. For more details, see "Strength of the Body of Evidence" and Appendix H references in the AHRQ review.

Pharmacological interventions are listed in Table D–1, and outcomes include the following:

- Functional outcomes (e.g., social, occupational)
- Health-related quality of life (including physical)
- Rates of response and/or remission
- Mortality (all-cause and/or specific)
- Reductions in self-harm, suicide, and suicide attempts
- Improvements in core illness symptoms, as indicated by scale score changes
- Overall/any adverse events (rate or proportion)
- Withdrawal due to adverse events

Psychosocial and other nonpharmacological interventions are listed in Tables D–2 to D–13, and outcomes include the following:

- Functional outcomes (e.g., social, occupational)
- Health-related quality of life
- Reductions in self-harm, suicide, and suicide attempts
- Rates of response and/or remission
- Improvements in core illness symptoms, as indicated by scale score changes
- Treatment discontinuation (typically reported as the number of patients lost to follow-up or leaving the study early)
- Rates of relapse
- Outcomes reported as adverse events related to the intervention

TABLE D–1. Pharmacological treatment

Outcome	Comparators	Number of studies and subjects	Study limitations	Consistency	Directness	Precision	Magnitude of effect: summary effect size (95% CI)	Strength of evidence (high, moderate, low, insufficient)
Social functioning	Olanzapine, risperidone, quetiapine IR	1 SR (2 RCTs; N=343 and 1 observational study; N=9,028)	Moderate; Observational evidence: moderate	Inconsistent; Observational evidence: unknown	Direct; Observational evidence: direct	Imprecise; Observational evidence: precise	Inconclusive; RCT 1: no significant differences on RFS or the SAS-SMI; RCT 2: change on SFS greater with olanzapine (+7.75) than risperidone (−0.92, P=0.0028); Socially active: OR 1.27 (1.05–1.54); olanzapine 84.6% vs. risperidone 82.4%	Insufficient
Social functioning	Paliperidone LAI (monthly) vs. risperidone LAI (biweekly)	1 SR (2 RCTs; N=452)	Moderate	Inconsistent	Direct	Precise	No statistically significant differences in PSP scale; Mean change from baseline: 16.8 paliperidone and 18.6 risperidone; least squares mean difference 0.5 (−2.14 to 3.12)	Low
Social functioning	Paliperidone XR vs. olanzapine	1 meta-analysis of selected studies	High	Unknown	Direct	Precise	No significant difference in PSP scale: mean change 7.8–12.2 in paliperidone dose groups vs. 8.7 in olanzapine group	Insufficient
Social functioning	Risperidone LAI vs. quetiapine IR	1 RCT; N=666	Moderate	Unknown	Direct	Precise	Risperidone LAI resulted in greater improvements in SOFAS at 6 months (differences in change 6.1 vs. 2.7, P=0.02), 12 months (9.5 vs. 6.1, P=0.009), and endpoint (6.6 vs. 1.1, P<0.0001)	Low

Outcome	Comparators	Number of studies and subjects	Study limitations	Consistency	Directness	Precision	Magnitude of effect: summary effect size (95% CI)	Strength of evidence (high, moderate, low, insufficient)
Employment outcomes	Older SGAs (olanzapine, risperidone, quetiapine, ziprasidone)	1 SR (2 RCTs, 3 observational studies; N=1,379)	Low Observational evidence: moderate	Inconsistent Observational evidence: consistent	Direct Observational evidence: direct	Imprecise Observational evidence: imprecise	No significant differences in rates of employment (mean 18% in CATIE phase 1)	Low
Function: employment	Haloperidol vs. risperidone	1 SR (1 RCT; N=100)	Moderate	Unknown	Direct	Imprecise	Inconclusive Proportion of patients with economic independence: RR 0.94 (0.68–1.29)	Insufficient
Function: employment	Perphenazine vs. olanzapine	1 SR (1 RCT; N=597)	Moderate	Unknown	Direct	Imprecise	Inconclusive Proportion with paid employment: RR 1.29 (0.70–2.38)	Insufficient
Function: employment	Perphenazine vs. quetiapine	1 SR (1 RCT; N=598)	Moderate	Unknown	Direct	Imprecise	Inconclusive Proportion with paid employment: RR 1.75 (0.90–3.43)	Insufficient
Function: employment	Perphenazine vs. risperidone	1 SR (1 RCT; N=602)	Moderate	Unknown	Direct	Imprecise	Inconclusive Proportion with paid employment: RR 1.38 (0.74–2.57)	Insufficient
Function: employment	Perphenazine vs. ziprasidone	1 SR (1 RCT; N=446)	Moderate	Unknown	Direct	Imprecise	Inconclusive Proportion with paid employment: RR 1.22 (0.60–2.51)	Insufficient
Occupation and residential status	Older SGAs (olanzapine, risperidone, quetiapine, ziprasidone)	1 SR (21 RCTs; N=771)	Moderate	Unknown	Direct	Imprecise	Inconclusive 75.5% and 75.3% had stable status, 3.8% and 3.1% had improved status (NS)	Insufficient

TABLE D–1. Pharmacological treatment (*continued*)

Outcome	Comparators	Number of studies and subjects	Study limitations	Consistency	Directness	Precision	Magnitude of effect: summary effect size (95% CI)	Strength of evidence (high, moderate, low, insufficient)
Global functioning (GAF)	Olanzapine *vs.* risperidone	1 SR (4 cohort studies; *N*=3,211)	High	Inconsistent	Direct	Precise	No difference Pooled WMD 0.61 (−1.78 to 2.99), I²=43%	Low
Global functioning (GAF)	Olanzapine *vs.* quetiapine	1 SR (2 RCTs; *N*=363)	Moderate	Consistent	Direct	Imprecise	Pooled WMD 1.14 (−4.75 to 7.02); Q=3.99, *df*=1, *P*=0.045	Low
Function: general	Haloperidol *vs.* olanzapine	1 SR (1 RCT; *N*=208)	Moderate	Unknown	Direct	Imprecise	Inconclusive GAF effect estimate: −4.00 (−13.70 to 5.70)	Insufficient
Function: encounters with legal system	Haloperidol *vs.* olanzapine	1 SR (1 RCTs; *N*=31)	Moderate	Unknown	Direct	Imprecise	Inconclusive Encounters with legal system: RR 3.20 (0.76–13.46)	Insufficient
Quality of life	Olanzapine *vs.* risperidone	1 SR (2 RCTs; *N*=492)	Moderate	Consistent	Direct	Precise	QLS change: 7 months 13.4 *vs.* 8.8 (*P*>0.074); 12 months 0.19 *vs.* 0.26 (*P*=0.53)	Moderate
Quality of life	Olanzapine *vs.* ziprasidone	1 SR (2 RCTs; *N*=740)	Moderate	Consistent	Direct	Precise	QLS change: 6–7 months 61.3 *vs.* 58.9 (*P*=0.36 using mixed-effect modeling); 12 months 0.19 *vs.* 0.26 (*PNR*)	Moderate
Quality of life	Olanzapine *vs.* quetiapine IR	1 SR (1 RCT; *N*=227)	Low	Unknown	Direct	Imprecise	QLS change: 12 months 0.19 *vs.* 0.09 (*P*>0.05)	Low
Quality of life	Olanzapine *vs.* asenapine	1 SR (1 RCT; *N*=464)	Moderate	Unknown	Direct	Imprecise	QLS change: 12 months 11.7 *vs.* 11.8 and 11.1 *vs.* 7.1 (multicountry study reported by hemisphere; *P*=NS)	Insufficient

TABLE D–1. Pharmacological treatment *(continued)*

Outcome	Comparators	Number of studies and subjects	Study limitations	Consistency	Directness	Precision	Magnitude of effect: summary effect size (95% CI)	Strength of evidence (high, moderate, low, insufficient)
Quality of life	Olanzapine vs. clozapine	1 SR (1 RCT; N=114)	Moderate	Unknown	Direct	Imprecise	SWN scale: at 26 weeks, olanzapine found noninferior to clozapine; difference 3.2 (4.2–10.5)	Insufficient
Quality of life	Risperidone vs. ziprasidone	1 SR (N=154)	Low	Unknown	Direct	Imprecise	QLS change: 12 months 0.19 vs. 0.26 (P>0.05)	Low
Quality of life	Risperidone vs. quetiapine	1 SR (1 RCT; N=189)	Low	Unknown	Direct	Imprecise	QLS change: 12 months 0.26 vs. 0.26 (P>0.05)	Low
Quality of life	Quetiapine XR vs. risperidone	1 RCT; N=798	Moderate	Unknown	Direct	Imprecise	SWN short form 20% response rate at 6 months: 65% vs. 68%; adjusted difference –5.7% (–15.1 to 3.7) but not meeting noninferiority criteria	Insufficient
Quality of life	Aripiprazole oral vs. aripiprazole LAI (monthly)	1 RCT; N=724	Moderate	Unknown	Direct	Precise	SF-36 12 months: mean changes in mental component 0.82 vs. 0.38; difference 0.44 (–1.24 to 2.12) and physical component 0.23 vs. –0.27; difference 0.50 (–1.11 to 2.11)	Low
Quality of life	Aripiprazole LAI vs. paliperidone palmitate LAI (monthly)	1 RCT; N=295	Moderate	Unknown	Direct	Imprecise	QLS change: 28 weeks 7.47 vs. 2.80; least squares mean difference 4.67 (0.32–9.02) Meets noninferiority criteria; does not meet minimally clinical important difference	Insufficient

TABLE D–1. Pharmacological treatment *(continued)*

Outcome	Comparators	Number of studies and subjects	Study limitations	Consistency	Directness	Precision	Magnitude of effect: summary effect size (95% CI)	Strength of evidence (high, moderate, low, insufficient)
Quality of life	Risperidone LAI vs. quetiapine	1 RCT; N=666	Moderate	Unknown	Direct	Precise	SF-12 physical and mental component scores and SQLS-Revision 4 scores improved from baseline in both groups but were not significantly different at endpoint, 24 months (SF-12 physical, P=0.09; SF-12 mental and SQLS-R4, P=NR)	Low
Quality of life	Haloperidol vs. olanzapine	1 SR (5 RCTs; N=816)	Moderate	Consistent	Direct	Precise	Inconclusive Effect sizes ranged from –3.62 to 0 using different measures; CIs were not significant	Moderate
Quality of life	Haloperidol vs. quetiapine	1 SR (1 RCT; N=207)	Moderate	Unknown	Direct	Imprecise	Inconclusive Effect estimate 0.00 (–1.38 to 1.38)	Insufficient
Quality of life	Haloperidol vs. risperidone	1 SR (2 RCTs; N=352)	Moderate	Inconsistent	Direct	Imprecise	Inconclusive Effect estimates ranged from –0.10 to 0.10; CIs were not significant	Insufficient

TABLE D–1. Pharmacological treatment *(continued)*

Outcome	Comparators	Number of studies and subjects	Study limitations	Consistency	Directness	Precision	Magnitude of effect: summary effect size (95% CI)	Strength of evidence (high, moderate, low, insufficient)
Quality of life	Haloperidol *vs.* ziprasidone	1 SR (2 RCTs; *N*=784)	High	Inconsistent	Direct	Imprecise	Studies favored ziprasidone in quality of life measures. One trial found effect favoring ziprasidone based on QLS: effect estimate –12.12 (–22.06 to –2.17); there was no difference in another trial in MANSA: effect estimate –0.10 (–1.48 to 1.28)	Low
Quality of life	Perphenazine *vs.* aripiprazole	1 SR (1 RCT; *N*=300)	Moderate	Unknown	Direct	Imprecise	Inconclusive. Proportion with 20% improvement: RR 4.74 (2.58–8.69)	Insufficient
Quality of life	Perphenazine *vs.* olanzapine	1 SR (1 RCT; *N*=597)	Moderate	Unknown	Direct	Precise	No difference. Effect estimate 0.00 (–0.16 to 0.16)	Low
Quality of life	Perphenazine *vs.* quetiapine	1 SR (1 RCT; *N*=598)	Moderate	Unknown	Direct	Precise	No difference. Effect estimate 0.10 (–0.07 to 0.27)	Low
Quality of life	Perphenazine *vs.* risperidone	1 SR (1 RCT; *N*=602)	Moderate	Unknown	Direct	Precise	No difference. Effect estimate –0.07 (–0.24 to 0.10)	Low
Quality of life	Perphenazine *vs.* ziprasidone	1 SR (1 RCT; *N*=446)	Moderate	Unknown	Direct	Precise	No difference. Effect estimate -0.07 (–0.27 to 0.13)	Low

TABLE D–1. Pharmacological treatment *(continued)*

Outcome	Comparators	Number of studies and subjects	Study limitations	Consistency	Directness	Precision	Magnitude of effect: summary effect size (95% CI)	Strength of evidence (high, moderate, low, insufficient)
Response	Network meta-analysis of olanzapine, risperidone, quetiapine IR, aripiprazole, clozapine, ziprasidone, asenapine, paliperidone, aripiprazole LAI (monthly), carpipramine, brexpiprazole, lurasidone	46 RCTs; $N=12,536$	Moderate	Consistent	Indirect	Precise	Two statistically significant differences between the drugs; both olanzapine (OR 1.71, 95% CI 1.11–2.68) and risperidone (OR 1.41, 95% CI 1.01–2.00) were significantly more likely to result in response than quetiapine IR	Low
Response	Fluphenazine vs. olanzapine	1 SR (1 RCT; $N=60$)	Moderate	Unknown	Direct	Imprecise	Inconclusive; RR 0.74 (0.51–1.07)	Insufficient
Response	Fluphenazine vs. quetiapine	1 SR (1 RCT; $N=25$)	Moderate	Unknown	Direct	Imprecise	Inconclusive; RR 0.62 (0.12–3.07)	Insufficient
Response	Fluphenazine vs. risperidone	1 SR (1 RCT; $N=26$)	Moderate	Unknown	Direct	Imprecise	Inconclusive; RR 0.67 (0.13–3.35)	Insufficient
Response	Haloperidol vs. aripiprazole	1 SR (5 RCTs; $N=2,185$)	Moderate	Inconsistent	Direct	Precise	No difference; RR 1.01 (0.76–1.34), $I^2=83\%$	Low
Response	Haloperidol vs. asenapine	1 SR (1 RCT; $N=335$)	Moderate	Unknown	Direct	Imprecise	Inconclusive; RR 0.82 (0.64–1.04)	Insufficient
Response	Haloperidol vs. clozapine	1 SR (2 RCTs; $N=144$)	Moderate	Inconsistent	Direct	Imprecise	Inconclusive; RR 0.64 (0.28–1.47), $I^2=72\%$	Insufficient
Response	Haloperidol vs. olanzapine	1 SR (14 RCTs; $N=4,099$)	Moderate	Inconsistent	Direct	Precise	Favors olanzapine; RR 0.86 (0.78–0.96), $I^2=55\%$	Low
Response	Haloperidol vs. quetiapine	1 SR (6 RCTs; $N=1,421$)	Moderate	Inconsistent	Direct	Precise	No difference; RR 0.99 (0.76–1.30), $I^2=77\%$	Low

TABLE D–1. Pharmacological treatment (*continued*)

Outcome	Comparators	Number of studies and subjects	Study limitations	Consistency	Directness	Precision	Magnitude of effect: summary effect size (95% CI)	Strength of evidence (high, moderate, low, insufficient)
Response	Haloperidol vs. risperidone	1 SR (16 RCTs; N=3,452)	Moderate	Consistent	Direct	Precise	No difference; RR 0.94 (0.87–1.02), I²=29%	Moderate
Response	Haloperidol vs. ziprasidone	1 SR (6 RCTs; N=1,283)	Moderate	Inconsistent	Direct	Imprecise	Inconclusive; RR 0.98 (0.74–1.30), I²=80%	Low
Response	Perphenazine vs. aripiprazole	1 SR (1 RCT; N=300)	Moderate	Unknown	Direct	Imprecise	Inconclusive; RR 0.95 (0.64–1.40)	Insufficient
Remission	Haloperidol vs. clozapine	1 SR (1 RCT; N=71)	Moderate	Unknown	Direct	Imprecise	Inconclusive; RR 0.16 (0.02–1.20)	Insufficient
Remission	Haloperidol vs. olanzapine	1 SR (3 RCTs; N=582)	Moderate	Consistent	Direct	Imprecise	Favors olanzapine; RR 0.65 (0.45–0.94), I²=54%	Low
Remission	Haloperidol vs. quetiapine	1 SR (1 RCT; N=207)	High	Unknown	Direct	Imprecise	Inconclusive; RR 0.72 (0.41–1.25)	Insufficient
Remission	Haloperidol vs. risperidone	1 SR (2 RCTs; N=179)	Moderate	Consistent	Direct	Imprecise	Inconclusive; RR 0.84 (0.56–1.24), I²=0%	Low
Remission	Haloperidol vs. ziprasidone	1 SR (3 RCTs; N=1,085)	High	Consistent	Direct	Precise	No difference; RR 0.89 (0.71–1.12), I²=12%	Low
Mortality (all-cause)	Olanzapine vs. risperidone vs. quetiapine	1 SR (1 retrospective cohort study; N=48,595)	Low	Unknown	Direct	Precise	No difference in all-cause mortality between risperidone and olanzapine (HR 1.09, 95% CI 0.79–1.49) or quetiapine (HR 0.75, 95% CI 0.53–1.07)	Low

TABLE D–1. Pharmacological treatment (continued)

Outcome	Comparators	Number of studies and subjects	Study limitations	Consistency	Directness	Precision	Magnitude of effect: summary effect size (95% CI)	Strength of evidence (high, moderate, low, insufficient)
Mortality (all-cause)	Clozapine, risperidone, olanzapine, and quetiapine vs. no treatment	1 SR (1 retrospective cohort study; N=6,987)	Low	Unknown	Direct	Imprecise	Clozapine and quetiapine had significantly lower risk of all-cause mortality (adjusted ORs 0.35, 95% CI 0.21–0.58 and 0.46, 95% CI 0.30–0.72), and risperidone and olanzapine were not statistically significantly different from control	Insufficient
Mortality (all-cause)	Asenapine vs. olanzapine	2 RCTs; N=2,174 (1 RCT reported 2 RCT studies)	Moderate	Consistent	Direct	Imprecise	Inconclusive RCT 1: 0.41% vs. 0.42% RCT 2: 0% vs. 0.77% RCT 3: 0.32% RR 2.49 (0.54–11.5)	Low
Mortality (all-cause)	Paliperidone palmitate LAI (monthly) vs. risperidone LAI	2 RCTs; N=752	Moderate	Consistent	Direct	Imprecise	Inconclusive RCT 1: 0.79% vs. 0.27% RCT 2: 0% vs. 0.45% RR 1.26 (0.21–7.49)	Low
Mortality (all-cause)	Quetiapine vs. risperidone	2 RCTs; N=1,057	Moderate	Consistent	Direct	Imprecise	Inconclusive RCT 1: 1.17% vs. 0.40% RCT 2: 0.72% vs. 0% RR 3.24 (0.72 to 14.6)	Low
Cardiovascular mortality	Olanzapine vs. risperidone vs. quetiapine	1 SR (2 retrospective cohort studies; N=55,582)	Low	Consistent	Direct	Precise	No significant differences between the drugs: HR 0.99 (0.37–2.67) and 0.76 (0.25–2.28), respectively	Low
Cardiovascular mortality	Clozapine vs. risperidone	1 SR (2 retrospective cohort studies; N=1,686)	Moderate	Unknown	Direct	Imprecise	Inconclusive No significant differences between drugs: 4.8% vs. 2.5%; RR 1.39 (0.61–2.53)	Insufficient

TABLE D–1. Pharmacological treatment *(continued)*

Outcome	Comparators	Number of studies and subjects	Study limitations	Consistency	Directness	Precision	Magnitude of effect: summary effect size (95% CI)	Strength of evidence (high, moderate, low, insufficient)
Self-harm: suicidal behavior, suicide	Clozapine vs. olanzapine in high-risk patients	1 SR (1 RCT; N=980)	Low	Unknown	Direct	Imprecise	Suicidal behavior: HR 0.76 (0.58–0.97)	Low
Self-harm: suicidal behavior, suicide	Clozapine vs. olanzapine in high-risk patients	1 SR (1 RCT; N=980)	Low	Unknown	Direct	Precise	Worsening on CGI-Suicide Severity: HR 0.78 (0.61–0.99)	Moderate
Self-harm: suicidal behavior, suicide	Clozapine vs. olanzapine in high-risk patients	1 SR (1 RCT; N=980)	Low	Unknown	Direct	Imprecise	Suicide deaths: no significant differences (5 clozapine, 3 olanzapine)	Low
Self-harm: suicidal behavior, suicide	Clozapine, risperidone, olanzapine, quetiapine, ziprasidone, aripiprazole	1 SR (2 retrospective cohorts; N=16,584)	Moderate	Consistent	Direct	Precise	Death by suicide lower with clozapine: OR 0.29 (0.14–0.63) compared with no treatment at 6 months and lower with clozapine (1.1%) than baseline (2.2%) or other drugs (range 2.1%–3.7%) at 1 year	Low
Self-harm: suicidal behavior, suicide	Clozapine, risperidone, olanzapine, quetiapine, ziprasidone, aripiprazole	1 SR (1 prospective cohort; N=10,204)	High	Unknown	Direct	Precise	Suicide attempts (6 months): no statistically significant difference between drugs	Insufficient

TABLE D–1. Pharmacological treatment (continued)

Outcome	Comparators	Number of studies and subjects	Study limitations	Consistency	Directness	Precision	Magnitude of effect: summary effect size (95% CI)	Strength of evidence (high, moderate, low, insufficient)
Self-harm: suicidal behavior, suicide	Clozapine, risperidone, olanzapine, quetiapine, ziprasidone, aripiprazole	1 SR (1 prospective cohort; N=20,489)	High	Unknown	Direct	Precise	Inconclusive Suicide attempts or death by suicide: aripiprazole vs. all others combined HR 0.69 (0.42–1.14)	Insufficient
Reduction in self-harm	Haloperidol vs. olanzapine	1 SR (1 RCT; N=182)	Moderate	Unknown	Indirect	Imprecise	Inconclusive Attempted suicide: RR 3.13 (0.13–76) Completed suicide: RR 3.13 (0.13–76)	Insufficient
Reduction in self-harm	Perphenazine vs. olanzapine	1 SR (1 RCT; N=597)	Moderate	Unknown	Indirect	Imprecise	Inconclusive Attempted suicide: RR 0.64 (0.06–7.06) Completed suicide: RR 3.86 (0.40–37)	Insufficient

Outcome	Comparators	Number of studies and subjects	Study limitations	Consistency	Directness	Precision	Magnitude of effect: summary effect size (95% CI)	Strength of evidence (high, moderate, low, insufficient)
Core illness symptoms	Oral SGAs (except carpipramine): meta-analysis of clozapine, amisulpride, olanzapine, risperidone, paliperidone, zotepine, haloperidol, quetiapine, aripiprazole, sertindole, ziprasidone, chlorpromazine, asenapine, lurasidone, and iloperidone	212 RCTs; $N = 43,049$	Moderate	Consistent	Indirect	Precise	Significantly better improvement with clozapine than the other drugs except olanzapine: SMDs on PANSS or BPRS –0.32 to –0.55 Olanzapine and risperidone superior to the other drugs, except for each other and paliperidone: SMDs –0.13 to –0.26 Paliperidone superior to lurasidone and iloperidone: SMD –0.17 All drugs superior to placebo: SMDs –0.33 to –0.88	Low
Core illness symptoms	Treatment-resistant patients: clozapine, risperidone, olanzapine, quetiapine, ziprasidone	Network meta-analysis (40 RCTs; $N = 5,172$)	Moderate	Consistent	Indirect	Precise	The only significant difference was that the mean change in the PANSS was greater with olanzapine than quetiapine: SMD –0.29 (–0.56 to –0.13)	Low
Core illness symptoms	Brexpiprazole vs. aripiprazole	1 open label study; $N = 97$	Moderate	Unknown	Indirect	Imprecise	Inconclusive PANSS: least squares mean difference –22.9 vs. –19.4 at 6 weeks from baseline; direct comparison not reported	Insufficient

TABLE D–1. Pharmacological treatment *(continued)*

Outcome	Comparators	Number of studies and subjects	Study limitations	Consistency	Directness	Precision	Magnitude of effect: summary effect size (95% CI)	Strength of evidence (high, moderate, low, insufficient)
Overall/any adverse events	Asenapine vs. olanzapine	5 RCTs (4 publications; N=2,189)	Moderate	Consistent	Direct	Precise	Pooled RR 1.00 (0.96–1.05), I²=9%	Moderate
Overall/any adverse events	Quetiapine vs. risperidone	7 RCTs; N=3,254	Moderate	Consistent	Direct	Precise	Pooled RR 1.04 (0.97–1.12), I²=56%	Moderate
Overall/any adverse events	Clozapine vs. olanzapine	2 RCTs; N=182	Moderate	Consistent	Direct	Imprecise	Pooled RR 1.15 (1.00–1.33), I²=0%	Low
Overall/any adverse events	Risperidone vs. olanzapine	5 RCTs; N=873	Moderate	Inconsistent	Direct	Precise	Pooled RR 1.02 (0.81–1.29), I²=77%	Low
Overall/any adverse events	Olanzapine vs. ziprasidone	5 RCTs; N=1,097 (6-week to 6-month durations)	Moderate	Inconsistent	Direct	Precise	Pooled RR 1.00 (0.86–1.16), I²=80%	Low
Overall/any adverse events	Olanzapine vs. quetiapine	3 RCTs; N=448	Moderate	Consistent	Direct	Imprecise	Pooled RR 0.90 (0.74–1.11), I²=30%	Low

TABLE D–1. Pharmacological treatment *(continued)*

Outcome	Comparators	Number of studies and subjects	Study limitations	Consistency	Directness	Precision	Magnitude of effect: summary effect size (95% CI)	Strength of evidence (high, moderate, low, insufficient)
Overall/any adverse events	Quetiapine XR vs. quetiapine IR and risperidone; risperidone vs. clozapine and aripiprazole; olanzapine vs. paliperidone; risperidone LAI vs. paliperidone and paliperidone palmitate LAI (monthly); and aripiprazole vs. aripiprazole LAI (monthly); additionally, there were 6 trials comparing asenapine and olanzapine	1 SR (28 RCTs; N=7,810)	Moderate	Consistent	Direct	Imprecise	No statistically significant differences were found in each comparison	Low

Outcome	Comparators	Number of studies and subjects	Study limitations	Consistency	Directness	Precision	Magnitude of effect: summary effect size (95% CI)	Strength of evidence (high, moderate, low, insufficient)
Overall/any adverse events	Oral aripiprazole vs. brexpiprazole, olanzapine, paliperidone, and risperidone LAI; ziprasidone vs. clozapine, risperidone, iloperidone, and lurasidone; risperidone vs. asenapine, carpipramine, and risperidone LAI; clozapine vs. quetiapine, quetiapine vs. risperidone LAI; olanzapine vs. olanzapine LAI and lurasidone; aripiprazole LAI (monthly) vs. paliperidone; and paliperidone palmitate LAI (monthly) vs. 3-month LAI	1 SR (31 RCTs; N=6,700)	Moderate	Unknown	Direct	Imprecise	No statistically significant differences were found in single studies of each comparison	Insufficient

TABLE D–1. Pharmacological treatment (continued)

Outcome	Comparators	Number of studies and subjects	Study limitations	Consistency	Directness	Precision	Magnitude of effect: summary effect size (95% CI)	Strength of evidence (high, moderate, low, insufficient)
Overall adverse events	Haloperidol vs. aripiprazole	1 SR (3 RCTs; N=1,713)	Moderate	Consistent	Direct	Precise	RR 1.11 (1.06–1.17), I²=0%; less with aripiprazole	Moderate
Overall adverse events	Haloperidol vs. risperidone	1 SR (8 RCTs; N=1,313)	Moderate	Consistent	Direct	Precise	RR 1.20 (1.01–1.42), I²=84%; less with risperidone	Moderate
Overall adverse events	Haloperidol vs. ziprasidone	1 SR (6 RCTs; N=1,448)	Moderate	Consistent	Direct	Precise	RR 1.13 (1.03–1.23), I²=31%; less with ziprasidone	Moderate

The APA Practice Guideline for the Treatment of Patients With Schizophrenia

TABLE D–1. Pharmacological treatment *(continued)*

Outcome	Comparators	Number of studies and subjects	Study limitations	Consistency	Directness	Precision	Magnitude of effect: summary effect size (95% CI)	Strength of evidence (high, moderate, low, insufficient)
Discontinuation due to adverse events	Network meta-analysis of aripiprazole, aripiprazole LAI (monthly), asenapine, brexpiprazole, cariprazine, clozapine, iloperidone, lurasidone, olanzapine, olanzapine LAI, paliperidone 3-month LAI, paliperidone, paliperidone LAI (monthly), quetiapine XR, quetiapine IR, risperidone, risperidone LAI, ziprasidone	89 RCTs (N = 29,678)	Moderate	Consistent	Indirect	Precise	Risperidone LAI had statistically significantly lower risk of withdrawals due to adverse events than asenapine (OR 0.50, 95% CI 0.23–0.97), clozapine (OR 0.26, 95% CI 0.10–0.67), lurasidone (OR 0.38, 95% CI 0.17–0.79), paliperidone (OR 0.43, 95% CI 0.17–0.98), paliperidone LAI (monthly) (OR 0.51, 95% CI 0.26–0.98), quetiapine XR (OR 0.42, 95% CI 0.21–0.78), risperidone (OR 0.48, 95% CI 0.23–0.92), and ziprasidone (OR 0.39, 95% CI 0.18–0.76) Olanzapine had lower risk than clozapine (OR 0.40, 95% CI 0.21–0.79), lurasidone (OR 0.58, 95% CI 0.36–0.98), quetiapine IR (OR 0.64, 95% CI 0.45–0.93), risperidone (OR 0.74, 95% CI 0.55–0.98), and ziprasidone (OR 0.59, 95% CI 0.43–0.84) Aripiprazole had lower risk than ziprasidone (OR 0.65, 95% CI 0.44–0.95), and iloperidone had lower risk than clozapine (OR 0.35, 95% CI 0.13–0.91)	Low

Outcome	Comparators	Number of studies and subjects	Study limitations	Consistency	Directness	Precision	Magnitude of effect: summary effect size (95% CI)	Strength of evidence (high, moderate, low, insufficient)
Withdrawal due to adverse events	Fluphenazine vs. olanzapine	1 SR (1 RCT; N=60)	Moderate	Unknown	Indirect	Imprecise	Inconclusive; RR 0.74 (0.51–1.07)	Insufficient
Withdrawal due to adverse events	Fluphenazine vs. quetiapine	1 SR (1 RCT; N=25)	Moderate	Unknown	Indirect	Imprecise	Inconclusive; RR 0.19 (0.01–3.52)	Insufficient
Withdrawal due to adverse events	Haloperidol vs. asenapine	1 SR (1 RCT; N=335)	Moderate	Unknown	Indirect	Imprecise	Inconclusive; RR 1.53 (0.74–3.16)	Insufficient
Withdrawal due to adverse events	Haloperidol vs. aripiprazole	1 SR (7 RCTs) plus 1 additional RCT; N=3,232	Moderate	Consistent	Direct	Precise	RR 1.25 (1.07–1.47), I^2=0%	Moderate
Withdrawal due to adverse events	Haloperidol vs. clozapine	1 SR (5 RCTs; N=719)	Moderate	Consistent	Direct	Imprecise	Inconclusive; RR 1.00 (0.66–1.50), I^2=0%	Low
Withdrawal due to adverse events	Haloperidol vs. olanzapine	1 SR (21 RCTs) plus 3 RCTs; N=5,708	Moderate	Consistent	Direct	Precise	RR 1.89 (1.57–2.27), I^2=0%	Moderate
Withdrawal due to adverse events	Haloperidol vs. quetiapine	1 SR (8 RCTs) plus 2 RCTs; N=1,759	Moderate	Consistent	Direct	Imprecise	Inconclusive; RR 1.97 (0.96–4.01), I^2=62%	Low

TABLE D–1. Pharmacological treatment *(continued)*

Outcome	Comparators	Number of studies and subjects	Study limitations	Consistency	Directness	Precision	Magnitude of effect: summary effect size (95% CI)	Strength of evidence (high, moderate, low, insufficient)
Withdrawal due to adverse events	Haloperidol *vs.* risperidone	1 SR (23 RCTs) plus 2 RCTs; *N*=4,581	Moderate	Consistent	Direct	Precise	RR 1.32 (1.09–1.60), I²=0%	Moderate
Withdrawal due to adverse events	Haloperidol *vs.* ziprasidone	1 SR (6 RCTs) plus 1 RCT; *N*=1,597	Moderate	Consistent	Direct	Precise	RR 1.68 (1.26–2.23), I²=0%	Moderate
Withdrawal due to adverse events	Perphenazine *vs.* aripiprazole	1 SR (1 RCT; *N*=300)	Moderate	Unknown	Direct	Imprecise	Inconclusive; RR 0.53 (0.27–1.05)	Insufficient
Withdrawal due to adverse events	Perphenazine *vs.* olanzapine	1 SR (1 RCT; *N*=597)	Moderate	Unknown	Direct	Imprecise	Inconclusive; RR 0.83 (0.58–1.19)	Insufficient
Withdrawal due to adverse events	Perphenazine *vs.* quetiapine	1 SR (1 RCT; *N*=598)	Moderate	Unknown	Direct	Imprecise	Inconclusive; RR 1.05 (0.72–1.55)	Insufficient
Withdrawal due to adverse events	Perphenazine *vs.* risperidone	1 SR (1 RCT; *N*=602)	Moderate	Unknown	Direct	Imprecise	Inconclusive; RR 1.54 (1.00–2.36)	Insufficient

TABLE D–1. Pharmacological treatment *(continued)*

Outcome	Comparators	Number of studies and subjects	Study limitations	Consistency	Directness	Precision	Magnitude of effect: summary effect size (95% CI)	Strength of evidence (high, moderate, low, insufficient)
Withdrawal due to adverse events	Perphenazine vs. ziprasidone	1 SR (1 RCT; N=446)	Moderate	Unknown	Direct	Imprecise	Inconclusive; RR 1.01 (0.65–1.58)	Insufficient

Abbreviations. BPRS=Brief Psychiatric Rating Scale; CATIE=Clinical Antipsychotic Trials of Intervention Effectiveness; CGI=Clinical Global Impression; CI=confidence interval; *df*=degrees of freedom; GAF=Global Assessment of Functioning; HR=hazard ratio; IR=immediate release; LAI=long-acting injectable; MANSA=Manchester Short Assessment of Quality of Life; NR=normal range; NS=not significant; OR=odds ratio; PANSS=Positive and Negative Syndrome Scale; PSP=Personal and Social Performance; Q=Cochran's Q test; QLS=Heinrichs-Carpenter Quality of Life Scale; RCT=randomized controlled trial; RFS=Role Functioning Scale; RR=relative risk; SAS-SMI=Social Adjustment Scale—Severely Mentally Ill version; SF=short form; SFS=Social Functioning Scale; SGA=second-generation antipsychotic; SMD=standard mean difference; SOFAS=Social and Occupational Functioning Assessment Scale; SQLS=Schizophrenia Quality of Life Scale; SR=systematic review; SWN=Subjective Well-being under Neuroleptic Treatment; WMD=weighted mean difference; XR=extended release.

TABLE D–2. Assertive community treatment (ACT)

Outcome	Comparators	Number of studies and subjects	Study limitations	Consistency	Directness	Precision	Magnitude of effect: summary effect size (95% CI)	Strength of evidence (high, moderate, low, insufficient)
Function	ACT vs. usual care	1 SR (3 RCTs) plus 1 RCT; N=118	Moderate	Consistent	Direct	Imprecise	No difference in social function compared with usual care Social function: MD 0.03 (−0.28 to 0.34)	Low
Trouble with police	ACT vs. usual care	1 SR (4 RCTs)	Moderate	Consistent	Direct	Imprecise	No differences in arrests (2 trials; OR 1.17, 95% CI 0.60–2.29), imprisonment (4 trials; OR 1.19, 95% CI 0.70–2.01), or police contacts (2 trials; OR 0.76, 95% CI 0.32–1.79)	Low
Housing and independent living	ACT vs. usual care	1 SR (3 RCTs) plus 1 RCT; N=118	Moderate	Consistent	Direct	Precise	Less likely to be not living independently (4 trials; OR 0.52, 95% CI 0.35–0.79) and to be homeless (4 trials; OR 0.20, 95% CI 0.09–0.47) Less likely to be homeless (4 trials; OR 0.24, 95% CI 0.12–0.48)	Moderate
Employment	ACT vs. usual care	1 SR (3 RCTs)	Moderate	Consistent	Direct	Precise	Less likely to be unemployed (OR 0.46, 95% CI 0.21–0.99)	Moderate
Quality of life	ACT vs. usual care	1 SR (1 RCT; N=125) plus 1 RCT; N=118	Moderate	Inconsistent	Direct	Imprecise	Quality of life was slightly better with ACT (MD −0.52, 95% CI −0.99 to −0.05) in one trial, but no differences were found in the other trial	Insufficient

TABLE D–2. Assertive community treatment (ACT) (continued)

Outcome	Comparators	Number of studies and subjects	Study limitations	Consistency	Directness	Precision	Magnitude of effect: summary effect size (95% CI)	Strength of evidence (high, moderate, low, insufficient)
Overall symptoms	ACT vs. usual care	1 SR (3 RCTs) plus 1 RCT; N=118	Moderate	Consistent	Direct	Precise	No differences were found in 4 trials (MD –0.14, 95% CI –0.36 to 0.08)	Moderate
Treatment maintenance (loss to follow-up)	ACT vs. usual care	1 SR (10 RCTs) plus 1 RCT; N=118	Moderate	Consistent	Direct	Precise	Significantly less loss to follow-up with ACT (OR 0.51, 95% CI 0.40–0.65) on the basis of 10 trials in the SR; significantly fewer patients "out of care" in the other trial (OR 0.10, 95% CI 0.03–0.33)	Moderate

Abbreviations. CI=confidence interval; MD=mean difference; OR=odds ratio; RCT=randomized controlled trial; SR=systematic review.

TABLE D–3. Cognitive-behavioral therapy (CBT)

Outcome	Comparators	Number of studies and subjects	Study limitations	Consistency	Directness	Precision	Magnitude of effect: summary effect size (95% CI)	Strength of evidence (high, moderate, low, insufficient)
Function: global function, short term (≤6 months since CBT initiation)	CBT vs. usual care	1 SR (3 RCTs) plus 5 RCTs; N=701	Moderate	Consistent	Direct	Precise	GAF (6 RCTs): MD 5.49 (1.85–9.14), I²=75%; excluding one outlier: 6.62 (4.68–8.56), I²=0% SOFAS (2 RCTs): MD 9.11 (6.31–11.91) Proportion with normal function (1 RCT): RR 2.21 (1.25–3.93)	Moderate
Function: global function, medium term (>6 months to 1 year since CBT initiation)	CBT vs. usual care	3 RCTs; N=465	Moderate	Inconsistent	Direct	Imprecise	Inconclusive GAF: 1 trial with 6-month posttreatment follow-up found no difference; another trial found effect favoring CBT SOFAS, SFS: No difference between groups	Insufficient
Function: global function, long term (>1 year since CBT initiation)	CBT vs. usual care	1 SR (4 RCTs) plus 4 RCTs; N=851	Moderate	Consistent	Direct	Imprecise	Inconclusive GAF: 1 SR found MD 4.20 (−0.63 to 9.03); another RCT found positive effect of CBT 3 RCTs found no difference in SOFAS, global function (scale not reported), and proportion of patients with normal function	Low
Function: basic living skills	CBT vs. usual care	1 RCT; N=76	Moderate	Unknown	Direct	Imprecise	No difference between groups	Insufficient
Function: employment outcomes	CBT vs. usual care	2 RCTs; N=522	Moderate	Inconsistent	Direct	Imprecise	Inconclusive 1 RCT of vocation-focused CBT favored CBT for hours worked and WBI score; another trial found no difference in proportion of patients with occupational recovery	Insufficient

TABLE D–3. Cognitive-behavioral therapy (CBT) (continued)

Outcome	Comparators	Number of studies and subjects	Study limitations	Consistency	Directness	Precision	Magnitude of effect: summary effect size (95% CI)	Strength of evidence (high, moderate, low, insufficient)
Quality of life	CBT vs. usual care	12- to 24-week follow-up; 2 RCTs; N=216	Moderate	Consistent	Direct	Imprecise	CBT led to improved quality of life 0 and 16 weeks after cessation of treatment on the basis of CHOICE, WEMWEBS, and WHOQOL-BREF scales	Low
Quality of life	CBT vs. usual care	18- to 24-month follow-up; 2 RCTs; N=489	Moderate	Consistent	Direct	Imprecise	CBT not different from usual care on WHOQOL and EUROQOL scales	Low
Suicide and suicidality	CBT vs. usual care	2 RCTs; N=307	Moderate	Consistent	Direct	Imprecise	Inconclusive; RR 0.68 (0.12–3.93) and RR 0.53 (0.12–2.79)	Insufficient
Core illness symptoms	CBT vs. usual care	1 SR (34 RCTs; N=2,989)	Moderate	Consistent	Direct	Precise	SMD −0.33 (0.47 to −0.19); subgroup with outcome assessment blinding SMD −0.15 (−0.27 to −0.03)	Moderate
Negative symptoms	CBT vs. usual care	2 SRs (34 RCTs; N=3,393)	Moderate	Inconsistent	Direct	Precise	SMD −0.13 (−0.25 to −0.01), I^2=48% (in this review, a negative estimate favors CBT); SMD 0.09 (−0.03 to 0.21), I^2=63% (in this review, a positive estimate favors CBT)	Low
Ability to maintain treatment	CBT vs. usual care	13 RCTs; N=1,847	Moderate	Inconsistent	Direct	Precise	No difference; RR 1.03 (0.96–1.10), I^2=64%	Low
Relapse	CBT vs. usual care	6 RCTs; N=1,090	Moderate	Inconsistent	Direct	Imprecise	Inconclusive; RR 0.80 (0.51–1.25), I^2=77% Subanalysis limited to relapse defined as "hospitalization" (3 RCTs): 0.70 (0.54–0.91), I^2=0%	Insufficient
Harms	CBT vs. usual care	1 RCT; N=150	Moderate	Inconsistent	Direct	Imprecise	None of the adverse events were related to treatment: 2 vs. 4 suicide attempts; 1 vs. 1 serious violent incident	Insufficient

Abbreviations. CHOICE=Choice of Outcome in CBT for psychoses; CI=confidence interval; EUROQOL=European Quality of Life scale; GAF=Global Assessment of Functioning; MD=mean difference; OR=odds ratio; RCT=randomized controlled trial; RR=relative risk; SFS=Social Functioning Scale; SMD=standard mean difference; SOFAS=Social and Occupational Functioning Assessment Scale; SR=systematic review; WBI=Work Behavior Inventory; WEMWEBS=Warwick-Edinburgh Mental Well-being Scale; WHOQOL=World Health Organization Quality of Life.

TABLE D–4. Cognitive remediation

Outcome	Comparators	Number of studies and subjects	Study limitations	Consistency	Directness	Precision	Magnitude of effect: summary effect size (95% CI)	Strength of evidence (high, moderate, low, insufficient)
Function	Cognitive remediation vs. usual care	1 SR (19 RCTs) plus 3 RCTs; N=1,323	Moderate	Consistent	Direct	Imprecise	In studies comparing with usual care, cognitive remediation resulted in a small positive effect on function that was not consistently statistically significant: effect size 0.16 (–0.16 to 0.49), SMD 0.56 (0.34–0.88), and SMD 0.41 (–0.10 to 0.91).	Low
Quality of life	Cognitive remediation vs. usual care	1 RCT; N=69	Moderate	Unknown	Direct	Imprecise	Quality of life was reported in only 1 trial, with no difference between cognitive remediation and usual care	Insufficient
Overall symptoms	Cognitive remediation vs. usual care	2 RCTs; N=153	Moderate	Consistent	Direct	Imprecise	Cognitive remediation improved total symptoms in 2 trials: SMD –0.62 (–1.01 to –0.24); 4 trials included in the Wykes review reported effect sizes ranging from 0.05 to 0.45 (CIs were not reported)	Low
Negative symptoms	Cognitive remediation vs. usual care	1 SR (18 RCTs; N=781)	Moderate	Consistent	Direct	Precise	Negative symptoms improved more in cognitive remediation groups: effect size –0.36 (–0.52 to –0.20); a negative effect size favors cognitive remediation	Moderate
Ability to maintain treatment	Cognitive remediation vs. usual care	3 RCTs; N=302	Moderate	Consistent	Direct	Imprecise	No difference in ability to maintain treatment in 3 RCTs of cognitive remediation	Low

Abbreviations. CI=confidence interval; RCT=randomized controlled trial; SMD=standard mean difference; SR=systematic review.

TABLE D–5. Family interventions

Outcome	Comparators	Number of studies and subjects	Study limitations	Consistency	Directness	Precision	Magnitude of effect: summary effect size (95% CI)	Strength of evidence (high, moderate, low, insufficient)
Function: occupational (unemployed), 1 year	Family intervention vs. usual care	1 SR (4 RCTs; N=230)	Moderate	Consistent	Direct	Imprecise	RR 1.09 (0.92–1.29)	Low
Function: occupational (unemployed), 2 years	Family intervention vs. usual care	1 SR (1 RCT; N=51)	Moderate	Unknown	Direct	Imprecise	RR 1.33 (0.84–2.10)	Insufficient
Function: occupational (unemployed), 3 years	Family intervention vs. usual care	1 SR (1 RCT; N=99)	Moderate	Unknown	Direct	Imprecise	RR 1.19 (0.92–1.55)	Insufficient
Function: living situation (cannot live independently), 1 year	Family intervention vs. usual care	1 SR (3 RCTs; N=164)	Moderate	Consistent	Direct	Imprecise	RR 0.83 (0.66–1.03)	Low
Function: living situation (cannot live independently), 3 years	Family intervention vs. usual care	1 SR (1 RCT; N=99)	Moderate	Unknown	Direct	Imprecise	RR 0.82 (0.59–1.14)	Insufficient
Function: living situation (cannot live independently, months in psychiatric facility), 5 years	Family intervention vs. usual care	1 RCT; N=73	Moderate	Unknown	Direct	Imprecise	10.87 vs. 21.18 months, P=0.04	Insufficient
Social functioning	Family intervention vs. usual care	1 RCT; N=69	Moderate	Unknown	Direct	Imprecise	No between-group differences	Insufficient

TABLE D–5. Family interventions (continued)

Outcome	Comparators	Number of studies and subjects	Study limitations	Consistency	Directness	Precision	Magnitude of effect: summary effect size (95% CI)	Strength of evidence (high, moderate, low, insufficient)
Quality of life	Family intervention vs. usual care	1 SR (1 RCT; N=50) plus 1 RCT not in SR; N=55	Moderate	Unknown	Direct	Imprecise	QLS: MD –5.05 (–15.44 to 5.34) EUROQOL: MD –7.38 (–22.07 to 7.31)	Insufficient
Depression	Family intervention vs. usual care	2 RCTs; N=124	Moderate	Consistent	Direct	Imprecise	RCT 1, 6 months: –1.0 (–12 to 22) vs. 0 (–15 to 17) RCT 1, 12 months: 3.0 (–15 to 17) vs. 0 (–14 to 17) RCT 2, 12 months: 3.35 (–2.64 to 9.34) RCT 2, 24 months: –0.11 (–6.91 to 6.68)	Low
Anxiety	Family intervention vs. usual care	1 RCT; N=55	Low	Unknown	Direct	Imprecise	12 months: –0.42 (–6.97 to 6.13) 24 months: –2.36 (–9.13 to 4.40)	Insufficient
Suicide	Family intervention vs. usual care	1 SR (6 RCTs; N=314)	Moderate	Consistent	Direct	Imprecise	RR 0.85 (0.24–3.02)	Low
Core illness symptoms	Family intervention vs. usual care	1 SR (2 RCTs; N=223)	Moderate	Consistent	Direct	Imprecise	SMD –0.46 (–0.73 to –0.20)	Low
Negative symptoms	Family intervention vs. usual care	3 RCTs; N=163	Moderate	Consistent	Direct	Imprecise	SMD –0.38 (–0.69 to –0.07)	Low
Leaving the study early (3–6 months)	Family intervention vs. usual care	1 SR (6 RCTs; N=504)	Moderate	Consistent	Indirect	Imprecise	RR 0.86 (0.50–1.47)	Low
Leaving the study early (7–12 months)	Family intervention vs. usual care	1 SR (9 RCTs; N=487) plus 4 RCTs; N=466	Moderate	Consistent	Indirect	Imprecise	RR 0.77 (0.64–0.93)	Low
Leaving the study early (13–24 months)	Family intervention vs. usual care	1 SR (6 RCTs; N=362)	Moderate	Consistent	Indirect	Imprecise	RR 0.82 (0.57–1.16)	Low

TABLE D–5. Family interventions *(continued)*

Outcome	Comparators	Number of studies and subjects	Study limitations	Consistency	Directness	Precision	Magnitude of effect: summary effect size (95% CI)	Strength of evidence (high, moderate, low, insufficient)
Leaving the study early (25–36 months)	Family intervention vs. usual care	1 SR (2 RCTs; N=90)	High	Consistent	Indirect	Imprecise	RR 0.59 (0.24–1.49)	Insufficient
Leaving the study early after 3 years	Family intervention vs. usual care	1 SR (1 RCT; N=63)	Moderate	Unknown	Indirect	Imprecise	RR 1.72 (0.71–4.16)	Insufficient
Poor compliance with medication	Family intervention vs. usual care	1 SR (4 RCTs; N=174) plus 2 RCTs; N=256	Moderate	Consistent	Indirect	Imprecise	RR 0.78 (0.65–0.92)	Low
Relapse (0–6 months)	Family intervention vs. usual care	1 SR (2 RCTs; N=167)	Moderate	Consistent	Direct	Imprecise	RR 0.62 (0.41–0.92)	Low
Relapse (7–12 months)	Family intervention vs. usual care	1 SR (16 RCTs; N=861) plus 4 RCTs; N=314	Moderate	Consistent	Direct	Imprecise	RR 0.67 (0.54–0.83)	Moderate
Relapse (13–24 months)	Family intervention vs. usual care	1 SR (9 RCTs; N=517)	Moderate	Consistent	Direct	Imprecise	RR 0.75 (0.58–0.99)	Low
Relapse (25–36 months)	Family intervention vs. usual care	1 SR (2 RCTs; N=147)	Moderate	Inconsistent	Direct	Imprecise	RR 1.05 (0.80–1.39)	Low
Relapse (5 years)	Family intervention vs. usual care	1 SR (1 RCT; N=63) plus 1 RCT; N=77	Moderate	Consistent	Direct	Imprecise	RR 0.82 (0.72–0.94)	Low
Relapse (8 years)	Family intervention vs. usual care	1 SR (1 RCT; N=62)	Moderate	Unknown	Direct	Imprecise	RR 0.86 (0.71–1.05)	Insufficient

TABLE D–5. Family interventions *(continued)*

Outcome	Comparators	Number of studies and subjects	Study limitations	Consistency	Directness	Precision	Magnitude of effect: summary effect size (95% CI)	Strength of evidence (high, moderate, low, insufficient)
Family burden not improved or worse	Family intervention vs. usual care	1 SR (1 RCT; N=51)	Moderate	Unknown	Direct	Imprecise	Social functioning: RR 2.40 (0.51–11.27) at 1 year RR 2.88 (0.64–12.97) at 2 years Subjective burden: RR 1.44 (0.60–3.46) at 1 year RR 0.58 (0.15–2.16) at 2 years	Insufficient
Nonsuicide mortality	Family intervention vs. usual care	1 SR (3 RCTs; N=113)	Moderate	Consistent	Direct	Imprecise	RR 0.96 (0.17–5.33)	Insufficient

Abbreviations. EUROQOL=European Quality of Life scale; MD=mean difference; QLS=Heinrichs-Carpenter Quality of Life Scale; RCT=randomized controlled trial; RR=relative risk; SMD=standard mean difference; SR=systematic review.

TABLE D–6. Intensive case management

Outcome	Comparators	Number of studies and subjects	Study limitations	Consistency	Directness	Precision	Magnitude of effect: summary effect size (95% CI)	Strength of evidence (high, moderate, low, insufficient)
Function	Intensive case management vs. usual care	1SR (3 RCTs) plus 1 RCT; $N=77$	Moderate	Consistent	Direct	Imprecise	Inconclusive Pooled MD 0.46 (–0.34 to 1.26); one subsequent trial also found no difference using a different scale	Low
Quality of life	Intensive case management vs. usual care	1SR (2 RCTs) plus 1 RCT; $N=77$	Moderate	Consistent	Direct	Imprecise	Inconclusive Pooled MD 0.09 (–0.23 to 0.42); one subsequent trial also found no difference between groups in quality of life using a different scale	Insufficient
Overall symptoms	Intensive case management vs. usual care	1SR (2 RCTs) plus 1 RCT; $N=77$	Moderate	Consistent	Direct	Imprecise	Inconclusive Pooled MD 0.46 (–3.67 to 4.60); one subsequent trial also reported no difference	Low
Loss to follow-up	Intensive case management vs. usual care	1SR (7 RCTs) plus 1 RCT; $N=77$	Moderate	Consistent	Direct	Precise	Less loss to follow-up with intensive case management compared with usual care: OR 0.70 (0.54–0.90)	Moderate
Imprisonment	Intensive case management vs. usual care	1 SR (5 RCTs)	Moderate	Consistent	Direct	Imprecise	No significant differences in imprisonment: OR 0.90 (0.45–1.82)	Low

Abbreviations. CI=confidence interval; MD=mean difference; OR=odds ratio; RCT=randomized controlled trial; SR=systematic review.

TABLE D–7. Illness management and recovery

Outcome	Comparators	Number of studies and subjects	Study limitations	Consistency	Directness	Precision	Magnitude of effect: summary effect size (95% CI)	Strength of evidence (high, moderate, low, insufficient)
Functioning	Illness self-management/self-management education intervention vs. usual care	1 SR (10 RCTs; N=409) plus 1 RCT; N=210	Moderate	Inconsistent	Direct	Imprecise	Inconclusive Heterogeneous methods for measuring various types of functioning were used, with 5 finding benefit and 6 not	Insufficient
Symptoms	Illness self-management/self-management education intervention vs. usual care	1 SR (5 RCTs; N=409)	Moderate	Consistent	Direct	Precise	BPRS, WMD: –4.19 (–5.84 to –2.54)	Moderate
Negative symptoms	Illness self-management/self-management education intervention vs. usual care	1 SR (3 RCTs; N=257)	Moderate	Consistent	Direct	Imprecise	PANSS negative –4.01 (–5.23 to –2.79)	Low
Relapse	Illness self-management/self-management education intervention vs. usual care	1 SR (3 RCTs; N=534)	Moderate	Consistent	Direct	Imprecise	Relapse (>10 interventions): N=233, OR 0.41 (0.21–0.79), P=0.008 Relapse (<10 interventions): N=269, OR 0.67 (0.39–1.15), P=0.014	Low

Abbreviations. BPRS=Brief Psychiatric Rating Scale; CI=confidence interval; OR=odds ratio; PANSS=Positive and Negative Syndrome Scale; RCT=randomized controlled trial; SR=systematic review; WMD=weighted mean difference.

TABLE D–8. Psychoeducation

Outcome	Comparators	Number of studies and subjects	Study limitations	Consistency	Directness	Precision	Magnitude of effect: summary effect size (95% CI)	Strength of evidence (high, moderate, low, insufficient)
Global functioning (GAF/GAS) at end of intervention	Psychoeducation vs. standard care	1 SR (1 RCT; N=41)	Medium	Unknown	Direct	Imprecise	Inconclusive; MD −2.64 (−12.74 to 7.46)	Insufficient
Global functioning (GAS) at 6 months	Psychoeducation vs. standard care	1 SR (1 RCT; N=92)	Medium	Unknown	Direct	Imprecise	Inconclusive; RR 0.83 (0.50–1.38)	Insufficient
Global functioning (GAF/GAS) at 1 year	Psychoeducation vs. standard care	1 SR (3 RCTs; N=260)	Medium	Consistent	Direct	Imprecise	MD −5.23 (−8.76 to −1.71), I^2=79%	Low
Global functioning (GAS) at 18 months	Psychoeducation vs. standard care	1 SR (1 RCT; N=92)	Medium	Unknown	Direct	Imprecise	Inconclusive; RR 0.90 (0.58–1.39)	Insufficient
Global functioning (GAF/GAS) at 2 years	Psychoeducation vs. standard care	1 SR (1 RCT; N=59)	Medium	Unknown	Direct	Imprecise	MD −6.70 (−13.38 to −0.02)	Insufficient
Global functioning (GAF/GAS) at 5 years	Psychoeducation vs. standard care	1 SR (1 RCT; N=60)	Medium	Unknown	Direct	Imprecise	Inconclusive; MD −3.80 (−8.04 to 0.44)	Insufficient
Social functioning (SAS-II) at end of intervention	Psychoeducation vs. standard care	1 SR (1 RCT; N=19)	Medium	Unknown	Direct	Imprecise	Inconclusive; MD −0.10 (−0.37 to 0.17)	Insufficient
Quality of life (QLS) at end of intervention	Psychoeducation vs. standard care	1 SR (1 RCT; N=114)	Medium	Unknown	Direct	Imprecise	MD −8.20 (−14.78 to −1.62)	Insufficient
Quality of life (QLS) at 3 months	Psychoeducation vs. standard care	1 SR (1 RCT; N=108)	Medium	Unknown	Direct	Imprecise	MD −9.70 (−17.22 to −2.18)	Insufficient
BPRS at 3 months	Psychoeducation vs. standard care	1 SR (1 RCT; N=19)	Medium	Unknown	Direct	Imprecise	Inconclusive; MD −0.06 (−0.53 to 0.41)	Insufficient
BPRS at 1 year	Psychoeducation vs. standard care	1 SR (1 RCT; N=159)	Medium	Unknown	Direct	Imprecise	MD −6.0 (−9.15 to −2.85)	Insufficient
Relapse with or without readmission: 9–18 months	Psychoeducation vs. standard care	1 SR (6 RCTs; N=720)	Medium	Consistent	Direct	Precise	RR 0.80 (0.70–0.92), I^2=54%	Moderate

TABLE D–8. Psychoeducation *(continued)*

Outcome	Comparators	Number of studies and subjects	Study limitations	Consistency	Directness	Precision	Magnitude of effect: summary effect size (95% CI)	Strength of evidence (high, moderate, low, insufficient)
Relapse without readmission: total	Psychoeducation *vs.* standard care	1 SR (3 RCTs; *N*=385)	Medium	Consistent	Direct	Imprecise	Inconclusive; RR 1.05 (0.84–1.31), I^2=60%	Low
Relapse without readmission: 1 year	Psychoeducation *vs.* standard care	1 SR (2 RCTs; *N*=303)	Medium	Consistent	Direct	Imprecise	Inconclusive: RR 1.16 (0.92–1.46), I^2=0.0%	Low
Relapse without readmission: 18 months	Psychoeducation *vs.* standard care	1 SR (1 RCT; *N*=382)	Medium	Unknown	Direct	Imprecise	Inconclusive; RR 0.5 (0.23–1.11)	Insufficient
Harms: mortality	Psychoeducation *vs.* standard care	1 SR (2 RCTs; *N*=170)	Medium	Consistent	Direct	Imprecise	Inconclusive; RR 0.53 (0.07–3.95), I^2=0.0%	Low

Abbreviations. BPRS=Brief Psychiatric Rating Scale; CI=confidence interval; GAF=Global Assessment of Functioning; GAS=Global Assessment Scale; MD=mean difference; QLS=Heinrichs-Carpenter Quality of Life Scale; RCT=randomized controlled trial; RR=risk ratio; SAS=Social Adjustment Scale; SR=systematic review.

TABLE D–9. Social skills training

Outcome	Comparators	Number of studies and subjects	Study limitations	Consistency	Directness	Precision	Magnitude of effect: summary effect size (95% CI)	Strength of evidence (high, moderate, low, insufficient)
Function	Social skills training vs. usual care	3 RCTs (4 publications); N=384	Moderate	Consistent	Direct	Imprecise	Significant improvement in scale scores during treatment for 6 months to 2 years (SMD range 0.65–1.60)	Low
Function	Social skills training vs. usual care	1 RCT; N=183	Moderate	Unknown	Direct	Imprecise	Social function not different from control after treatment cessation (1 study; SMD 0.24, 95% CI –0.05 to 0.53)	Insufficient
Overall symptoms	Social skills training vs. usual care	2 RCTs; N=201	Moderate	Consistent	Direct	Imprecise	Inconclusive PANSS: SMD –1.50 (–1.92 to –1.09) and –0.81 (–1.22 to –0.40) BPRS (mixed population): SMD –0.04 (–0.33 to 0.25)	Low
Overall symptoms	Social skills training vs. usual care	1 RCT; N=183	Moderate	Unknown	Direct	Imprecise	Inconclusive Mixed population (55% schizophrenia), no significant effect on symptoms (BPRS): SMD –0.04 (–0.33 to 0.25)	Insufficient
Negative symptoms	Social skills training vs. usual care	3 RCTs (4 publications); N=384	Moderate	Consistent	Direct	Imprecise	Negative symptoms improved with social skills training vs. usual care on the basis of PANSS negative and SANS: SMD range –0.45 to –1.30 at 6 months to 2 years	Low
Negative symptoms	Social skills training vs. usual care	1 RCT; N=183	Moderate	Unknown	Direct	Imprecise	Negative symptoms were better with social skills training than usual care 1 year after treatment discontinuation: SMD –0.45 (–0.74 to –0.15)	Insufficient
Ability to maintain treatment	Social skills training vs. usual care	2 RCTs; N=384	Moderate	Consistent	Direct	Imprecise	No difference: 1 year: RR 1.10 (0.92–1.31) 2 years: RR 1.01 (0.88–1.16)	Low
Relapse	Social skills training vs. usual care	1 RCT; N=82	Moderate	Unknown	Direct	Imprecise	Inconclusive; RR 0.50 (0.18–1.36)	Insufficient

Abbreviations. BPRS=Brief Psychiatric Rating Scale; CI=confidence interval; PANSS=Positive and Negative Syndrome Scale; RCT=randomized controlled trial; RR=relative risk; SANS=Scale for the Assessment of Negative Symptoms; SMD=standard mean difference.

TABLE D–10. Supported employment

Outcome	Comparators	Number of studies and subjects	Study limitations	Consistency	Directness	Precision	Magnitude of effect: summary effect size (95% CI)	Strength of evidence (high, moderate, low, insufficient)
Functional (occupational): number in competitive employment	IPS vs. standard services	1 trial; N=204	Moderate	Unknown	Direct	Imprecise	75% vs. 27.5%, P<0.001	Low
Functional (occupational): number in competitive employment	Supported employment (primarily IPS) vs. vocational training or usual care	1 RCT; N=1,273	Moderate	Consistent	Indirect for this review question	Precise	IPS vs. vocational training or usual care: 55% vs 34%, P<0.001	Moderate
Functional (occupational): number in competitive employment	All comparators						Subgroup analysis of only patients with schizophrenia: 22% vs. 12%, P<0.001 with mixed effects logistic regression	Moderate
Functional (occupational): days to first competitive employment	IPS vs. standard services	1 trial; N=204	Moderate	Unknown	Direct	Imprecise	Days to first job: 196.63 vs. 218.84, P=0.019	Low
Functional (occupational): worked more than 20 hours per week	IPS vs. standard services	1 trial; N=204	Moderate	Unknown	Direct	Imprecise	Worked >20 hours per week: 33.8% vs. 13%, P=0.001	Low
Functional (occupational): worked more than 20 hours per week	Supported employment (primarily IPS) vs. vocational training or usual care	1 RCT; N=1,273	Moderate	Consistent	Indirect for this review question	Precise	IPS vs. vocational training or usual care Working ≥40 hours per month: 51% vs. 39%, P<0.001	Moderate

TABLE D-10. Supported employment (continued)

Outcome	Comparators	Number of studies and subjects	Study limitations	Consistency	Directness	Precision	Magnitude of effect: summary effect size (95% CI)	Strength of evidence (high, moderate, low, insufficient)
Functional (occupational): worked more than 20 hours per week	All comparators							Moderate
Functional (occupational): wages earned	IPS vs. standard services	1 trial; N=204	Moderate	Unknown	Direct	Imprecise	$2,078/month vs. $617.59/month, P<0.001	Low
Functional (occupational): wages earned	Supported employment (primarily IPS) vs. vocational training or usual care	1 RCT; N=1,273	Moderate	Consistent	Indirect for this review question	Precise	IPS vs. vocational training or usual care $122/month vs. $99/month, P=0.04	Moderate
Functional (occupational): wages earned	All comparators							Moderate
Functional (occupational): weeks worked (mean)	IPS vs. standard services	1 trial; N=204	Moderate	Unknown	Direct	Imprecise	Total weeks worked: 29.72 vs. 5.45, P<0.001	Low
Functional (occupational): weeks worked (mean)	Supported employment (primarily IPS) vs. vocational training	1 SR; N=2,265	Moderate	Consistent	Indirect for this review question	Precise	Supported employment vs. vocational training days employed: mean difference 70.63 (43.22–98.04)	Moderate
Functional (occupational): weeks worked (mean)	All comparators							Moderate

Abbreviations. CI=confidence interval; IPS=individual placement and support; RCT=randomized controlled trial; SR=systematic review.

TABLE D–11. Supportive therapy

Outcome	Comparators	Number of studies and subjects	Study limitations	Consistency	Directness	Precision	Magnitude of effect: summary effect size (95% CI)	Strength of evidence (high, moderate, low, insufficient)
Global functioning	Supportive therapy vs. standard care	1 SR (2 RCTs; N=289)	Moderate	Consistent	Direct	Imprecise	Inconclusive GAF-M: n=29; MD 1.40 (–5.09 to 7.89) GAS: n=260; MD –2.66 (–6.20 to 0.88)	Low
Social functioning	Supportive therapy vs. standard care	1 SR (1 RCT; N=260)	Moderate	Unknown	Direct	Imprecise	Inconclusive SFS: MD –0.67 (–7.05 to 5.71)	Insufficient
Quality of life	Supportive therapy vs. standard care	1 SR (1 RCT; N=260)	Moderate	Unknown	Direct	Imprecise	Inconclusive RSES: MD –1.21 (–2.85 to 0.43) WBS: MD –2.73 (–6.04 to 0.58) GHQ: MD –2.45 (–2.41 to 7.31)	Insufficient
Relapse	Supportive therapy vs. standard care	1 SR (1 RCT; N=54)	Moderate	Unknown	Direct	Imprecise	Inconclusive Medium-term follow-up (13–26 weeks): RR 0.12 (0.01–2.11) Long-term follow-up (>26 weeks): RR 0.96 (0.44–2.11)	Insufficient
Core symptoms	Supportive therapy vs. standard care	1 SR (2 RCTs; N=167)	Moderate	Unknown	Direct	Imprecise	Inconclusive PANSS: Short term (13–26 weeks, n=131), MD –4.42 (–10.13 to 1.29) Long term (>26 weeks, n=36): MD 4.70 (–6.71 to 16.11)	Insufficient
Negative symptoms	Supportive therapy vs. standard care	1 SR (1 RCT; N=47)	Moderate	Unknown	Direct	Imprecise	Inconclusive Short term: mean 10.19 vs. 10.73 Long term: mean 9.90 vs. 11.46 (no statistical analysis because of skewed data)	Insufficient
Discontinuing treatment	Supportive therapy vs. standard care	1 SR (4 RCTs; N=354)	Moderate	Consistent	Direct	Imprecise	Inconclusive; RR 0.86 (0.53–1.40)	Low

Abbreviations. CI=confidence interval; GAF-M=Global Assessment of Functioning modified; GAS=Global Assessment Scale; GHQ=Global Health Quotient; MD=mean difference; PANSS=Positive and Negative Syndrome Scale; RCT=randomized controlled trial; RR=relative risk; RSES=Rosenberg Self-Esteem Scale; SFS=Social Functioning Scale; SR=systematic review; WBS=Well-Being Scale.

TABLE D–12. Early interventions for patients with first-episode psychosis

Outcome	Number of studies and subjects	Study limitations	Consistency	Directness	Precision	Magnitude of effect: summary effect size (95% CI)	Strength of evidence (high, moderate, low, insufficient)
Functional: global (GAS, GAF)	1 SR, 1 RCT; N=369 (2-year data only) plus 2 RCTs; N=744, N=98	Moderate	Consistent	Direct	Precise	GAS and GAF results only Team-based CSC resulted in higher functioning scores Pooled WMD: 3.88 (0.91–6.85), I²=64%	Moderate
Functional: work or school	1 SR, 1 RCT (OPUS-Scandinavia); N=547 plus 2 RCTs; N=744, N=125	Moderate	Consistent	Direct	Precise	Significantly more people (22%) are working or in school with team-based CSC Pooled RR 1.22 (1.01–1.47)	Moderate
Functional: housing status	1 SR, 1 RCT; N=547 plus 1 RCT; N=128	Moderate	Consistent	Direct	Imprecise	No significant difference between groups Pooled RR 1.06 (0.86–1.30)	Low
Health-related quality of life	2 RCTs; N=92, N=403	Moderate	Consistent	Direct	Precise	Team-based CSC resulted in greater quality of life ratings as endpoint Pooled effect size 0.84 (0.14–1.55), P=0.02 Cochran's Q=7.43 P=0.0064 (significant heterogeneity)	Moderate
Core illness symptoms (PANSS)	3 RCTs; N=99, N=403, N=1,184	Moderate	Inconsistent	Direct	Precise	No clinically important difference between groups in endpoint scores Pooled WMD of all 3 RCTs –2.53 (–5.45 to 0.39), I²=55% Sensitivity analysis removing a study with a 5.9-point difference at baseline resulted in a very small but statistically significant difference and no heterogeneity Pooled WMD of 2 RCTs –1.40 (–2.25 to –0.55); Cochran's Q =0.0014 (df=1), P=0.97	Low

TABLE D–12. Early interventions for patients with first-episode psychosis (continued)

Outcome	Number of studies and subjects	Study limitations	Consistency	Directness	Precision	Magnitude of effect: summary effect size (95% CI)	Strength of evidence (high, moderate, low, insufficient)
Core illness symptoms (Calgary Depression Scale)	2 RCTs; $N=99$, $N=205$	Moderate	Consistent	Direct	Precise	No significant difference between groups in endpoint scores Pooled WMD −0.44 (−1.08 to 0.20); heterogeneity: Cochran's Q=0.528157 ($df=1$), $P=0.4674$	Moderate
Discontinuation of treatment	2 RCTs; $N=1,239$, $N=136$	Moderate	Consistent	Direct	Precise	Team-based CSC had a significantly greater rate of treatment retention compared with standard care Pooled RR 1.27 (1.16–1.38); Cochran's Q=0.03 ($df=1$), $P=0.86$	High
Rates of relapse	2 RCTs; $N=1,239$, $N=122$	Moderate	Consistent	Direct	Imprecise	Participants in team-based CSC were significantly less likely to relapse than those in standard care Pooled RR 0.64 (0.52–0.79), Cochran's Q=0.024 ($df=1$), $P=0.88$	Moderate

Abbreviations. CI=confidence interval; CSC=coordinated specialty care; df=degrees of freedom; GAF=Global Assessment of Functioning; GAS=Global Assessment Scale; PANSS=Positive and Negative Syndrome Scale; RCT=randomized controlled trial; RR=relative risk; SR=systematic review; WMD=weighted mean difference.

TABLE D–13. Co-occurring substance use and schizophrenia

Outcome	Number of studies and subjects	Study limitations	Consistency	Directness	Precision	Magnitude of effect: summary effect size (95% CI)	Strength of evidence (high, moderate, low, insufficient)
Function: global function (integrated models of care vs. treatment as usual: GAF; 6 months)	1 SR (1 RCT; N=162)	Moderate	Unknown	Direct	Imprecise	Inconclusive; MD 1.10 (–1.58 to 3.78)	Low
Function: global function (integrated models of care vs. treatment as usual: GAF; 18 months)	1 SR (1 RCT; N=176)	Moderate	Unknown	Direct	Imprecise	Inconclusive; MD 1.00 (–1.58 to 3.58)	Low
Function: global function (integrated models of care vs. treatment as usual: GAF; 24 months)	1 SR (1 RCT; N=166)	Moderate	Unknown	Direct	Imprecise	Inconclusive; MD 1.70 (–1.18 to 4.58)	Low
Function: global function (integrated models of care vs. treatment as usual: GAF; 30 months)	1 SR (1 RCT; N=164)	Moderate	Unknown	Direct	Imprecise	Inconclusive; MD –0.60 (–3.56 to 2.36)	Low
Function: global function (integrated models of care vs. treatment as usual: GAF; 36 months)	1 SR (1 RCT; N=170)	Moderate	Unknown	Direct	Imprecise	Inconclusive; MD 0.40 (–2.47 to 3.27)	Low
Function: global function (nonintegrated: mean RFS score; 6 months)	1 SR (1 RCT; N=50)	Moderate	Unknown	Direct	Imprecise	Inconclusive; MD –0.78 (–2.91 to 1.35)	Insufficient
Function: global function (nonintegrated: mean RFS score; 6 months)	1 SR (1 RCT; N=29)	Moderate	Unknown	Direct	Imprecise	MD –2.67 (–5.28 to –0.06)	Insufficient
Ability to maintain treatment (6 months)	1 SR (3 RCTs; N=134)	Moderate	Consistent	Direct	Imprecise	Inconclusive; RR 1.23 (0.73–2.06)	Insufficient
Ability to maintain treatment (18 months)	1 SR (3 RCTs; N=134)	Moderate	Consistent	Direct	Imprecise	Inconclusive; RR 1.35 (0.83–2.19)	Insufficient

Abbreviations. CI=confidence interval; GAF=Global Assessment of Functioning; MD=mean difference; RCT=randomized controlled trial; RFS=Role Functioning Scale; RR=relative risk; SR=systematic review.